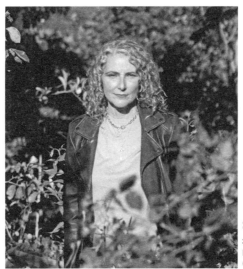

Dr. Jen Gunter is the internationally bestselling author of *The Vagina Bible* and *The Menopause Manifesto* and a board-certified obstetrician and gynecologist with more than three decades of experience. Born in Winnipeg, Manitoba, she now practices medicine in San Francisco, California. The recipient of the 2020 NAMS Media Award from The North American Menopause Society, her writing has appeared in *The New York Times, The Globe and Mail, Glamour* and *Chatelaine*. She is the star of *Jensplaining,* a CBC Gem video series that highlights the impact of medical misinformation on women. Her TED Talk on menstruation was the third most viewed talk of 2020, and she hosts the podcast *Body Stuff with Jen Gunter* from the TED Audio Collective. Dr. Gunter is widely known as a fierce advocate for women's health; the *Guardian* called her "the world's most famous—and outspoken—gynecologist." She believes an empowered patient requires facts to advocate for their body.

BY DR. JEN GUNTER

The Preemie Primer
The Vagina Bible
The Menopause Manifesto
Blood

BLOOD

THE SCIENCE,
MEDICINE, AND MYTHOLOGY
OF MENSTRUATION

DR. JEN GUNTER

PIATKUS

PIATKUS

First published in the US and Canada in 2024 by Citadel Press Books,
an imprint of Kensington Publishing Corp., and Random House Canada,
a division of Penguin Random House Canada
First published in Great Britain in 2024 by Piatkus

PUBLISHER'S NOTE: The reader is advised that this book is not
intended to be a substitute for an assessment by, and advice
from, an appropriate medical professional(s).

A CIP catalogue record for this book
is available from the British Library.

ISBN 978-0-34942-762-1

Printed and bound in Great Britain by
Clays Ltd, Elcograf S.p.A.

Papers used by Piatkus are from well-managed forests
and other responsible sources.

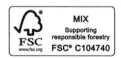

MIX
Supporting
responsible forestry
FSC® C104740

Piatkus
An imprint of
Little, Brown Book Group
Carmelite House
50 Victoria Embankment
London EC4Y 0DZ

An Hachette UK Company
www.hachette.co.uk

www.littlebrown.co.uk

To Anyone Who Has Ever Wondered
"What the . . ."

Contents

The Menstrual Cycle Is the Wheel That Drives Humanity

Evolution demands that all species solve the equation of converting energy from the world around them into the next generation. Living things, from bacteria to blue whales, solve this equation in different and often ingenious ways based on their biology, environmental pressures, the care required for offspring to reach maturity, and even social structure. For example, some organisms reproduce asexually, some deposit unfertilized eggs that will hopefully get fertilized, and some have very long gestations, like an elephant, which carries its calf—which will ultimately weigh approximately 110 kg (243 pounds) at birth—for twenty-two months.

Reproducing a human is a massive biological effort. Energy-wise, it's on par with the limits of the most extreme sports, for example, running 5,000 km (3,000 miles) over 120 days or cycling the Tour de France. Walking upright—being bipedal—results in a relatively smaller pelvis, which makes for a physically challenging and sometimes physically traumatic delivery, considering the relatively large head of a human fetus. Human infants are relatively helpless, a phenomenon known as secondary altriciality, so they require a significant amount of care, including breastfeeding, which is also metabolically demanding, and our ancestors had no choice but to pay this metabolic price and provide that physical care.

For humans, the platform that orchestrates turning this energy into offspring is the menstrual cycle, a unique trait seen in only a few species. To make human reproduction work, half the population needs to have a highly specialized biology that can be, repeatedly, hormonally rewired for a potential pregnancy, as well as bleed hundreds of times and each time repair itself without scar tissue. And while biologically this is an evolutionary marvel, it's also a source of aggravation, pain, and suffering for many, because retrofitting a body for a potential pregnancy and then bleeding for several days four hundred or so times over a lifetime can have medical consequences. At times it can be a faulty system, but individual discomfort or injury isn't evolution's concern, and in fact, evolution's motto might be best summed up as "good enough."

Unfortunately, instead of a world where those who bear the physical burdens of reproduction—whether they reproduce or not—have equal footing, we have the opposite. The Ancient Greeks, the originators of Western medicine, labeled the female body as inferior, and the act of menstruation has been viewed as proof that women have troublesome physiology and are by nature dirty and toxic. Many religions and cultures have long carried that same torch based on the erroneous belief of impurity and the idea that menstrual blood is filthy and contains actual toxins that poison the body (and especially men, if they were to touch it). Women have been banned from places of worship, from preparing food, from having sex, and even from their own homes based on the supposed polluting powers of menstrual blood. And lest we think that was the medicine of yore, there was more than one letter published in 1974 in *The Lancet*, a leading medical journal, hypothesizing that there might be sound medical beliefs to support the notion that menstrual blood was toxic and that menstruating women could wilt flowers. I know, 1974!

I just can't get my head around the concept of believing that menstruating women could wilt plants. If this were true, it wouldn't be a curse; it would be a weapon. After all, if they could, wouldn't they have used that power to lay waste to entire crops, bringing kings, emperors, and governments to their knees? Yet the fact that no woman has ever done this, or even used magical plant-wilting abilities to own a little land of her own, was not proof enough of its absurdity. But that is the patriarchy: facts are irrelevant; it's the world order that matters.

As women were long viewed as lesser and more troublesome versions of men, the idea that their differences might be important and might warrant specific study to offer them better care was largely absent from medicine.

What happened instead was that medicine was created for men and then retrofitted poorly for women. For many years, studying the reproductive tract mattered mostly for improving pregnancy outcomes, rather than improving the lives of those who lived with those reproductive tracts. It wasn't until 1993 (yes, 1993) that including women in medical studies became a requirement for government-funded research in the United States. And diseases unique to the reproductive biology attached to ovaries and a uterus are woefully underfunded compared with diseases that more commonly affect the other half of the population. We can blame medicine, and we should, but our governments provide the funding for much of this work.

The practice of viewing female physiology as both toxic and lesser throughout the ages has left a damaging legacy of inadequate research, dismissal by a patriarchal medical system, an uncaring society, and insufficient education about how the female body works. The consequences are that people struggle to get care, and the gaps in medicine are subsequently exploited by a rogue's gallery of medical charlatans from the wellness industrial complex. When I scroll Instagram or TikTok, I'm horrified at the disinformation about the menstrual cycle and associated medical conditions that is perpetually propagated. There are creators claiming that menstrual blood can tell you about hormone levels, or that a "normal" period is less than three days in length and painless, or that eating raw carrots daily is essential to detoxifying dangerous estrogens, or that menstrual blood can be used as a face mask to treat acne because it has stem cells and special "healing" chemicals. To someone who knows science, this all comes off as ignorance masquerading as confidence. Look: if menstrual blood had magical healing powers, the vagina and vulva would age at a slower rate, courtesy of four hundred or so regenerative "menstrual spa" therapies.

The truth is, many people haven't received enough information to distinguish medicine from mythology, and disinformation is often simple and sexy, so it sells. Offering seemingly simple solutions is easy when you aren't constrained by facts or the truth. And let's be clear here: almost every claim offered by these menstrual charlatans is unstudied and unregulated, which is the antithesis of feminism. Feminism demands bodily autonomy, and that can be achieved only with facts. You cannot make an empowering decision about your health when the information you have been given is false. Lying about the body is a hallmark of the patriarchy, and no amount of wrapping it with a pink bow or abusing words like *natural* can change that fact.

The best strategy, whether it's dealing with a dismissive medical provider or sorting through endless menstrual misinformation on Instagram or TikTok, is a robust education, and that is the purpose of this book. I want you to have a solid knowledge of the menstrual cycle and the medical conditions and therapies associated with that cycle so you can be empowered. One aspect that is beyond the scope of this book is infertility; in my opinion, that is best addressed by a board-certified reproductive endocrinologist.

Also, a word about language. Not all women menstruate, and not everyone who menstruates is a woman. Women born without a uterus, trans women, women who have had a hysterectomy, and women who no longer menstruate because of medical conditions or menopause are all women. Some trans men and gender nonbinary people menstruate. So how do we find terms that can encompass all these experiences? Some have used the words *menstruator* or *person with a uterus* but I dislike distilling people down to body functions or parts, and some people don't menstruate and some don't have a uterus but still ovulate and so still have a menstrual cycle, so these terms don't cover the totality of experiences. Another term that is used is *pregnancy capable*, but that sounds like we're reducing people to a potential incubator. In addition, not everyone with a uterus has any desire to be pregnant, while others have tried very hard to be pregnant and are not, and to them *pregnancy capable* might be jarring or hurtful. I'm also concerned that describing people by their reproductive capabilities seems to mostly apply to only half of the population, as *ejaculator* and *potential impregnator* are largely absent from our current lexicon.

To me, the answer is clear: use the term *people* whenever possible when discussing the menstrual cycle. I trust people who are reading this book know what sections relate specifically to them and which ones aren't applicable. If a study or an article being used as reference describes the subjects as women, then that is how they will be described in these pages, and if they use a different term, then that will be used. When discussing history or the influences of society, the term *women* will generally be used, because the pathway of inadequate research and medical gaslighting started with the patriarchal concept that a female body that menstruated was a defective variant of a male body. And while jumping from *people* to *women* to perhaps even *those who menstruate* may seem an odd editorial choice to some, I feel it works well to honor the past while considering how we move forward.

I've been a gynecologist since 1995, and I've seen a lot of change during that time. We have amazing new therapies that weren't possible when I trained and in my early years of practice. When I attended medical school in the 1980s, the idea that the human papillomavirus (HPV) caused cervical cancer was just a hypothesis, and now we can prevent cervical cancer with a vaccine against HPV. We now know so much more about so many conditions. I've also seen things that should have changed remain sadly stagnant. Research is slower than it should be, many people still struggle to access quality care, politicians in many parts of the world are still weaponizing reproductive health for political gain, and social media provides a playground for disinformation.

For me, the answer to advocating in the doctor's office, or insisting our political leaders do better, or sifting through the misinformation on social media, is to provide a source of quality information. I think back to my own experiences. I suffered from terrible menstrual diarrhea (yes, there is no good menstrual diarrhea, but while the qualifier might seem unnecessary, if you've had menstrual diarrhea, you get it). I thought I was uniquely broken because no one ever discussed this, not even Judy Blume. It wasn't until I was a medical student, when we had a lecture about prostaglandins and I learned they could cause diarrhea and were released during menstruation, that I had my light-bulb moment. I wanted to stand up and scream, "SAY WHAT NOW?" Of course period diarrhea was a thing! I raced down after the lecture to ask the professor if the two might be connected, and his answer made it clear that he hadn't really thought about it, but yes.

I promptly negotiated my way into the OB/GYN clinic, scooped up some sample packs of oral contraceptive pills, and by the next cycle was as close to menstrual nirvana as possible—minimal cramping and diarrhea. The next year in medical school, I learned you could take the pill every day and not have a period, and like magic, my periods were gone—except it was courtesy of medical research and some ingenuity on my own part. Before starting the pill, I had to plan my life around my menstruation, because when the diarrhea was bad, I might need a bathroom fifteen times a day. Now I could just live my life.

There are several important take-home messages here. The first is that knowledge about my body and the available medications allowed me to make an informed decision and act on it. The second is that having quality knowledge about the menstrual cycle since age twenty, when I started medical school, meant I was essentially immune to the disinformation found everywhere, so I had nothing to unlearn. And the final one is the tenacious nature of menstrual shame. When I later found out that menstrual diarrhea affects 12 percent of people who menstruate, I was stunned. This phenomenon has at times ruined my life. Once, before my hormonal contraception era, I was lucky enough to go to New York City and visit the Metropolitan Museum of Art, but I spent the entire time in the bathroom with menstrual diarrhea. Why did I have to wait until I was in medical school to find out that I suffered from something that was common and could be treated? Why did I have to wait so long to find out that I was not in this alone?

Even now, when I mention menstrual diarrhea in a lecture (and you bet I do: letting everyone know about this phenomenon has become one of my missions), there's always someone who approaches me afterward to tell me they thought they were the only one. Same thing when I post on social media: I get direct messages from people who thought they were alone in this. How's that for gaslighting? Six percent of the world's population will at one point in their lives experience menstrual diarrhea (when everyone is counted, those who menstruate and those who don't), but it's still something few people know about? And yet 8 percent of Americans have asthma, and I'm sure every person old enough to read this book has heard of asthma.

One of my favorite experiences is when people who have read either *The Vagina Bible* or *The Menopause Manifesto* tell me they found the information enlightening and empowering. I hear stories of how people advocated for an IUD, got physical therapy to treat pain with sex, or weren't afraid to start vaginal estrogen because of words I wrote. That's why I am writing this book—not just for diarrhea education, of course, but for all of it. Because if you have or have had a menstrual cycle, or you know someone who menstruates, or you have benefited from menstruation, you should know about it. (Let's be real: everyone has benefited from menstruation; otherwise, you wouldn't be alive to read this book.) And if your menstrual cycle is troubling you, I want you to understand the science behind it and the therapies that are available so you can be empowered and advocate for yourself when needed.

The menstrual cycle really is the wheel that drives humanity, and it's time to kick shame and lack of knowledge about it to the curb.

Part 1

THE MENSTRUAL CYCLE, A PRIMER

1

Why Menstruation?

As a teen I often went by myself to buy pads. Tagging along with my parents to the grocery store was an experience to be avoided at all costs, as their behavior in public was often mortifying, and not in the way most kids think. My father wouldn't go by himself to pick up the pads, and my mother had dramatic mood swings, so it was easier and safer for me to fly under the radar as much as possible and figure things out on my own. So I'd ride my bike or walk to the drugstore myself and get a box of forty-eight pads, which was usually enough to handle my bleeding with a few to spare so I wouldn't be caught unawares with my next cycle. My preferred brand of menstrual products was Kotex Super Plus, because that pad was huge. It was like wearing a box of Kleenex between my legs—suboptimal from a comfort standpoint, but the only solution for the first three days of bleeding. Any other pad, and I would leak everywhere.

The first night of every period I had to get up at least once to change my pad, and even then, it almost always soaked through onto the towel that I'd put down for backup. Looking back on that time now, as a gynecologist, I am fully aware that this was excessive bleeding that should have prompted a visit to a compassionate doctor, but at the time I had no reference to go by and no idea what was considered heavy bleeding. While I learned something about menstruation from Judy Blume, as did many girls of my era, the actual volume of blood was never discussed anywhere that I recall, and I would sooner have entered a cage with a tiger while wearing a dress made of meat than discuss menstruation with my mother.

When I eventually did visit a physician, it was because I had tried to donate blood my first year of college, when I was eighteen, and was turned away because my iron level was low. I went to see my doctor on the advice of the nice nurse from the Winnipeg Red Cross. However, my doctor did not do any blood work to confirm that my iron level or blood counts were low. She told me it was normal for a woman to have low iron and gave me the grand advice to eat liver. She was both a doctor and a woman, so I had no reason to doubt her authority, although I didn't eat more liver. And so I remained anemic until I eventually started the birth control pill.

When I think back on those days in the late seventies, in my mind's eye that box of forty-eight pads was huge—so large I could barely hold it under one arm. I wondered if my memory was exaggerating in the same way I might by telling my kids I had to walk through chest-deep snow to school all winter, uphill both ways. But thanks to the miracle of the Internet, I was able to track down the dimensions of that exact box, and it was about the size of a carry-on suitcase.

In the summer, I always biked to pick up my pads, because it was Winnipeg and the bike riding season was short. Riding back from the drugstore on my ten-speed bike, wearing a menstrual pad the size of a small box of Kleenex, balancing a suitcase-size box of pads on my hip, I would think deep thoughts about menstruation, because this seemed ridiculous. How did our ancestors cope? I'd barely escaped the agony of menstrual belts, and assumed things were much worse before those were invented. As amazing as I thought an adhesive strip was, what prior horror would have made menstrual belts seem liberating by comparison?

I often wondered why we menstruated. It seemed like a very intrusive bodily function. When I compared my periods to other things that were essential for human life, such as breathing or eating, it seemed problematic on an entirely different scale. Nothing else leaked by design. Why have such a burdensome system? What is the actual biological point of menstruation? Getting pregnant is obviously part of it, but the blood loss seemed to me like a big waste of resources.

When it comes to evolution, determining absolutes is hard, but it turns out we have some pretty good ideas about why we menstruate. And I wish teenage Jen had known what I am about to explain to you.

Menstruation Is Rare

Menstruation is the regular shedding of the superficial lining of the uterus, known medically as the endometrium, and it's part of the menstrual cycle. Menstruation is a rare phenomenon in the animal kingdom, experienced only by humans, most other primates, a few species of bats, the elephant shrew, and the spiny mouse. All told, less than 2 percent of mammals menstruate, although it's possible that number could be slightly on the low side, given that behaviors can be altered in captivity, and it can be challenging to observe more reclusive mammals and those with inaccessible habitats. (You must admit, it had to have taken some *Mission: Impossible*–style science to figure out which bats menstruate!) Instead of a menstrual cycle, most mammals have estrus, which does not involve cyclic bleeding from the uterus. Dogs do bleed, but it is from the vagina and is not biologically the same as menstruation.

Placental mammals—such as horses, dogs, cats, mice, and of course humans—are probably what come to mind if you're asked to name a mammal. Mammals with a placenta are known as eutherians (marsupials, like kangaroos, have placentas, but they are very different, so they are not considered placental mammals). The small collection of eutherian mammals that menstruate seems like an odd grouping. Are we more closely related to bats than we think?

All eutherian mammals, those that menstruate and those that don't, evolved from a common ancestor that didn't menstruate. Along the way, as evolution took its twists and turns and different species developed, menstruation evolved—and not just once, because the mammals that menstruate didn't all branch off together from a common ancestor. Rather, menstruation evolved four separate times, once for humans and other primates, again for bats, again for the spiny mouse, and yet again for the elephant shrew. A biological feature evolving independently multiple times suggests it adds value for survival. But what value does menstruation add to the survival of a species? This is a question I'm sure many of us have asked while curled up with cramps or dealing with a bout of period diarrhea or balancing a ginormous box of pads on a ten-speed bike.

When most of us think of menstruation, we think of the blood. What might blood leaving the uterus accomplish? One early theory was that bleeding was needed to wash out bacteria and viruses that hitched along with sperm. But there isn't anything especially clean about dog or horse sperm versus human or bat, meaning menstruating mammals don't have a unique spermal swill to manage. Also, if such a biohazard were delivered along with the sperm that the only way to have a cleanup on aisle uterus when fertilization didn't happen would be to dump the entire menstrual lining, what exactly happens when there is a pregnancy? It's hard to see how this microorganism could be so bad for the uterus but beneficial to a developing embryo. It just doesn't make sense, and unsurprisingly this theory has since been discarded.

Instead of focusing on the bleeding, let's take a step back and look at what happens inside the uterus *before* menstruation. For pregnancy to be successful for any mammal, both those that menstruate and those with estrus, the endometrium must undergo decidualization, a biologically complex and irreversible transformation. In humans, decidualization occurs approximately seven to ten days after ovulation, and it's during this narrow window when implantation is possible. The decidualized endometrium is filled with storage sugars and lipids and provides nutrients for the embryo until the placenta can take over. It also protects the embryo from the pregnant person's immune system, because a fetus is 50 percent foreign DNA and would otherwise be rejected like a transplanted organ with an incomplete match. Without decidualization, there can be no successful pregnancy. And decidualization may be the answer to why we humans and our primate, bat, mouse, and shrew pals are the only members of Club Menstruation.

Explaining Decidualization via Baking

What exactly *is* decidualization? I appreciate that this may be a new term for many, so before we go any further, let's get familiar with it. The word *decidua* is from the Latin *decidere*, meaning "to die, fall off, or detach," and decidualized endometrium is indeed cast off with menstruation and also after delivery. Decidualization may seem like a nebulous concept, so I like to explain it using the analogy of baking a soufflé. It may seem weird at first, but trust the process.

Making a soufflé involves a precision not seen in most other baking. With pie crusts or cakes, there is wiggle room. For example, if your pie dough is too wet, you can add flour. If you take a cake out of the oven too early, you can test it and put it back in to bake some more. Not so with a soufflé. I started baking them a few years ago. I admit I was a little intimidated at first, because in a restaurant it's one of those menu items with an asterisk and stern instructions about ordering it immediately, giving it an aura of mystery and skill. But I watched my partner make us a lovely cheese soufflé for dinner and that demystified the process, giving me some confidence to try it myself. Now I am proud to say that I have mastered multiple kinds of soufflés. My lemon soufflés are divine. (Chrissy Teigen even commented on them once on Twitter!)

With a soufflé, there are several key steps that must happen in a specific order. First the eggs must be separated and the whites whipped without a drop of yolk, then the soufflé must be baked at just the right temperature for an exact length of time. Take the soufflé out too soon, and it's soggy and hasn't risen; too late, and it's deflated like a sad soccer ball. But if you've done everything correctly, you have a beautiful, fluffy, delicious concoction that seems more alchemy than biochemistry.

Decidualization is similar in many ways: just as our baking project requires the correct ingredient preparation, oven temperature, and time to bake, decidualization requires the correct hormone levels in a precise sequence. The hormone changes that prepare human endometrium in the first part of the menstrual cycle are analogous to the soufflé prep. The progesterone released after ovulation, which is responsible for decidualization, is like baking the soufflé. Once the endometrium has undergone decidualization, there is a narrow ideal window for implantation, just as a narrow window separates a show-stopping soufflé from a mess of poorly scrambled eggs or a deflated egg pancake. If a pregnancy happens, soufflé for all my friends! But if it doesn't, the uterus is left with a decidualized endometrium that cannot be turned back into a non-decidualized endometrium. The cells of the endometrium were physically transformed by the progesterone when they were decidualized, and that was a one-way trip, just as a soufflé can't be turned back into a bowl of egg whites and another one of egg yolks. It's not possible to put more endometrium on top of a decidualized endometrium, just as you can't bake one soufflé on top of another. And you can't keep the decidualized endometrium on ice, because all the hormones released in the next menstrual cycle need non-decidualized endometrium on which to act. Keeping the decidualized endometrium through to the next cycle isn't possible.

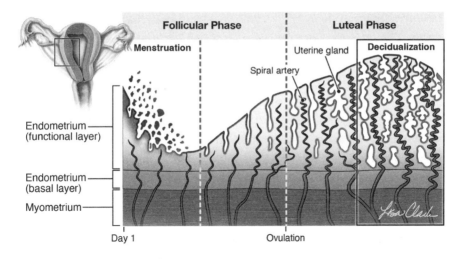

Figure 1 • *Decidualized Endometrium (Illustration by Lisa A. Clark, MA, CMI)*

The uterus has two options to get back to a clean slate for the next cycle: either reabsorb the decidualized endometrium or dump it. Decidua isn't clotted blood; it's a real change to the endometrial cells. It can look a lot like strips of liver or other tissue. People sometimes see decidualized tissue with their menstrual blood and think, "Was I pregnant and am I miscarrying?" or "Is part of my uterus coming out?" That's how much it can look like human tissue. Given the amount of decidua and its flesh-like consistency, the option of the body breaking it down and reabsorbing it really isn't compatible with how we work, biologically speaking. It would take an apparatus as complex as the digestive tract to deal with it, so getting rid of it—meaning menstruation—is the only option.

Timing Is Everything

You might be wondering, if it isn't possible to reabsorb decidualized endometrium and the only option is to let it go, then why do animals with estrus not menstruate? Doesn't their endometrium also undergo decidualization? It's a great question! Yes, their endometrium undergoes decidualization, but the answer lies with the trigger. Animals with estrus have what is known as induced decidualization, because it's induced by the embryo implanting. If there is no embryo, the irreversible changes don't happen. With estrus, think of the embryo as a dinner guest who orders the dessert soufflé with their meal.

If no one shows up to order the soufflé, cleaning up the unbaked egg mix is easy. The endometrium can be reabsorbed because it never underwent those irreversible changes.

With a menstrual cycle, decidualization happens whether there is an embryo or not, because the trigger is the progesterone released with ovulation. This is known as spontaneous decidualization—the soufflé is going to be baked whether a guest, meaning an embryo, is coming or not. For humans, an embryo connects with an already decidualized endometrium. If there is no embryo, the only way to start the cycle again is to get rid of the decidualized endometrium with menstruation, or—to finish our rather long baking analogy—clean out the soufflé dish and start again. Meaning menstruation. Decidualized endometrium is removed when chemical changes triggered by falling levels of progesterone cause blood vessels that supply the endometrium to rupture, and the bleeding, along with inflammatory chemicals, causes the layer of decidualized endometrium to peel off or split from the uterus.

The question isn't "Why did we evolve to bleed?"; rather, we should be asking "Why is spontaneous decidualization so important that the loss of blood and the hassle of menstruation are worth the trade-off, evolutionarily speaking?"

Whoa. Right?

So what *is* the benefit of spontaneous decidualization?

Placental Management

Humans and other menstruating mammals have a hemochorial placenta, a fancy way to say that the fetal placenta directly contacts the blood vessels in the uterus. In most non-menstruating mammals, there are at least a few cells between the placenta and maternal blood. To get to the point where it is bathing in blood from the uterus, the placenta must invade the muscle of the uterus and destroy some of the blood vessels it encounters to make contact so the transfer of nutrients can occur.

Humans have the most invasive placentas of all mammals, and this invasiveness must be managed, because if it goes awry, the placenta can easily damage the uterus. It can burrow too deep into the muscle of the uterus, a condition called placenta accreta, which, fortunately, is rare. Placenta accreta can lead to excessive bleeding with delivery because the placenta can't separate properly from the lining of the uterus. If the placenta invades deep enough, it can grow through the uterus into the organs in the belly, such as the bladder, bowel, and even liver. This is called placenta percreta, and it can result in catastrophic bleeding. It is impossible to explain to someone who has not witnessed a cesarean section with placenta percreta the extent of the bleeding—blood banks at smaller hospitals can run out of blood trying to keep up. Now, thanks to MRI scans and advanced ultrasounds, we can often diagnose placenta percreta before delivery and take advance precautions to reduce the risk of hemorrhage, but we didn't have any of that when I trained. That moment of terror when you open the abdomen for a C-section and see placental tissue growing everywhere is the stuff of nightmares.

The point here is, while the invasiveness of the placenta is good from the standpoint of nutrient and oxygen delivery for the fetus, if it gets out of control, it can be harmful to the pregnant person/mammal. One way to manage invasiveness is to have, ready and waiting for the embryo, a thick endometrium with the skill set to handle an invasive placenta, meaning spontaneous decidualization. The human decidualized endometrium is among the thickest. In fact, some have referred to the battle between the thickness of the decidualized endometrium and the invasiveness of the human placenta as an evolutionary arms race.

Testing the Embryo

This theory might be upsetting to someone who has had a miscarriage, but to others the explanation might be helpful. You know yourself and what you are ready for. I'm giving this warning in case it's something you might not be in a space to read and might prefer to skip over.

Human embryos have a high rate of genetic malformations, and evolutionarily speaking, it isn't practical to invest limited biological resources in a pregnancy destined for a poor outcome. One way this equation can be solved is by selecting embryos with a better chance of survival, and so the high rate of genetic anomalies typical in human pregnancies is counterbalanced by the fact that only 20 to 30 percent of conceptions result in a live birth. Much of this embryo selection is guided by the decidualized endometrium waiting for the embryo. The theory is that the decidualized endometrium acts as a biosensor of embryo quality. If a problem is detected, an inflammatory response can be triggered to end the pregnancy.

Support for this theory comes from research showing that the decidualized endometrium mounts a stress reaction when a significantly abnormal embryo implants. In addition, encountering a thick decidualized endometrium means the embryo must work harder to invade sufficiently to implant, essentially providing a test of embryo fitness.

It's about Resource Curation . . . We Think

Spontaneous decidualization creates an environment geared for reproductive success, meaning an endometrium that can handle the invasiveness of a human placenta as well as embryo curation. The preparations necessary for implantation are driven by the progesterone released during ovulation, meaning for mammals that menstruate, reproductive choice is coded into the system.

In animals with an estrus cycle, meaning no menstruation, the embryo itself triggers decidualization, so the body cannot choose, metaphorically speaking, whether the pregnancy is worth the resource allocation.

The theories boil down to optimizing pregnancy outcomes. As we'll see in later chapters, many aspects of the menstrual cycle are ultimately about resource curation, as human pregnancy, lactation, and caring for a child until it is self-sufficient—steps that are required to pass along genetics—are resource-heavy undertakings.

Ultimately, this is a theory, although there is lots of supporting data. It's always possible, with new techniques, that what we believe now may change; such is the meandering path of science. But it seems as close to certain as science can be that menstruation is a by-product of the menstrual cycle and not the point. The bleeding is technically a waste of resources, but in the grand evolutionary scheme, it works because it allows spontaneous decidualization, which in turn helps humans produce healthy offspring.

Regardless, this system requires the half of the population who menstruate to "suck it up." I'm sure teenage Jen would have shouted, "Ha! I knew it."

Why Do We Call It Menstruation?

I'm often asked why *menstruation* includes the word *men*, but this is one rare example in medicine when the patriarchy wasn't blustering in and mansplaining. Many ancient cultures associated menstruation with the moon, and to make that connection they would have observed that menstruation came approximately once a lunar month, which is 29.5 days. While we now know that menstruation is not related in any way to the moon, this historical association with a monthly occurrence is reflected in the words we use today. *Menses*, the medical term for menstrual blood, is from the Latin *mēnsis*, for "month." *Period* is from the Latin *periodus* and/or the Greek *periodos*, which means "a recurring or repeated cycle of events." In this book, I'll use the term *menstrual cycle* for all the hormonal changes that bring about menstrual bleeding and for the bleeding itself (basically, the whole kit and kaboodle), and *menstrual bleeding, bleeding, blood, menstrual blood, menstruation*, and *period* for the bleeding. As this is a book on menstruation, assume *blood* means *menstrual blood*. If the bleeding has any other cause, I'll be sure to specify!

While this book will stick with medical terms, you can absolutely call your menstrual bleeding whatever you want. That time of the month, Aunt Flo, surfing the crimson tide, moon time, the curse, the visitor, my girl, Carrie, the English have landed, and shark week are all euphemisms I've heard, and I marvel at the creativity and wryness and even slyness behind many of them. My personal favorites are "checking into the Red Roof Inn" (likely regional to the United States) and "there are communists in the funhouse," which, according to Urban Dictionary, is Danish in origin. According to a 2016 survey by Clue, the period tracking app, there are over five thousand euphemisms used around the world for menstruation.

It's important to acknowledge that the creativity behind these phrases was often a result of the inability to discuss menstruation openly. Much of the silencing is patriarchal, as if the very biology that drives humanity is dirty. Euphemisms are "polite" ways to get around the unseemly act of bleeding, or "women's things," although I love the subversiveness of a euphemism like shark week—it's far more graphic than "menstruation" or simply saying "I'm bleeding."

Imagine if it were socially acceptable to say, when someone asks you how you are doing, "Well, I've changed my fourth pad today" or "I just passed a clot the size of a quarter" or "Actually, it feels like I have a hot poker in my vagina and I still made it to this meeting that absolutely could have been handled by email." Maybe more people would take menstruation seriously. I still remember when I asked my ninth grade teacher if I could go to the bathroom and he said no, because he was one of those teachers who thought a full bladder was conducive to learning. But I didn't need to urinate; I needed to change my pad. I wanted to avoid a critical pad incident, so I walked up to his desk and said,

"I have my period and I need to change my pad." I didn't think anything of it. I would ask for a tissue if I had a runny nose, and it's not as if snot is pixie dust. I wouldn't have announced to the class that I needed to change my pad (and it sucks that that hasn't really changed much, even though it's more than forty years later), but I was talking to an adult man who taught ninth grade. Surely the concept that some girls might need menstrual products wasn't news to him. But the color drained from his face, and he was overtaken by a look of horror as he waved me to the classroom door. He let me go, but with a stern warning that I should never use those words again. I was going to say, "So I should use semaphore, then?" but thought better of it.

Use terms that speak to you and that you feel safe saying, but it's also good to know the medical words so you can communicate clearly about your body. And spend some time learning what terms people in other cultures use to describe menstruation, to revel not just in their inventiveness but also in their similarity to the words you might use. It's almost as if menstruation is a cultural Rosetta stone.

There has been a recent attempt to rename many medical terms associated with the female body. Some are eponymous, named after the men who first described them, which is unfair, as women were not allowed to contribute to the naming of organs. Imagine if society had been equal; we would have seen many parts named after learned female physicians and anatomists. But even worse than the mansplaining of many body parts is that some were given misogynistic names by these supposedly learned men. For example, *pudendum* is from the Latin "to shame," and *vagina* is from the Latin for "sheath," because *penis* is from the Latin for "sword." As if. We should be using non-pejorative, non-sexist language, and really, the uterus and ovaries and their workings aren't something these men discovered—they were there all along. Renaming some structures isn't revisionism; it has the worthy goal of removing judgment from body parts. And quite frankly, it's setting the record straight. Also, it seems wise to rename things based on what we know now versus terminology that reflected cutting-edge medicine in 1562.

In this book, I will focus on these new terms where they exist. Given the origin of the word *menses* (and all of its derivatives, such as *menstrual cycle* and *menstruation*) and *period*, these words are not inherently problematic. In fact, *menses* feels like a nod to the ancient matriarchs of menstruation, because the first person to make a connection between menstruation having a cycle like the lunar cycle would undoubtedly have been a woman.

Bottom Line

- Less than 2 percent of mammals menstruate. They include humans, most other primates, some species of bats, the spiny mouse, and the elephant shrew.
- Menstruation is associated with spontaneous decidualization, meaning the progesterone produced after ovulation triggers an essential and irreversible change in the endometrium that is essential for a successful pregnancy.
- Menstruation itself doesn't appear to be a beneficial adaptation; rather, it's a trade-off that allows spontaneous decidualization to occur so that a decidualized endometrium is waiting for an embryo.
- One main theory regarding the evolution of menstruation is that, with spontaneous decidualization, the endometrium plays a role in embryonic quality assurance, thus improving reproductive outcomes.
- Another theory is that spontaneous decidualization controls the unique invasiveness of the human placenta.

2

Menstrual Cycle 101

The menstrual cycle, meaning the hormonal changes as well as the bleeding, is typically broken down into two phases, or parts: the follicular phase, which is from the first day of bleeding to ovulation, and the luteal phase, which is from ovulation until the next period. This terminology reflects what is happening in the ovary. The follicular phase is when the follicles (the eggs) are developing and producing estrogen and ends the day before the LH (luteinizing hormone) surge. Some people break the follicular phase down further, adding menstruation as a distinct phase, but from a practical standpoint this isn't necessary. Also, it doesn't make sense medically, because menstruation isn't a unique hormonal phase—the bleeding occurs while the hormonal changes for the next cycle are starting. If menstruation is pulling the sheets off a bed because the guests didn't arrive, the next menstrual cycle is ironing another set of sheets at the exact same time to ensure the bed is ready for the next potential set of houseguests. The day of the LH surge marks the start of the luteal phase, and during this time the leftover cells from the follicle organize into a structure called the corpus luteum, which produces progesterone, controlling the process of decidualization covered in Chapter 1.

These two phases of the menstrual cycle are sometimes called proliferative and secretory, reflecting what is happening in the endometrium (the lining of the uterus). During the proliferative (follicular) phase, the endometrium is proliferating, or growing, under the influence of estrogen; during the secretory (luteal) phase, the cells of the endometrium become filled with storage sugars and lipids and they release a glycogen-rich secretion, largely influenced by progesterone. If a pathologist looks at a sample of endometrium under the microscope, they may describe what they see as either proliferative or secretory. *Proliferative* tells the health care provider that the endometrium has been exposed to estrogen, and *secretory* tells us that either ovulation has occurred or the person has taken progesterone or a progesterone-like medication. Decidualization occurs toward the end of the secretory phase.

I'll use the terms *follicular* and *luteal* to describe the phases of the menstrual cycle. A good way to remember their order of occurrence is by the first letter: the *f* stands for both follicular and first, and the *l* stands for both luteal and last.

Ovulation, the Menstrual Engine

The ovaries sit on either side of the uterus, next to the oviducts—what we used to call the Fallopian tubes because they were first described by Gabriele Falloppio. In the 1500s, Falloppio also performed one of the earliest clinical trials, evaluating the impact of linen condoms on sexually transmitted infections, so there is no denying his contribution to medicine. However, *oviducts* is a better term, as they are literally the ducts that transport the ovum (mature egg) to the uterus. *Ovary* is a fine term, as it shares a common root with many ancient languages that means "egg." An older term for ovaries is *stones*, and they do look like small white stones. I'm not suggesting we start referring to ovaries as stones in textbooks, but it does make me think of a phrase used to describe someone as daring: "They've got balls." Perhaps "They've got stones" might be an even better expression.

By puberty, the ovaries are home to approximately four hundred thousand tiny structures called primordial follicles, which are oocytes (immature eggs) surrounded by supporting cells. These primordial follicles are in a type of hibernation, nestled in the supporting tissue of the ovary and waiting for their invitation to Club Ovulation. Only some of them will be selected, as getting into the club isn't guaranteed—think of a bouncer choosing a few potential candidates for entry. How primordial follicles are selected isn't fully known, but once they are, they get ready for the party, meaning they gradually transform into antral follicles, which are follicles with the potential to ovulate. The journey from primordial follicle to antral follicle takes about a year, and this process is underway constantly from puberty to menopause. Many primordial follicles that get the initial signal don't make it to antral follicle status; instead, they disintegrate and are lost along the way.

The antral follicles are the ones that make it past the velvet rope outside the club, hoping to get inside—they get the chance to try to ovulate. At the beginning of the menstrual cycle, a hormone called follicle-stimulating hormone, or FSH, is released by the pituitary gland, and it does exactly what you think: it stimulates these antral follicles. Some of them develop—or, using our analogy, get access to the club—and they hit the dance floor, firing up their hormone-producing engines and starting to produce estrogen and other hormones.

The menstrual cycle requires a two-way communication path between the brain and the ovaries, and estrogen is one of the languages used to communicate. As the follicles develop, estrogen and other hormones are produced, which tell the brain to increase production of FSH. One follicle wouldn't raise estrogen levels quickly enough, so having many follicles contributing to estrogen production early in the cycle is a work-around. The follicle destined to ovulate is selected early in the cycle, by days five to seven, and to the best of our knowledge this choice appears to be a lottery. This follicle quickly dominates in size and estrogen production; hence it's called the dominant follicle. The other follicles disintegrate.

We used to think there was just one VIP group of four to fourteen follicles that was given the opportunity to join the ovulation party, but we now know that there is often more than one wave. It's the dominant follicle from what ends up being the last wave that ovulates. About a thousand primordial follicles are pulled out of hibernation for every one that ovulates, so as far as ovulation is concerned, it takes a village.

In addition to communicating with the brain about the status of the follicles, estrogen from the developing follicles instructs the cells in the basal, or bottom, layer of the endometrium to start dividing. Think of the endometrium as a brick wall where each brick is a cell and estrogen is the bricklayer. The lining of the uterus thickens, and the new top layer of tissue is known as the functional layer. Coiled blood vessels called spiral arteries, which are shaped like pig's tails, grow up from the basal layer (a bit like ivy into a brick wall); they are essential because all this new tissue and a prospective embryo need oxygen and nutrients.

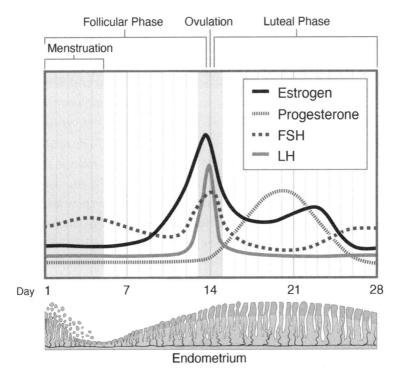

Figure 2 • *Hormone Levels and the Menstrual Cycle (Illustration by Lisa A. Clark, MA, CMI)*

Eventually the estrogen gets to a level where it causes the messaging in the brain to change, and the pituitary gland begins to release luteinizing hormone (LH). Levels rise rapidly, called an LH surge, which is essential for several reasons:

- It encourages the maturation of the oocyte so the egg is ready for fertilization.
- It triggers ovulation about eight to ten hours after the peak level of LH.
- It initiates follicle luteinization, during which the follicular tissue left behind after ovulation is converted into the corpus luteum, which produces progesterone.

Luteinization of the follicle requires new blood vessels, which quickly grow into the ovary, bringing large amounts of blood and hence the cholesterol needed to make progesterone. Sometimes the process is overzealous, causing bleeding into the corpus luteum, something known as a hemorrhagic corpus luteum.

The progesterone released by the corpus luteum stabilizes the lining of the uterus, a bit like mortar with bricks, but this is just an analogy, because it doesn't act exactly like mortar. Progesterone slows the effect of estrogen on the lining, causes the spiral arteries to grow in length and to coil even more, and triggers decidualization, that necessary change for implantation. And it acts like a brake on the pituitary gland, reducing FSH and LH so that no more follicles will develop or get a signal to ovulate, because at this point the body doesn't want to invest energy in ovulation. Remember, groups of primordial follicles are constantly being selected to develop into antral follicles, so the ability to turn off the signaling that recruits antral follicles is important.

After ovulation, the egg, now called an ovum, is swept up by kelp-like projections called fimbriae at the end of the oviduct. It's in the oviduct where fertilization with sperm occurs. In the event of fertilization, the ovum makes its way to the uterus. If it implants, it sends hormonal signals to the corpus luteum to maintain high levels of progesterone, keeping that brake on ovulation, as throughout the pregnancy primordial follicles will continue to get called up to join the roster of follicles with the potential to ovulate. It can take one to two weeks for progesterone to fully suppress the system, so during this window it is theoretically possible that another antral follicle could "escape" and ovulate. If two pregnancies occur this way, the initial one and then another one within the next two weeks, it is known as superfecundation, where fraternal twins are conceived on different days. Superfecundation is very rare.

If fertilization doesn't happen, then the corpus luteum shrinks and stops producing progesterone according to its preprogrammed life span, which is typically twelve to fourteen days (but can range from eleven to seventeen days). The rapid drop in progesterone at the end of the corpus luteum's natural life span causes two key menstrual events: it destabilizes the lining of the uterus, resulting in menstruation, and it releases the hormonal brake on the brain so the cycle to recruit antral follicles can begin again.

Do the Ovaries Alternate Ovulation from Cycle to Cycle?

We used to believe that ovulation alternated between ovaries from cycle to cycle: the right ovary would ovulate one cycle, then the left ovary the next cycle, and so on. But newer research suggests it may be more random, without a pattern. Ovulation can even happen from one ovary for several cycles, then switch to the other. If one ovary is removed, the remaining ovary will pick up the slack, so to speak, and ovulate each cycle.

Interestingly, the ovum doesn't always travel down the oviduct on the same side as the ovary it was released from. We first realized this when it became apparent that some people who were getting pregnant had only one oviduct and one ovary, on opposite sides! This swap is called transmigration, which absolutely sounds like a magic spell. It seems unbelievable—at least if you're picturing a reproductive system that is almost T-shaped, with the ovaries at the end of either arm of the T. In that image, each ovary appears to be far away from the opposite oviduct. In reality, for most people the oviducts and ovaries hang down behind the uterus, so they are closer together than you might think. Even so, it's amazing to think of a tiny ovum heading out on its own and crossing over to the other oviduct without getting smushed or chemically damaged. Talk about an incredible journey! It's a bit like *Jurassic Park*: life finds a way.

The exact signaling that leads to the egg being picked up by the oviduct on the opposite side is poorly understood. It's not as if we can put a tracker on an ovum and monitor its migration, like we can with a shark. But thanks to data from pregnant people with only one oviduct, we now know something about the frequency of transmigration. Ultrasound can identify which ovary ovulated, because the corpus luteum—the hormonally active tissue left behind after ovulation—is easy to see. In this situation, where there is one oviduct, transmigration may be as common as 30 percent. It's impossible to know whether it happens at the same rate for people with two ovaries and two oviducts. But considering that oviducts can be damaged by infection, it makes sense that the system has a built-in backup plan.

Why Does Ovulation Hurt?

Some people have visions of the follicle bursting open with ovulation, but it isn't under pressure. Enzymes cause the tissue to dissolve, and so the ovum doesn't have a dramatic entry, as it were, from the ovary. Why, then, do many people report pain with ovulation? It's a good question, as ovulation pain, also known as mittelschmerz (which, surprisingly, is not named after a Dr. Mittelschmerz but is German for "middle pain"), affects up to 40 percent of people and often occurs in every cycle. It's typically short-lived, lasting less than twelve hours. The discomfort can vary in intensity from a mild cramp to agonizing pain, and it is felt on the same side as the developing follicle. It can lead some people to erroneously receive a diagnosis of a ruptured cyst when what they have is severe pain linked to ovulation.

Pain with ovulation coincides with the highest level of LH, meaning the follicle is still growing but hasn't yet ovulated. Meaning it isn't due to ovulation itself; rather, the pain is believed to be caused by contracting muscle tissue in the ovary triggered by chemicals known as prostaglandins. It is perhaps more accurate to think of it as mid-cycle menstrual cramps. This is a great example of how understanding more about the hormones in the menstrual cycle and about anatomy (the fact that there is muscle in the ovaries) can help reframe what is happening to your body and empower you to make decisions. Also, knowing that ovulatory pain coincides with the LH surge, meaning right before ovulation, means you are being given a biological signal that ovulation is about to occur, which may be helpful in timing intercourse for pregnancy.

Thinking Outside of the Twenty-Eight Days

You may have noticed that the menstrual cycle is described in phases, and not halves, and that is because the follicular and luteal phases are rarely the same length. The idea of halves comes from an "idealized" cycle length of twenty-eight days, where the luteal phase was believed to be a strict fourteen days. But twenty-eight days isn't the most common length, or even the average.

How did twenty-eight days as the length of the menstrual cycle become canon, even though it's false a good percentage of the time? For most of history, people thought of menstruation as monthly, meaning a lunar month of 29.5 days. Seeing a connection between the lunar cycle and menstruation didn't mean the ancients expected the waxing or waning of the moon to drag people into menstruation the way its gravitational pull controls the tides (although "king tide," or perhaps "queen tide," might be another good euphemism for menstrual bleeding). Rather, they thought of menstruation as coming and going like the phases of the moon, and timed its appearance based on its occurring once a lunar month. To be clear, the moon isn't related to menstruation in any way. There is data to back this up, but common sense also tells us that if the moon controlled menstruation as it does tides, everyone would menstruate at the same time.

Now is probably as good a time as any to dispel the urban legend that in days of yore humans rarely menstruated. This myth is based on a common belief that the historical hardships of life, pregnancy, breastfeeding, and famine inhibited menstruation. But if menstruation were rare in our history, multiple ancient societies would not have connected it with the lunar cycle, and we wouldn't have all these words that literally translate to "once a month" or "monthly." Why would you link one or two periods a year with a lunar cycle? It just doesn't make sense. Moreover, if menstruation rarely happened, then pregnancy too would be rare. We know that only 20 to 30 percent of conceptions (meaning an egg and sperm meeting) result in pregnancy, and historically only about 50 percent of children lived to the age of reproduction. If there had been only one or two ovulations a year, it's unlikely there would have been enough offspring to maintain the population.

It's clear from their writings that the Ancient Greeks expected menstruation once a month. They believed women were overly moist, their flesh was too spongy, and they retained too much fluid. The fact that they leaked blood in a cyclic and regular fashion was proof of their physical inferiority. (Men, on the other hand, were in perfect balance.) Menstruation was seen basically as an overflow valve for bad plumbing, and its absence was medically concerning, as the extra moisture could build up and cause harm. Plus, regular menstruation was known to be important for fertility, so the Ancient Greeks had all kinds of recipes that were meant to restore it. If menstruation had been uncommon, its absence simply wouldn't have been cause for concern.

Did women historically have fewer periods? Most likely, as they had more pregnancies and likely breastfed longer. But overall, enough menstruated regularly that it was universally accepted as a once-a-month cycle.

Most historical medical writings weren't overly concerned with the precise number of days in the menstrual cycle—if menstruation occurred monthly, that seemed healthy. Although interestingly, in *The Midwives Book*, published in 1691, midwife Jane Sharp wrote that the courses (as menstruation was known then) came once a month, which she listed as "27 daies [*sic*] and odd minutes," which is a strange number.

My hypothesis is that the rigid twenty-eight days of perfection comes from the Victorians, who seem perpetually to be the source of prudishness and conformity. Variance of a few days from cycle to cycle is normal, but that's messy, so better to gaslight everyone into a regimented standard of twenty-eight days. I imagine Victorian physicians listening to women explaining their cycles and then picking up a steel-nibbed pen and saying, "My dear, I think you meant two fortnights." And then, once we learned about ovulation and hormones, it seemed as if the luteal phase was fourteen days, which fit nicely with a twenty-eight-day cycle.

When in doubt, blame the Victorians.

So if it's not twenty-eight days, what *is* a typical menstrual cycle, timewise? One of the first large-scale studies on menstrual regularity, published in 1967, encompassed thirty years of data from 2,700 women. After the first few years, there was significant participant attrition, and by the final year there was but one lone stalwart remaining. I imagine her as an explorer, daring to go where others wouldn't, arm raised defiantly, yelling, "For science!" Collecting data for a study for thirty years is hard-core, so kudos and thank you to her (and, of course, all the other participants). This study's data placed the typical menstrual cycle in a range of twenty-six to twenty-nine days, and the authors noted, "There is no justification for the widespread belief that women normally vary in menstrual interval about a value of 28 days."

We now have more knowledge about the menstrual cycle, thanks to recent studies looking at hormone levels (which adds accuracy about the phase of the cycle), as well as data collected by menstrual tracking apps. These apps provide an opportunity to gather an enormous amount of data, although it's prudent to consider that they may not accurately reflect the general population, as there might be differences between people who choose to use a tracking app and those who don't. These kinds of studies, where data is collected as the menstrual cycle is happening, are important because many people are less reliable than they think when it comes to remembering the first day of their last menstrual period. For example, 15 to 45 percent of pregnant people don't accurately recall the date of their last menstrual period, as revealed by ultrasound dating. There is no shame in forgetting when your period started (look, I can't remember what I had for breakfast two days ago), and it doesn't mean that people don't know their own body, but it's important to recognize that studies that ask people to recall their last cycle or cycles are prone to inaccuracies.

We now believe the average length of the menstrual cycle is twenty-nine days for those between ages twenty and forty (one study put it at 28.9 days and the other 29.3, so very close to the 29.5-day lunar calendar, but not spot-on). One thing to keep in mind is that while averages may be useful for communicating data in studies, they tell us very little about the individual human experience. For example, if we say the average menstrual cycle is twenty-nine days, it could mean that 100 percent of people have a twenty-nine-day cycle or that 50 percent of people have a thirty-four-day cycle and 50 percent have a twenty-four-day cycle. For this reason, it is better to think about the menstrual cycle in terms of the normal range, which can be anywhere from twenty-four to thirty-eight days. Some sources use twenty-one to thirty-five days as the normal range, but we'll use twenty-four to thirty-eight here as that is the range used by FIGO (The International Federation of Gynecology and Obstetrics). Variations in cycle length of up to seven days (up to nine days for those age twenty-five and younger) from cycle to cycle are not a cause of alarm, meaning one cycle could be twenty-five days and the next twenty-nine days and that would not signify any medical concern. Most of the variation in cycle length is built into the follicular phase. Think back to the waves of follicles in that phase: more waves mean a longer follicular phase and hence a longer cycle overall.

Cycles tend to be longer for people closer to age twenty, then they gradually get shorter, and then lengthen out again in the few years before menopause, when it is not uncommon to go two to three months between periods. The average length of menstrual bleeding is five days, but anything from one day to seven is considered typical. The heaviest bleeding is typically on day 2.

We don't understand why some people have shorter menstrual cycles and others longer ones. However, a shorter cycle appears to be linked with an earlier onset of menopause and with endometriosis. It's not clear why this association exists, but it's something to know about.

Is Menstruation a Vital Sign?

Yes and no. But not in the way you might think. Meaning, it's complicated.

Vital signs are measurements that provide important information about health. For example, a heart rate that is too fast or too slow can be a sign of heart disease. However, people can also have heart disease with a normal heart rate. And some people have a slow heart rate and don't have heart disease. And if people are on medications that affect heart rate, we can still assess the health of their heart. Like most things in medicine, the situation matters immensely.

Some time ago, menstruation was introduced as a vital sign. This was aimed primarily at teens and their health care providers, to stress the importance of education about menstruation, as teens are often unaware of what a typical period entails. Consider my experience as a teen, where I had no concept that my bleeding was heavy and assumed it was something to suck up. After all, television and the movies were filled with lots of innuendo about the hardship of being a woman. Education about basic biology is lacking in most schools, and many health care providers dismiss people with menstrual concerns, so the framing of menstruation as a vital sign was and is an important step toward education and empowerment. As we'll learn in later chapters, heavy, irregular, missed, and painful periods can all be signs of medically concerning conditions (and of course deserve treatment). You can only know whether your situation is abnormal if you know what is considered medically normal.

Unfortunately, some corners of the Internet that promote what I call Big Natural Menstruation—sites that are often inhabited by naturopaths, period coaches, and others who sell unregulated supplements to fix "broken" periods—have corrupted the messaging about menstruation as a vital sign into a false narrative that you can't possibly know how healthy you are if you are taking hormonal contraception and not having what I can only describe as a RealPeriod™. The barely veiled implication is that "real women" ovulate, and their bleeding is an offering that shows they are "in tune" with nature or God (the word choice varying depending on the person's worldview and political affiliation). Apparently, not being able to monitor health via menstruation during pregnancy is not a concern, because if you are pregnant you have leveled up, as far as nature or God is concerned.

While there are medical situations where it is preferable for menstrual monitoring to not take hormonal contraception, there are also many medical situations where hormonal contraception is the most evidence-based therapy, and of course for many it is the contraception of choice. But the influencers who peddle the so-called real period narrative seem unconcerned with facts or nuance. It's also important to point out that many of the people railing against contraception in this manner are themselves selling supplements that are grossly undertested if they are tested at all. Their hypocrisy here knows no bounds. And if you look a little closer, you will find that many are forced birthers, and there is also a significant anti-vaccine overlap. Meaning these are not folks from whom you should be getting health advice. This is a quest for a so-called real period at all costs, not education, and it is dismissive of the medical benefits of contraception. When these people say "You can only properly track your health if you don't take the pill," I hear "We're totally okay if you get endometrial cancer as a result of your irregular ovulation and lack of progesterone" or "It's fine that you suffer from terrible cramps once a cycle" or "If you get pregnant, it's your own fault" (side note: I've yet to see anyone from Big Natural Menstruation who provides abortions). The implication is, if you can't control your symptoms or conditions or prevent pregnancy by taking supplements, following a restrictive diet, and/or charting your cycle, you aren't trying hard enough. It's as if we aren't living in the twenty-first century.

The truth is, while menstrual disturbances can be a sign of health concerns (as you will learn in later chapters), they are rarely the only sign. Moreover, hormonal contraception is often the best therapy for many conditions and has been extremely well tested.

What's in a Name?

A typical menstrual cycle revolves around ovulation, so it is often referred to as an ovulatory cycle. However, it's important to recognize that this term doesn't apply to everyone. Many people have bleeding but aren't ovulating (the mechanisms behind this are covered in Part 3). Medically, there are reasons why it's important to know whether bleeding is due to ovulation, so there are some who want to label menstruation with hormonal contraception as a withdrawal bleed instead of a menstrual bleed.

I am not a fan of othering some bleeding. Someone who has a period with the birth control pill is bleeding because of the withdrawal of progestin (a progesterone-like hormone), and someone who is ovulating is bleeding because of the withdrawal of progesterone. They are *both* withdrawal bleeds. And if we decide to tie the definition of menstruation to ovulation, which the pill prevents, then what do we call menstruation that occurs without ovulation? As I'll discuss in later chapters, there are many medical reasons why people between puberty and menopause may have a period without ovulating. Do we tell a thirteen-year-old who has just started menstruating that their bleeding isn't really a period because during the first year or two they are likely not ovulating regularly? Do we tell people with polycystic ovarian syndrome, a condition characterized by irregular bleeding that often occurs without ovulation, that they aren't really menstruating? Even cycles that appear "regular" may not involve ovulation.

For me, the answer isn't clunky terminology that can easily be abused by the so-called real period charlatans selling period coaching and supplements. I advocate for referring to all bleeding between puberty and menopause as menstrual bleeding or menstruation (or whatever euphemism you like), because it all shares the same basic physiologic trigger: something has destabilized the lining of the uterus. I also believe it's important to educate yourself so that you understand *your* cycle in the context of your own health and any medication you may be taking, so you know when to be concerned and why and how to self-advocate. (Hence this book!)

Bottom Line

- The average menstrual cycle is twenty-nine days, but it is better to think of it as a range of twenty-four to thirty-eight days, which can fluctuate in length by up to seven days from cycle to cycle.
- The body goes through about a thousand primordial follicles to get one to the point of ovulation.
- The first part of the menstrual cycle is when waves of antral follicles develop, eventually resulting in one dominant follicle that becomes the egg. The follicular phase is driven by follicle-stimulating hormone (FSH) and characterized by the production of estrogen.
- When estrogen levels are high enough, they cause the brain to release luteinizing hormone (LH), and when those levels surge, ovulation is triggered and large amounts of progesterone are released to decidualize the endometrium.
- Menstruation is considered a vital sign in the sense of the importance of knowing what is typical and what is concerning. This doesn't mean everyone who isn't tracking their cycle is missing out.

3

The Brain-Brain-Ovary Connection

How does the body know to keep menstrual time? It's something, right?

The menstrual cycle has two clocks. One keeps time for the follicles, regularly guiding some primordial follicles from hibernation to the potential to ovulate. This is a long cycle that occurs over months and months, and the exact messaging is unknown. However, there is another clock, one that produces the hormones to stimulate the follicles that have been awakened. This cycle, the one that governs the menstrual cycle, is a bit like a relay race, except instead of a baton being passed from person to person, it's a message being passed from organ to organ via hormones. The message must originate somewhere, and with menstruation, the story starts deep in the brain.

Menstruation that results from ovulation depends on a communication superhighway between two areas of the brain—the hypothalamus and the pituitary—and the ovaries (medically this is called the hypothalamic-pituitary-gonadal axis, or HPG axis, as the ovaries are also gonads). I like to think of it as the brain-brain-ovary connection. Understanding the basics of this communication pathway will open up much about the menstrual cycle that might have previously seemed mysterious or weird. The impact of diet, stress, sleep, and many medications, and even how many contraceptives work, can be easily explained once you are familiar with the menstrual superhighway.

The hypothalamus, one of the body's key command centers, is located deep in the brain. If your body is Goldilocks, it's the job of the hypothalamus to keep most things in the "just right" range. It receives all kinds of complex information and then makes adjustments on the fly involving many vital functions, such as hunger, thirst, weight, temperature, sleep, emotion, pain, the immune response to infection, sexual behaviors, and, yes, menstruation. One example of how these shared connections work is the link between body temperature and menstruation. A slightly higher temperature favors implantation, which is why body temperature rises during ovulation. Sometimes I think of a very tired but knowledgeable cast of characters living in the hypothalamus, similar to the plot of the Pixar movie *Inside Out*. When the reproduction tech gets the call that ovulation is ready, they yell at the temperature tech, "Time to rev up the furnace!"

When it comes to the hypothalamus and menstruation, instead of brightly colored imaginary avatars, the messenger is a hormone called gonadotropin-releasing hormone (GnRH). GnRH doesn't work directly on the ovaries; rather, it triggers the pituitary gland (also in the brain) to release hormones called gonadotropins. Admittedly, the name *gonadotropin-releasing hormone* is a bit of a mouthful, but it tells you exactly what it does. GnRH is released in pulses, the frequency depending on the phase of the menstrual cycle. These pulses are what's key, because the signals to the pituitary are encoded in the pulse frequency and the amount of hormone in the pulses. I like to think of GnRH pulses as a metronome for the cycle.

Why should you know about GnRH pulses? It might seem esoteric; after all, most of us don't think much on a day-to-day basis about the inner workings of our brains. But it's fascinating that human reproduction is based on what amounts to Morse code from a set of specialized nerve cells. It may sound like a fragile system—I mean, tiny hormone pulses that code a message? Yet all mammals use GnRH pulses, so evolutionarily speaking it's ancient, and systems that don't work well or are easily corrupted are typically weeded out by evolution. It isn't surprising that animal studies suggest normal fertility can be maintained even when only 10 percent of the specialized neurons that produce GnRH remain.

Initially, researchers thought the nerve cells that released GnRH set the beat, if you will, like a pacemaker in the heart. However, we now know there is another set of neurons, called KNDy neurons, that send instructions to the GnRH neurons. The KNDy neurons make substances called kisspeptin, neurokinin B, and dynorphins, so KNDy, pronounced "candy," is an acronym. You don't need to know these terms (there is no multiple-choice quiz at the end of the book), but aren't you interested to know why these neurons are called "candy" and why two of the substances sound like regular medical terms but one includes the word *kiss*? The first of these signaling substances was identified by researchers at the University of Pittsburgh in Hershey, Pennsylvania, who named it in honor of the Hershey's Kiss. Hence the whole candy theme, and this is why scientists are scientists and not standup comedians.

The KNDy-hypothalamus system is especially sensitive to estrogen and progesterone, and these hormones can act like both a gas pedal and a brake pedal, depending on the levels. Hormones have such a profound impact on the hypothalamus-KNDy system that animal studies have shown if a male monkey is castrated and then has an ovary implanted, and if that ovary is triggered to ovulate by pharmaceutical hormones, the hormones produced by the now-functioning ovary basically retrofit GnRH pulses in the brain to follow the female pattern. We also know that giving estrogen to trans women changes their GnRH pulses so they become more like those of cisgender women.

The KNDy-hypothalamus system constantly receives feedback from the body, such as daylight, temperature, stress, and calorie intake, and it adjusts accordingly. What you need to remember about all this is that hormones and multiple chemical signals are acting directly on the hypothalamus and by way of the KNDy neurons to regulate menstruation in a highly complex manner. GnRH has been running fertility, not just for humans but for all mammals, for tens of thousands of years. This is an ancient system that is immune to the smoothie hacks promoted by medical influencers on Instagram and TikTok. The idea that kale, acai berries, and special supplements for $29.99 ($24.99 if you get the subscription) can somehow override or "fix" this system is ridiculous. Unless, of course, those supplements or smoothies contain hormones, which some do, as they are unregulated (and you definitely want to avoid those!).

GnRH from the hypothalamus has one job: to communicate with the pituitary gland, which is a small but mighty hormone command center. It releases several hormones, including the hormone that triggers the thyroid gland to make thyroid hormone, prolactin for breastfeeding, and gonadotropins, the hormones that stimulate the follicles in the ovary, follicle-stimulating hormone (FSH) and luteinizing hormone (LH). Faster pulses of GnRH trigger FSH, and slower pulses trigger LH. FSH and LH are also important in the production of sperm and testosterone, but they were named before scientists knew that fact. Just another point in favor of renaming certain terms.

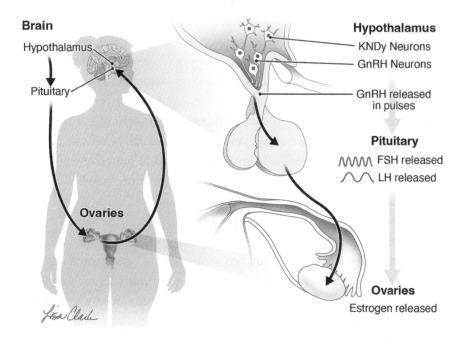

Figure 3 • *The Hypothalamic-Pituitary-Gonadal Axis (Illustration by Lisa A. Clark, MA, CMI)*

What Happens During Breastfeeding?

Lactation is perhaps the most metabolically taxing endeavor a human body can undertake. To produce 750–1000 ml (25–34 ounces) of milk requires 500–600 extra calories a day, and this intake must be sustained over months. Some of the energy for milk production comes from fat stores, but most comes from the food eaten that day. The metabolic drive for lactation is so strong that energy goes toward making milk regardless of nutritional status, so essentially lactation parasitizes the body. Because pregnancy is also metabolically demanding, a system to prevent pregnancy during breastfeeding is beneficial so that all resources can support breastfeeding.

When a baby breastfeeds, suckling sends signals to the hypothalamus, disrupting GnRH pulses, and this has a profound effect on LH, which affects the development of follicles and prevents ovulation. There are likely other mechanisms involved as well. Breastfeeding-induced lack of ovulation is known as lactational amenorrhea, and it can be very effective contraception for several months. People who breastfeed exclusively (meaning no supplementation with water) or who breastfeed almost exclusively (meaning infrequent water or juice), who don't go long periods of time between feedings, whose infant is less than six months old, and who have no menstrual bleeding (excluding post-delivery bleeding, which can last up to fifty-six days after delivery) can expect a pregnancy rate of 1 to 2 percent over six months with lactational amenorrhea. Unfortunately, pumping breast milk is not an adequate substitution for suckling. In one study that also included pumping, the pregnancy rate over six months was 5 percent.

Suckling also triggers the release of the hormone prolactin from the pituitary. Prolactin is important in milk production but doesn't seem to play a significant role in the suppression of ovulation.

After six months of breastfeeding, the absence of menstruation becomes an unreliable predictor of lactational amenorrhea, so an additional source of contraception is recommended for people who don't want another pregnancy at that time. A subsequent pregnancy is most likely to have a good outcome when the interval between birth and getting pregnant the next time is at least 18 months.

Without breastfeeding, once the placenta is delivered, the hormonal suppression of GnRH pulses (aka the hand brake on ovulation) is released, and menstruation typically resumes four to six weeks after delivery, although the first few cycles often don't involve ovulation. Some follicles develop and produce estrogen, but ovulation isn't triggered. As the follicles regress, the withdrawal of estrogen destabilizes the endometrium and menstruation occurs. The average time to the first ovulation after delivery is about forty-five days, but there is a wide range of experiences.

Interestingly, research shows that an increase in body mass index (BMI) during lactation occurs shortly before the return of ovulation, which makes sense because once energy is available to accumulate as fat stores (because lactation isn't consuming it all), that means there are calories to divert for a potential pregnancy.

Menstruation for Transmasculine People

Some trans men and nonbinary people with ovaries and a uterus may choose to start testosterone therapy for its masculinizing effects. Testosterone also interferes with the brain-brain-ovary connection, suppressing GnRH, so it provides another benefit by suppressing ovulation and decreasing estrogen. Ovulation typically stops within two months if testosterone levels are in the typical "male" range, and after six months of appropriately dosed testosterone therapy, menstruation should stop. Most people using testosterone therapy have adequate suppression of ovarian function, meaning they don't continue to produce high levels of estrogen from their ovaries, but some do, and they may need to add in other therapies to fully suppress estrogen (unless, of course, they decide to have their ovaries surgically removed).

The effect of testosterone on ovulation hasn't been adequately studied, meaning we don't yet have the data to say how effective testosterone may be as a contraceptive. Because many trans and nonbinary people have difficulty securing care or paying for medications, there may be unanticipated breaks in their therapy, increasing the odds of unplanned pregnancy for those who have sex that puts them at risk of it. Current advice is that people who take testosterone should use contraception if they have sex that involves a risk of pregnancy. Testosterone should be stopped prior to pregnancy because it can cause a female fetus to masculinize.

The long-term impact of testosterone on the follicles is unknown, but we currently believe the effects are reversible, so if trans men and nonbinary people who want to get pregnant stop taking testosterone and their levels return to the "female" range, there is no medical contraindication to pregnancy. More study is needed here.

Another consideration with testosterone is its effect on the uterus. Up to 10 percent of people taking testosterone may experience uterine bleeding, likely due to the testosterone suppressing estrogen enough that, as far as the endometrium is concerned, it's like menopause, meaning there is no estrogen to stimulate the lining. Think back to the brick wall analogy and the lower layer of endometrium. Without estrogen, this layer can become very thin and may bleed. Although testosterone is converted to estrogen by an enzyme called aromatase, overstimulation of the endometrium from this conversion doesn't seem to be an issue. Transmasculine people who have bleeding with testosterone should report it to their health care provider so they can determine if it is a side effect of the testosterone, if there is another cause, or if the testosterone dose is not high enough.

Is Cycle Syncing Real?

Many people have heard the myth that menstrual cycles can "sync up," meaning if two or more people who menstruate spend enough time together in relatively close confines, their menstrual cycles will get closer together and eventually run on the same schedule. We often hear stories of how this has happened with sisters or friends or officemates. The idea of menstrual cycle syncing has been around for a long time. I heard it when I was growing up in the 1980s, but I'm sure it predates me by centuries. The main study that is offered in support of this theory has some serious flaws, so it really can't be considered. The menstrual period tracking app Clue analyzed data in 2017 and was unable to find any evidence supporting the phenomenon.

Consider the brain-brain-ovary connection we've just reviewed. It's an ancient system that relies on GnRH pulses related to a person's own hormonal milieu and environmental cues. There is no external nonhormonal source that can override what is happening in the body in some mysterious way. KNDy neurons and GnRH pulses from one person can't affect another, nor can FSH, LH, or estrogen. Some proponents of menstrual syncing claim that pheromones—chemicals that can travel through the air and affect reproductive function—are the cause. After all, in some species, male animals can trigger female animals to ovulate via pheromones. There's a catch here, though: humans don't have a functional vomeronasal organ, which is the apparatus needed to detect pheromones. No one who has advanced the concept of cycle syncing has proposed a biologically plausible mechanism for it, which is needed for a working hypothesis. Menstrual miasma (she waves her hands in the air) drifting through the ether from one person to another just doesn't cut it.

And then there is the question of the biological value of a woman coordinating menstrual cycles with another woman. The menstrual cycle is about resource curation and optimizing reproduction. It seems to me it would be detrimental if everyone were to ovulate at the same time; the window for conception among a given group of people would be very narrow, reducing the group's overall ability to conceive.

My theory is that this belief is a holdover from when people thought women could cast hexes and spells. Remember, almost everything written about menstruation was penned by men, and magical ideas about it (and about women in general) often reflected their fear that women were witches. And so it became folklore and then gospel. But honestly, if any women had magic, I highly doubt they would waste it on a parlor trick like syncing menstrual cycles.

I know some of you are shaking your head right now, sure this has happened to you. I worked with an OB/GYN who was positive she could drag female coworkers into menstruation with her. But she only remembered the days when she was menstruating at the same time as someone else and seemed to forget those times when she and her supposed co-menstruators were on different schedules. This is a phenomenon known as recall bias—romanticizing or forgetting select pieces of information (it doesn't have to be intentional, but selective memory is common). Remember, menstrual cycle length can be anywhere from twenty-four to thirty-eight days, and a seven-day swing from cycle to cycle is normal, so it's likely that if you follow two people's menstrual calendars for a year, there will be two or three cycles where they start menstruating within one or two days of each other. It's statistics, not magic.

Vaccines and Menstruation

Many women reported via social media that they had a significant change in their menstrual cycle after receiving a COVID-19 vaccine. The changes included early periods, late periods, skipped periods, heavy periods, and more painful periods. The first step for health care providers in such a situation is to look to the medical literature to see what previous vaccine studies have shown . . . and it was infuriating and disappointing to find only one, low-quality study of women who had received the vaccination for human papillomavirus (HPV) in Japan, which suggested a possible link between the vaccine and heavy and/or irregular bleeding. But this study had a lot of issues and can't be relied upon for much, except to say maybe there was a link. Maybe.

Fast-forward to now. Fortunately, several groups of researchers took the reports of menstrual disturbances seriously and conducted good-quality studies. As of December 2022, there are two large sets of data from apps that track cycles (the Natural Cycles app and the Apple Watch), as well as a small prospective study and several surveys (of varying quality). The Natural Cycles/Apple data is perhaps the best, because people were tracking their menstrual cycles before and after vaccination, so the researchers went back and pulled data that was collected in real time, which allowed them to compare the participants' postvaccine menstrual experience with their prevaccine baseline. The Natural Cycles app study looked at over fourteen thousand vaccinated individuals and more than four thousand controls, and the Apple Watch study had over eight thousand vaccinated participants and more than one thousand unvaccinated controls. The control group was important to make sure there wasn't something else affecting everyone's menstruation—stress, for example—that could cause a change that was then mistaken for a vaccine effect.

Overall, the studies noted a postvaccination lengthening of the menstrual cycle by less than one day. Keeping in mind that a seven-day change in length between cycles (measured from day 1 to day 1) is normal, such a minor change is not medically concerning. The cycle length also quickly reverted to baseline. In the Natural Cycles study, the menstrual cycle was on average 0.55 day longer after the first dose of an mRNA vaccine and 0.29 day longer after the second. With the Apple Watch study, it was a difference of 0.50 day and 0.39 day for the first and second dose respectively. So the results were very similar, which is reassuring.

When researchers looked more closely at the data, they found that the change in menstrual cycle was observed primarily in people who had received two vaccine doses during the same cycle. These people experienced an average temporary lengthening of the cycle by 3.7 days, which returned to normal by the second cycle. A change in cycle length of eight days or more, something that *would* be medically significant, seemed to also be confined to people who had received two doses in a single cycle; 13.5 percent had an increase in cycle length of eight days or more, versus 5 percent for the unvaccinated control group. Meaning that, overall, about 8 percent of people who get two doses of an mRNA vaccine during a single cycle can expect that cycle to be longer than expected, but it will revert to baseline.

What about the reported experience of heavier periods? The Pharmacovigilance Risk Assessment Committee (PRAC) of the European Medicines Agency concluded that there is "reasonable possibility" that heavy menstrual bleeding is linked to the vaccine. As of December 2022, this assessment isn't based on a publicly available peer-reviewed study, so I haven't seen the data. As of this writing (and understanding that this could change, as it is an active area of research), the best data here is from the Norwegian Young Adult Cohort, a group of people ages eighteen to thirty already enrolled in a study evaluating the impact of the COVID-19 pandemic. In this group, approximately 7 percent of people reported heavier bleeding in their cycle after vaccination with an mRNA vaccine, and this returned to baseline by the next cycle.

We don't yet know how to link up the cause and effect for the minority of people who have a slightly longer cycle postvaccination. However, an effect on the corpus luteum is almost certainly not the cause. To lengthen the cycle, the life of the corpus luteum would have to be extended, and it's hard to come up with a vaccine-related mechanism that could accomplish that feat. Damaging the corpus luteum would shorten the cycle. It would also lead to miscarriages, but there is a lot of data on the safety of the vaccine in pregnancy, and there has been no increase in miscarriages or any negative outcome in pregnancy.

The most likely cause of postvaccine cycle lengthening is via the brain-brain-ovary connection at the beginning of the cycle, because this effect was almost exclusively seen when two doses were received in one cycle. With doses three or four weeks apart, the first dose would almost certainly have been given in the first week of the cycle, when GnRH pulses are telling FSH to stimulate the pool of follicles hoping to get recruited for ovulation. Think of how you may have felt after a vaccination. Many people feel crummy for a day, some have a fever, and some get swollen lymph nodes. This is all due to a temporary activation of the immune system. Basically, the body gets riled up and then realizes there's no threat, so it settles back down. Remember, the hypothalamus is the command center, taking in all kinds of information about temperature, stress, and illness, to name a few stimuli. It is biologically plausible that, for some people, the temporary immune system activation is enough to affect GnRH pulses. It might take a little longer for the brain to get the follicles in gear, and the effect would be a slight lengthening of the cycle.

As for heavy bleeding, the act of menstruation is controlled injury and repair that starts and stops the bleeding, and this process involves inflammation. It's possible that temporary inflammation from the vaccine could cause changes that result in a heavier cycle for some people. As we don't have much data on heavy periods, science is really in the hypothesis-generating phase in this area.

What we can take away from the studies is that any postvaccine menstrual cycle changes quickly revert to baseline, which is reassuring and expected. Remember, the GnRH system is an ancient and robust one—it takes a significant amount of damage to disrupt it. It evolved to be suppressed for long periods of time (pregnancy) and then pop back online. Doctors can prescribe medications to shut the system down, but when they are stopped, the cycle returns as if nothing had happened.

Another important lesson is that, because bleeding issues are common, it's essential to have cycle data before and after vaccination; otherwise, we can't distinguish between causation and correlation. In one of the studies, almost 38 percent of people surveyed reported a menstrual irregularity in the month before they were vaccinated. And before the COVID-19 vaccines were introduced, we were seeing exactly the same kinds of bleeding issues that some people are now attributing to the vaccine.

What about people who report that their periods have remained irregular for months after vaccination? More than 22,000 people and 375,000 menstrual cycles were tracked between the Natural Cycles and Apple Watch studies, and this phenomenon didn't emerge. While we need to learn more, if people are experiencing a significant change in their menstrual cycle that persists for more than two cycles, the currently available science tells us there is likely a cause other than vaccination.

Going forward, I hope menstrual tracking will become a routine part of vaccine research, as is temperature tracking and checking the lymph nodes. And as more data becomes available, we will hopefully learn more about the mechanisms responsible for menstrual cycle changes and heavier bleeding.

Bottom Line

- The menstrual cycle is a complex, coordinated sequence of events driven by pulses of the hormone GnRH, which are released from the hypothalamus in the brain.
- GnRH pulses are disrupted by exclusive breastfeeding, preventing ovulation. This is called lactational amenorrhea.
- Although testosterone therapy suppresses ovulation, trans and nonbinary people should not rely on it as a method of contraception.
- Menstrual cycle syncing is not a real phenomenon. Although the system of GnRH pulses can be affected by such factors as medications, fever, and access to sufficient calories, it isn't influenced by someone else's menstrual cycle.
- Vaccination against COVID-19 can produce a small, reversible change in the menstrual cycle that isn't medically concerning. Because the change is most pronounced when two doses of the vaccine are given within one cycle, it seems likely (to the best of our current knowledge) that there is a temporary effect on GnRH.

4

The Basics of Bleeding

Menstruation is the only scarless healing in the human body.

I know, right? It's amazing when you think of it that way.

Every cycle, much of the lining of the uterus sloughs off, and in many ways it's like skinning a knee. When you skin your knee, several layers of skin are removed and there is bleeding from the raw wound beneath; with menstruation, the superficial layer of the uterine lining detaches, exposing blood vessels that bleed. Yet unlike skinning your knee, menstruation can occur over and over again—possibly even 450 times—and each time heal as if nothing has happened. While it isn't magic, it is magical, and it demonstrates the marvel of evolution.

The Magician

This magic happens in the uterus, which is an organ, meaning it's a collection of tissues that form a structural unit with a specific function. Here, that function is reproduction. This doesn't mean the purpose of everyone with a uterus is baby making, but knowing the evolutionary design is helpful for explaining function.

The word *organ* comes from the Latin *organum*, which means "instrument" or "tool," so that is a fairly excellent etymology. And what an incredible organ the uterus is, unique in many fascinating ways. Even now, with more than thirty years of my life spent in OB/GYN, I am amazed at the uterus's dynamic nature. I don't believe any other organ in the body can perform so many diverse tasks while also simultaneously undergoing so many physical changes. During pregnancy, it must create new muscle cells, and by forty weeks the individual muscle cells are themselves tenfold bigger than before pregnancy. Then, after delivery it must repair without scarring and quickly return to a pre-pregnancy size, which requires selectively targeting some of the new muscle cells for death, a process called apoptosis. It's a sight to behold when the uterus contracts to half its size in a matter of minutes immediately after delivery. And then, six weeks later, when you see that patient back for a postpartum visit, the uterus is almost back to its pre-pregnancy size. It never quite shrinks back down all the way. It's like taking clothes out of the sealed plastic wrapping they arrive in when ordered online—if you decide to return the item, try as you might, you can never quite fold it back down to its original size.

In addition to the wonder of decidualization (discussed in Chapter 1) and repairing itself during each menstrual cycle without scarring, the uterus creates different kinds of cervical mucus. One kind protects the endometrium, and another allows sperm to pass through the cervix, assists in sperm transport and guiding the embryo to implantation, and is crucial for development of the placenta. It makes me think of the old television show *That's Incredible!* which ran from 1980 to 1984. Each week, people performed outrageous feats or showcased unusual talents or mind-blowing new technology, and there were sometimes even reenactments of paranormal events (now that I am writing this, it reminds me of a large portion of TikTok). Maybe it needs to be rebooted: *That's Incredible, Uterine Edition!*

The uterus is shaped a bit like an upside-down bottle and it's about 7.5 cm (3 inches) long and 5 cm (2 inches) in width at the widest section, weighs about 70 g (2.5 ounces), and is a little bit bigger for those who have been pregnant. The top of the uterus (which would be the bottom of the bottle) is known as the fundus; the body of the uterus is the main bulk of the bottle; the isthmus is where the body tapers to the neck of the bottle; and the cervix is the neck (the word *cervix* is even from the Latin for "neck"). I know that many people, doctors included, often say "the uterus and cervix," but that is like saying "your hand and thumb." Your thumb is part of your hand, and the cervix is part of the uterus. The cervix protrudes into the vagina, and the opening to it is called the os, which is from the Latin for "mouth."

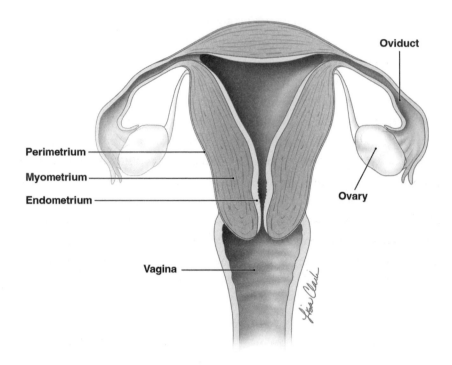

Figure 4 • *The Uterus (Illustration by Lisa A. Clark, MA, CMI)*

The shape of the uterus varies significantly among mammals. Many have a bicornuate uterus, meaning it divides at the top into two sections, or horns. Ancient humans were familiar with mammalian anatomy through the butchering of meat for food and religious sacrifice. But they were not familiar with human anatomy, as dissection was rarely performed, so the human uterus was often erroneously believed to have two horns as well. This may be why some ancient fertility symbols have two horns. Compared to our relatives in the mammalian kingdom, humans have a relatively simple uterine design with no special compartments. Think of how different a giraffe is from a human on the outside—it's no surprise that there is equal variation with internal structures like the uterus.

The wall of the human uterus is made up of three layers:

- *The endometrium:* The inner layer, often called the lining. It's composed of an inner basal layer and an outer, or superficial, functional layer. It's the functional layer that sloughs off with menstruation.

- *The myometrium:* The muscle of the uterus.
- *The perimetrium:* The outer layer, a thin layer of specialized tissue sometimes called the serosa. Think of it as plastic wrap around the bottle in our analogy.

The uterus is held in place between the rectum and the bladder by a large ligament called the broad ligament, which wraps around the front and back. The Ancient Greeks thought the uterus could roam around the body, putting pressure on organs and causing a plethora of ailments. They thought of it as a wild animal within a wild animal—the latter animal being a woman. One of the original purposes of vaginal steaming, which you may have heard rebranded as "yoni steaming," was to use fragrant herbs to coax the naughty uterus back into place. Sometimes they were not so fragrant (think disemboweled puppy stuffed with herbs). Simply because a practice is ancient does not make it medically worthwhile.

While the uterus doesn't wander, some people report that their cervix feels lower at different times of the menstrual cycle. This hasn't been studied, but there are several potential explanations. When the cervix is filled with mucus, its feel and size may change. It's also possible that during the luteal phase, when levels of progesterone and relaxin (another hormone) are high, the ligaments may relax a little, causing the cervix and uterus to drop slightly for some people who are predisposed.

The myometrium, the muscle of the uterus, is made up of millions of muscle cells intertwined with connective tissues that support, protect, and provide structure within the uterus. The individual muscle cells can be thought of as twigs, and the connective tissue as the twine that holds them together. There are also blood vessels, lymphatic vessels, and nerves. At the top of the uterus, the myometrium is mostly muscle, but heading down toward the cervix, the muscle fibers begin to mix with connective tissue, and by the cervix the muscle has been replaced entirely by connective tissue.

The myometrium is a type of smooth muscle, meaning it operates behind the scenes, without the brain's conscious involvement. Smooth muscle throughout the body is constantly working, performing all kinds of tasks, such as expanding and contracting within the walls of blood vessels to deliver blood to different parts of the body based on need; opening and closing the airways in your lungs; and squeezing the uterus during menstruation to help stop menstrual bleeding. Try as you might, you cannot think your bowels into contracting more often or turn uterine contractions on and off to control bleeding like a tap (although that would be useful—evolution needs to get on that). If our brains had to consciously think about moving stool in our intestines, making blood vessels dilate, or triggering blood to leave our bodies during menstruation—all tasks completed by smooth muscle on autopilot—we might never have had the brain space to crawl out of the primordial soup.

Since the invention of improved imaging techniques to look inside the body, like modern MRI and ultrasound machines, we now have a much greater understanding of how the muscle of the uterus contracts. Until these machines were invented, the only way to know what was happening was to insert a pressure catheter into someone's uterus, which they would wear for hours or longer. Not only is that expensive research, and uncomfortable for the gracious volunteers, but inserting the catheter could stimulate contractions, possibly affecting the results. Another option was extracting a human or animal uterus and hooking it up in the lab with electricity and monitors (think of a setup for creating Frankenstein's monster, but with a uterus), stimulating it with electricity or chemicals, and measuring activity. The issue here is that the way the uterus contracts in a lab, away from the chemical soup of hormones in the human body, may be different from the way it contracts inside the body. And of course, an animal uterus may not be designed for menstruation (most animals have estrus), and the ones we often study evolved to gestate a litter, so they may contract in very different ways. Lack of funding and misogyny (why should we study that?) always play huge roles in our lack of knowledge about the uterus and vagina—and about women's health care in general—but sometimes we don't know the answers because of research roadblocks. (Although it's true that with enough money, many roadblocks could turn into speed bumps.)

When people think of the uterus contracting, they often visualize a solid block of muscle squeezing, but there are actually three different layers of muscle in the uterus. The inner layer wraps around the uterus in a circle, directly supporting the endometrium. It contracts in a wave-like fashion that makes me think of those tall, waving, brightly colored inflatables outside of car dealerships. These contractions are present throughout the menstrual cycle, and their frequency increases as ovulation approaches; the hypothesis is that they move sperm up toward the oviducts. After ovulation, this inner layer of muscle also contracts to help guide the embryo to an ideal spot for implantation, and then the contractions stop with implantation. If there is no successful implantation, the muscle activity increases again when menstruation starts, and the directions of the waves reverse to help with the egress of endometrium and blood. That's incredible!

The middle layer, discovered recently, connects the inner and outer layers and has muscle fibers that are interlaced to form a web-like pattern. This layer also has a network of blood vessels. And in the outer layer, which is the thickest, the muscle fibers are arranged in a longitudinal or up-and-down pattern.

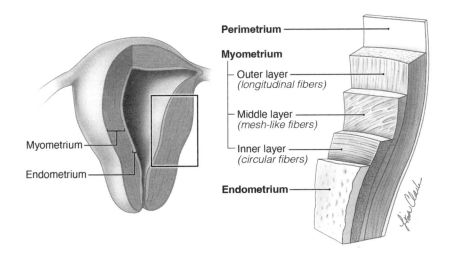

Figure 5 • *The Myometrium (Illustration by Lisa A. Clark, MA, CMI)*

During menstruation all three layers contribute to the contractions that move the blood out, and the pressure generated can reach 200 mmHg. That number likely means nothing to most non-OB/GYNs, but it is also the amount of pressure generated with uterine contractions during labor. Think of a blood pressure cuff when it is inflated to its tightest and is quite painful—that, too, is around 200 mmHg. Yeah, ouch. And during labor it's estimated that gram per gram, the myometrium is likely the strongest muscle in the body.

The Bleeding

By convention, day 1 of bleeding is the first day of the menstrual cycle, no matter how light the flow, although I understand why some people might not consider this intuitive. Since the bleeding happens because a pregnancy hasn't occurred, shouldn't it mark the end of the cycle? There are two issues here. First, the last day of bleeding is not reliable, as many people who have menstruated and had a "gotcha" day when they thought they were done can attest. To communicate about a cycle that is mostly invisible, we need a fixed day that is obvious. In addition, the hormonal changes of the next cycle—pulses of GnRH triggering FSH and rousing another wave of follicles—happen at the same time as menstruation.

The triggering event for menstruation with ovulation is the withdrawal of progesterone when the corpus luteum essentially runs out of gas. This causes a rapid increase in inflammatory cells, enzymes, and a chemical called nitric oxide. The net result is that the spiral arteries (coiled blood vessels) that have grown into the functional (top) layer of the endometrium constrict, reducing blood flow and causing the cells in the layer to die. The spiral arteries also rupture, and the endometrium fills with blood and inflammatory fluid; this bleeding helps to dislodge the dying functional layer, which cleaves off like a scab, leaving the basal layer. As this top layer of endometrium peels away, there is more bleeding from the now exposed blood vessels.

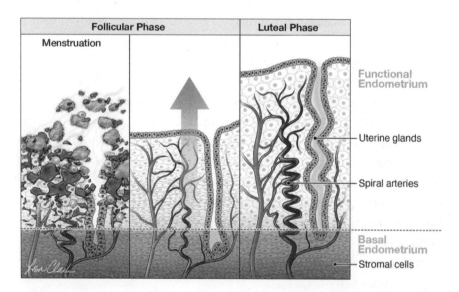

Figure 6 • *Changes with Menstruation (Illustration by Lisa A. Clark, MA, CMI)*

I think some people envision pools of blood in the uterus, sloshing around waiting for the signal to bleed. Because the uterus can feel heavy before menstruation, it's a logical assumption. Menstrual blood starts with blood from the ruptured vessels (it's about 75 percent arterial blood and 25 percent venous), decidualized endometrium, and inflammatory fluid and stem cells from the endometrium. As this mix passes through the cervix, it picks up cervical mucus, and then some vaginal discharge joins the jetsam. All this fluid together is considered menstrual blood, but it's only about 50 percent blood. Menstrual blood doesn't clot as well as other blood—if it did, it wouldn't flow freely out of the uterus, which would be problematic. A substance called fibrinolysin reduces the ability to clot, but it's not 100 percent effective, so it's not uncommon to see small clots, and occasionally larger clots with heavy bleeding.

This cascade of events also triggers prostaglandins, chemicals that govern inflammation, to be released from the endometrial cells, helping the blood vessels to spasm, which slows the bleeding and helps the blood clot. Prostaglandins cause the uterus to contract, which is felt as menstrual cramps. The inner layer of muscle helps to push the blood down the uterus and out the cervix, and contractions in the outer muscle layer put pressure on the blood vessels, which helps to stop the bleeding (just as, when you pinch your nose to stop it bleeding, you are compressing blood vessels, which helps them clot off). Prostaglandins can also induce contractions in the muscles around the vagina, which help to move blood downward; these contractions of the vaginal muscles are why some people feel cramping in their vagina.

When progesterone levels drop and the menstrual cycle starts up again, estrogen production kicks in, helping to rebuild the lining of the uterus from the basal layer and stop the bleeding. So the next cycle helps to repair the damage from the previous one. To go back to the brick wall analogy for the endometrium, at the end of menstruation what is left is like single bricks on the ground, with some spaces for blood vessels in between, like tufts of grass, where the decidualized endometrium was pulled away. Estrogen triggers the production of new endometrium, repairing these holes. Stem cells in the uterus, as well as specialized immune cells, help with this process, so the endometrium heals without scarring.

From time to time, I see posts on social media about the healing power of menstrual blood—for example, people using it as a facial to treat acne or reduce wrinkles. Some of this is likely just for shock value, but I'm sure there are people who think that because there are stem cells in menstrual blood, it has healing properties. However, simply applying stem cells to the skin's surface isn't any kind of therapy. During each menstrual cycle for several decades, those of us who used tampons or menstrual cups or discs got blood on our hands changing menstrual products, and most people who menstruate get blood on their vulva and inner thighs—never mind that the vagina is bathed in menstrual blood. If there were magical healing or anti-aging powers with topical application, we'd know.

What about the amount of bleeding? There is no lower limit on what is considered normal; basically, a spot of blood counts as a period. The upper end of the normal range is 80 ml (2.7 ounces) of blood for the entire menstrual cycle. Menstrual bleeding can last up to seven days, but five days or less is most common. Most of the blood loss, about 90 percent, happens in the first three days.

I know many people are thinking, "Say what now? Most cycles are less than 80 ml? That hardly seems possible!" This number wasn't pulled out of the air by a dismissive patriarchy; it is the result of several well-done studies to document the typical range. If you are throwing major side-eye right now because you think your bleeding is heavier and science has it all wrong, I can offer three possibilities: blood is only about half of menstrual fluid, meaning 50 ml of blood loss will be about 100 ml of fluid; actually your bleeding may indeed be heavier, and hopefully Chapter 13 will help you figure out why; or it looks like you are losing more blood than you actually are. It only takes a few milliliters (half a teaspoon) of blood in the toilet to give the appearance that there is more blood than water in the bowl.

Blood by Other Means

What I've just described is an ovulatory cycle, meaning estrogen and progesterone are produced in sequence by the process of ovulation. But as mentioned in Chapter 2, bleeding can happen without ovulation. How is this possible? There are two essential ingredients for bleeding from the uterus: some estrogen (so there is endometrium) and something to destabilize that endometrium. For example, as a follicle develops, it produces estrogen, but if ovulation doesn't happen (for any of a variety of reasons), the follicle will eventually stop producing estrogen and the levels will drop, destabilizing the uterine lining and causing bleeding. Medically, menstrual bleeding in the absence of ovulation is called anovulatory bleeding. As there is no way to tell for certain without blood work whether an individual bleed is ovulatory or anovulatory, conventionally we refer to all bleeding as menstrual bleeding.

Imagine a table set with a nice tablecloth (I'm partial to a red checkered cloth, like in a Parisian bistro) and dishes. The cloth and dishes are the top layer of the endometrium. An ovulatory bleed is analogous to using the tablecloth to lift everything off the table cleanly. Anovulatory bleeding is a cat knocking the dishes off the table. Some cats excel at knocking everything off quickly, dragging the tablecloth along for the ride; others may toy with the setup, knocking dishes off sporadically. The mayhem is unpredictable because in this analogy we are dealing with cats. So it is with anovulatory bleeding: the bleeding may be heavier than expected, it may seem typical, or it may be lighter. It can seem fairly regular or it can be wildly unpredictable. Basically, it's dealer's choice.

Does the Color of Menstrual Blood Matter?

The color of menstrual blood seems to be a Rorschach test for menstrual influencers. Depending on their point of view, bright red can mean high body temperature or the normal beginning of menstruation. Dark purplish red can mean endometriosis. But purple or blue blood is a sign of too much estrogen. Gray blood can be a sign of bacterial vaginosis. Pink blood means low estrogen. But pink blood is also the result of being on the pill. And the first day of bleeding. Dark-brown blood is also from the pill. And old blood.

I mean . . .

A lot of this comes from magazines and online sites wanting content. Other times it's companies selling menstrual products, trying to provide provocative content for page clicks. And sometimes it comes from people who have supplements and/or diets to sell, and who are often fearmongering about the pill.

First, menstrual blood is never purple or blue. It's also not gray. If you have a serious infection and there is pus pouring out of your uterus and you happen to be bleeding, the pus may mix with menstrual blood, leading someone to think, "Oh wow, there is pus in my menstrual blood." I would be shocked if anyone confused this for gray period blood. If this happens, call your health care provider immediately; if you can't reach them, you should seek urgent care.

The color of menstrual blood doesn't have any meaning cycle-wise because hormones don't change the color of blood. (If they did, when you have blood drawn at different times of the cycle it would be different colors!) Hemoglobin, the oxygen-carrying protein in blood, contains iron, which reflects red light, making blood look red—this has nothing to do with estrogen. Once blood leaves blood vessels, the color changes from bright red to crimson and eventually to an almost chocolate brown (which can sometimes be so dark it's almost black). This color shift occurs because of exposure to the oxygen in the air, which oxidizes the iron in hemoglobin from ferrous iron ($Fe2+$) to ferric iron ($Fe3+$). Oxidization converts hemoglobin to methemoglobin, which is dark brown. That is why a blood stain eventually turns a dark reddish brown.

Whether menstrual blood is bright red or crimson or chocolate colored depends on how oxidized it is when you first see it. Bright red blood has likely come straight out, but if the blood pools in the vagina for any length of time, even though the vagina is a low-oxygen environment, there is still enough to oxidize it. Spotting can produce what seems like light pink bleeding, which is a small amount of blood mixed with cervical mucus, but spotting can also be dark brown. Pink spotting is not related in any way to levels of estrogen or any other hormone.

The Immune System and the Endometrium

Because the inside of the uterus is connected to the outside world via the vagina, the endometrium must be able to respond to infections. The vagina is filled with bacteria, sperm is not sterile, and people who are sexually active may be exposed to sexually transmitted infections, so the immune system in the uterus must be able to mount a defense against microbes (such as bacteria and viruses) but tolerate sperm.

However, the immune system in the uterus doesn't just fight off viruses and bacteria; it is an integral part of the complex signaling of menstrual bleeding and repair each cycle. It's involved in embryo selection, the development of the placenta, and the growth of blood vessels during pregnancy. And there's more: it's also essential to the immune tolerance that is needed for an embryo, which has 50 percent foreign DNA. Normally the immune system rejects foreign DNA, which is why people who receive organ transplants need medications to suppress it.

In addition to specialized immune cells, the endometrium has a microbiome: a community of healthy bacteria that defend against other microbes by competing for space and food—basically hogging all the resources. This is a symbiotic relationship: the host houses and feeds the beneficial bacteria, and in return, the healthy bacteria provide some light housekeeping. What is different for the microbiome in the uterus, as opposed to the one in the gut, is that it must constantly adapt to changing levels of hormones, as well as a physically changing space with complex chemical changes.

Does Menstrual Blood Have an Odor?

If you had never heard of menstruation and were dropped into an American drugstore, you wouldn't be faulted for thinking that menstruation stinks. In fact, you'd probably think it's worse than foot odor or diarrhea. Why else would they sell shelves upon shelves of vulvar washes with names that sound like vacation cocktails, such as Sunset Delight and Coconut Breeze, along with douches, scented vaginal suppositories, and scented menstrual products? Even some vulvar moisturizers mention odor!

This false lesson about menstruation being foul-scented, in desperate need of abatement, isn't uniquely American by a long shot, but I'm not sure any other cultures excel quite as much at profiting financially from it. Many cultures consider menstrual blood to be one of the most foul, polluting odors there is, and some even require women to segregate themselves or avoid preparing meals during menstruation. There are religions that bar women from temples during menstruation or provide specific instructions on how they should clean themselves before they can have sex with their husbands again. While this disdain of menstrual blood isn't universal, it's very common, and it is misogyny. If you want to control half the population, a good place to start is to tell them—beginning when they are children—that they inherently stink or are polluting.

Human blood does have a smell, sometimes described as metallic. The smell is caused by the chemical trans-4,5-epoxy-(E)-2-decenal. When blood meets skin, there is a chemical reaction between the iron in the blood and the lipids (fat) that are normally present on the skin's surface, and this produces a chemical called oct-1-en-3-one, which also emits a metallic and musty smell. Theories about the smell of blood are interesting. Some say that there are those who like it, possibly because it represents food; others suggest that humans dislike the smell of blood because it represents injury. Whether people can differentiate the smell of menstrual blood specifically hasn't been studied, and no, there are no special repulsive menstrual pheromones. Humans can't detect pheromones because, as discussed in Chapter 3, we lack a vomeronasal organ.

Given the lack of quality data, I can only offer my experience. I've walked into a small exam room with poor ventilation thousands of times while someone is menstruating, and I've never detected an odor. I can't tell whether someone is on their period unless they tell me, or I do an exam and see the blood. If you lift a pad soaked with menstrual blood up to your nose, there may be a smell of blood, in the same way that you might smell it if you had a nosebleed or if blood got all over your hands and then you put your hands up to your nose.

Might some people be more sensitive to certain smells at certain times of the menstrual cycle? Although this has been investigated, the studies are conflicting. When I interviewed Dr. Asifa Majid, an expert on smell and culture, for my podcast, *Body Stuff*, she told me the research didn't support "any changes in women's abilities to detect smells in different phases of their cycle," but she also admitted that there is probably not enough research for a definitive answer.

What *can* happen during menstruation is a shift in vaginal bacteria. The vagina is dominated by bacteria, mostly lactobacilli, that help maintain health, and part of their job is keeping harmful bacteria in check. There is a complex interaction between the vaginal microbiome, menstruation, and estrogen, and the vaginal microbiome is what affects the vagina's scent. During days 1 to 5 of the cycle, meaning during menstruation and maybe one to two days after, depending on the length of the cycle, potentially harmful bacteria are at their highest level, possibly because a component of menstrual blood preferentially feeds them, or because estrogen levels are at their lowest at this time of the cycle and estrogen is basically fertilizer for good bacteria. The vaginal pH is briefly higher during the very early follicular phase (days 1 to 5), but it recovers quickly when the lactobacilli get the minor bacterial imbalance back under control. It's possible that some people are more sensitive, smell-wise, to this minor flux in the ecosystem, or that some people have a more dramatic swing in bacteria before the system self-corrects.

These changes in the microbiome at the beginning of the cycle are believed to be why some people get bacterial vaginosis right after their period. It's possible that people who are concerned about odor have bacterial vaginosis and are mistaking it for the smell of menstruation. If you believe you have an odor, you should see a provider who is skilled in diagnosing and managing vaginal concerns (much more on bacterial vaginosis and vaginal and vulvar odor can be found in my book *The Vagina Bible*).

I see social media posts of people who promote using vaginal boric acid to restore the vaginal pH after menstruation. Sometimes this is also promoted to treat odor. Boric acid does not work by changing the pH—it is an antiseptic, meaning it kills bacteria in the vagina, both unhealthy bacteria and good bacteria, so it could end up making the issue worse in the long run. In addition, when we put an acid in the vagina, it only changes the pH for a few hours because vaginal acidifiers don't work. Now that you know this, consider blocking accounts that promote using boric acid in this way, as they are spreading disinformation (and are also often coincidentally selling boric acid). If they don't know how boric acid works, or know that its use is medically incorrect in this situation, what else don't they know?

What should you do if you are concerned about an odor during or shortly after menstruation? Instead of turning to scented products or embarking on a potentially harmful regimen of douching or using other products that claim to treat odor or balance pH (which is impossible), see a health care provider like me, who specializes in vaginitis, as we will evaluate you for odor. If your doctor doesn't diagnose bacterial vaginosis, ask them if they detect an odor. They should tell you. If they don't detect one, hopefully that will be reassuring. At this point in the visit, I usually bring up all the negative messaging about menstrual odor that my patient has likely been exposed to since she was very little. I ask if her partner is saying awful things about her smell, because I have seen this type of emotional abuse before, where a man tells his partner that she stinks. To be clear, the women in these cases had no medical conditions; their partners were just abusers. And so we discuss what's normal, I screen for intimate partner violence, and I always remind people that if someone says something unkind about your body, it is they who have the problem.

Finally, for someone who doesn't have bacterial vaginosis but is truly bothered by what they perceive as an odor with menstruation, it wouldn't be wrong to use hormonal contraception to suppress the menstrual cycle and menstruation, to see if that improves quality of life.

Can You Kick-Start a Period?

It's not uncommon to see claims that taking this herb or that supplement (which the promoters invariably sell) can bring on a period, basically kick-starting menstruation. The older name for a product that could supposedly accomplish this feat is an emmenagogue.

It's important to know some history here. A hundred or so years ago there were plenty of advertisements for tonics that were basically DIY gynecology in a bottle. Heavy bleeding, painful bleeding, too frequent bleeding, and, yes, absent bleeding—all could be fixed with the potion of wonder. In this context, "bringing on a missed period" was typically a euphemism for abortion. Today, these magic menstrual potions are not about abortion; rather, they are about "resetting" the menstrual cycle, either to treat infertility or irregular cycles or to bring on a period early when you are just so bloated and wish it would start already. These claims make me want to scream, "That's not how this works! That's not how any of this works!"

In Chapter 3, you read about how a set of pacemaker neurons in the brain coordinates with multiple hormonal signals to bring about a menstrual cycle. There is no plant or supplement that can trigger menstruation in this way.

If the endometrium is exposed to estrogen and then progesterone, or a progesterone-like medication is taken to mimic what happens during the luteal phase and then this medication is stopped, bleeding will occur thanks to withdrawal from the progesterone or progesterone-like medication. This is called a progesterone withdrawal test, and it tells us that the endometrium has been exposed to estrogen (because estrogen is needed to create the lining that can be triggered to bleed by priming it with progesterone and then stopping that medication), but it doesn't reset anything, meaning it doesn't kick-start FSH or the follicles waiting in the wings for the next cycle.

And while I know it seems like some things do trigger an early period—a trip to the gynecologist, taking a vacation, wearing white pants—that is simply correlation, not causation.

Is It Safe to Have Sex While You Are Bleeding?

Yes.

Undoubtedly, the myth that you can't have sex while menstruating is intertwined with the history in many cultures and religions of promoting menstruation as not just foul and polluting, but also particularly poisonous to a penis. Some cultures and religions forbid sex during menstruation. I've also seen barely veiled modern attempts at reviving the myth with research of dismal quality that suggests harm to the person who is menstruating. This "research," and I use that term loosely, should be ignored.

Have sex on your period if you want to, and don't if you don't want to. The only practicality to consider is the potential mess. For those who might be interested, a menstrual disc (reusable or disposable) may help reduce the flow of blood during sex with vaginal penetration. They can shift during sex, so this isn't going to prevent 100 percent of leaks, but some people find them useful. There are special menstrual towels for the bed made from the same absorbent fabric as period underwear, but they are pricey. And then there is my old favorite, the navy-blue towel that you lay down on the bed (aka the sex towel). I'm convinced that is its origin story, as dark blue camouflages blood so well. This is purely for laundry reasons. If you have white or cream towels and all the bloodstains don't get removed, now you have stained towels. But with navy blue, who is the wiser?

Exactly.

Bottom Line

- The uterus has three layers, the endometrium (the lining), the myometrium (the muscle), and the perimetrium (the outer layer).
- The myometrium has two layers. The inner one assists with sperm and embryo transport, as well as the movement of menstrual blood. The outer layer is essential for stopping menstrual bleeding and in contractions to deliver a fetus and placenta.
- The uterus generates the same amount of pressure with menstrual cramps as it does during labor contractions.
- Up to 80 ml (2.7 ounces) of blood is typically lost per menstrual cycle.
- The color of menstrual blood has nothing to do with hormones, there is no evidence to support menstrual blood odor, and many myths related to the supposed uncleanliness of menstrual blood have their roots in patriarchal religions.

5

Reproductive Hormones: A Handbook

Hormones are chemical keys encoded with a message, and they work by interacting with receptors on cells, which are the locks that allow the message into the cell. Without the right receptor, a hormone is as useless as me trying to write in a language that I don't know and that uses a different alphabet, so none of the letters or characters are familiar to me.

A wide variety of messages can be created by hormones. For example, the message could be telling the cell to divide, to make an enzyme, or even to increase the production of hormone receptors.

A Word on the Binary Ideology

There are many different steroid hormones in the human body. The ones that affect the menstrual cycle—estrogens, progesterone, and androgens—are known as reproductive or sex steroids. We'll get into what they do shortly. It's true that, with enough estrogen, most people, regardless of sex or gender or whether they have ovaries or testicles, will develop some characteristics that have traditionally been associated with being female, such as breasts. It is also true that, with enough testosterone (an androgen), most of those same

54

people will develop facial hair and their voice will deepen, characteristics traditionally associated with being male. Because estrogen was first extracted from ovaries and testosterone from testicles, it's understandable how they became part of the feminine-masculine gender binary.

While it is also true that a person with ovaries makes much more estradiol (the main estrogen) than testosterone, both hormones are important. Think of a recipe for making bread. It typically calls for flour, water, yeast, and salt, but you need much more flour than yeast; in my preferred recipe, there are about 3½ cups of flour and 1 teaspoon of yeast. Even though flour dominates the recipe volume-wise, without the relatively small amount of yeast I would get a doorstop, not a loaf of bread. The tiny amount of yeast is just as important as the massive amount of flour. It's the combination that counts. That analogy holds true for estrogens and androgens. I wonder how we in medicine might have viewed these hormones if we had always known that the ovaries also produce testosterone.

Unfortunately, our perception of sex hormones has been contaminated by the long-held incorrect view that sex and gender are the same and that they are binary, and the toxic belief that women are weak, breeding creatures and men are strong, superior beings. Honestly, that's not too far removed from the Ancient Greek belief that men were perfect and women were shoddily constructed, leaky creatures that were overly moist.

But having higher or lower levels of reproductive hormones doesn't make someone a woman or a man. Women in menopause, who stop producing large amounts of estrogen, are still women. A girl is still seen as a girl even when she isn't yet producing large amounts of estrogen. A trans woman is a woman whether she takes estrogen or not. And a woman with polycystic ovarian syndrome and higher levels of testosterone is still a woman. A man who has breast tissue because liver disease has increased his levels of estrogen is still a man.

I believe the way around the societal misuse and abuse of hormones, and the habit of tying them to problematic binaries, is to simply learn what they do and focus on the fact that there is nothing at all binary about so-called sex steroids. We should do away with calling them sex steroids and rename them reproductive steroids. After all, their primary function is to act on the reproductive organs. I refuse to call my ovaries or uterus a sex organ, because I don't use either of them to have sex.

Reproductive Steroids 101

When most people hear the word *steroid*, they probably think of doping scandals at the Olympics and the illegal or quasi-legal substances used in sports. But a steroid is simply a chemical with carbon-hydrogen bonds arranged in four rings (the description is a bit of a letdown, I know). Steroids are ancient molecules that have been keeping creatures alive for hundreds of millions of years. They play two very important roles: they make up our cell membranes and they are signaling molecules, meaning hormones.

Reproductive steroids are made from cholesterol. You've likely heard about the cholesterol in food, such as eggs or beef. It's a type of fat found only in animal products, although if you are a strict vegan and consume no animal products, your body makes cholesterol from the carbon in your food, as cholesterol is essential for life. A lot of cholesterol travels through the body bound to a carrier protein called low-density lipoprotein, or LDL, which is often referred to as "bad cholesterol" because elevated levels of LDL are linked with cardiovascular disease. However, we need some LDL, as it is the main delivery vehicle for the cholesterol used to make reproductive steroids.

Reproductive hormones are found in nature, and they can also be made in a lab. There are a few key concepts here, and they are important because the terms *natural* and *synthetic* are frequently misused, often by those who think every medical issue can be treated with supplements, cleanses, diets, and coaching. In fact, abuse of these terms is one of my red flags. When you see people promoting a product because it's "natural" or denigrating one because it's "synthetic," you are seeing marketing, not medicine.

A natural hormone is either made by the body or is found in nature and extracted unchanged from an animal or plant source (think of boiling salt water to get salt—the salt was always there; boiling just removed the water). The word *natural* would be considered a "god term," which is a word we assign a positive connotation to. People tend to think that anything "natural" is good, which is why the word is used so often in marketing everything from laundry detergent to hormones. However, as far as hormones are concerned, the natural estrogen made by the body can kill you by causing breast cancer or cancer of the endometrium. I could prescribe estradiol, an exact replica of the hormone made by the ovaries, and if I gave you a high enough dose, you might have a stroke. Meaning "natural" does not mean safe.

According to the *Cambridge Dictionary*, "Synthetic products are made from artificial substances, often copying a natural product." If I asked you to name a synthetic product, you might say fake fur, or plastic, or nylon. And when this term is applied to hormones used in medicine, as it often is, you might think synthetic hormones are bad for you. After all, we know ingesting plastics is bad, and they are synthetic. However, where hormones are concerned, *synthetic* means a novel compound that is similar in many ways, but not every way, to a natural hormone. These novel compounds are often altered to increase effects or to reduce side effects of the natural hormone. That doesn't mean a synthetic hormone is either good or bad. What tells us if something is safe is not whether it is natural or synthetic, but research. One big issue, though, is that *synthetic* is a "devil term," a word we automatically assign a negative connotation to. This is important to know, as *synthetic* is used as a chemical slur implying that a medication must be harmful, when the term is simply a way to describe a novel hormone.

Follicles in the ovary make estradiol, but estradiol can also be made in a lab from compounds not found in the human body. The lab process of making estradiol is either semi-synthesis (meaning the starting compound is found in nature) or synthesis (meaning the hormone is made from chemicals not found naturally). I want to point out that no one is simply grinding up yams to make hormones (although that's often the implication when they are advertised as "natural"). What matters is that estradiol can come from the ovaries or estradiol can be made in a lab by semi-synthesis or by synthesis, and the body can't tell the two apart.

Having natural hormones made by semi-synthesis and synthesis is important because no one wants to take an extract of powdered human ovaries. And having synthetic hormones is important because natural hormones aren't always capable of safely achieving the desired effect.

How can you tell what a hormone is made from? Estradiol, estrone, progesterone, and testosterone are the main hormones produced by the body that will be discussed throughout this book. The names don't tell you if these were made by the body or in a lab; the context does. If they are being used medicinally—for example, being taken as a pill or delivered via a vaginal ring—they were made by either semi-synthesis or synthesis. And if the name isn't estradiol, estrone, progesterone, or testosterone (or any other hormone made by the body), then it is a novel compound made by semi-synthesis or synthesis.

Estrogens

There are three estrogens produced by the human body: estradiol, estrone, and estriol. Estradiol is the most potent of the three, and it is the main estrogen produced from puberty to menopause. Most of the estradiol in the blood travels bound to a carrier protein called sex hormone binding globulin (SHBG); only the free hormone that remains unbound is active and available to interact with tissues. Besides the ovaries, other tissues, such as adipose (fat) tissue, the endometrium, the liver, the brain, bone, and muscles, make estradiol and estrone, but in much smaller quantities. The estrogen made there only acts locally on the tissues; it isn't meant to travel to the brain or the uterus. Estrone is made in large quantities in the liver as part of the metabolism, or breakdown, of estradiol for removal. Estriol is primarily produced during the metabolism of estradiol and estrone, meaning it is a waste product. It is also produced in large amounts by the placenta during pregnancy.

The early research on estrogen in the 1920s and early '30s was done on hog ovaries, amniotic fluid, and urine from pregnant women (to name a few sources), and there are a variety of different estrogens in these source materials. As no one had agreed on a nomenclature system, a flood of names was created, such as ovarian follicular hormone, oestrin, thelykinin, and folliculin, although none of these hormones were pure extracts of one estrogen, but rather a combination. Eventually, the different estrogens in human follicles were purified, and the three estrogens that we know today were identified and given the names dihydrotheelin (estradiol), theelin (estrone), and theelol (estriol). The root *theely-* is Greek, indicating femaleness. (I know, sigh.) But by this point so many drug companies had already sent their impure extracts to market, and there were so many generic terms and name brands, that it was all one hot mess.

Recognizing the name confusion (although I am sure they didn't say "one hot mess"), in 1936 the Council on Pharmacy and Chemistry decided a unifying name was needed for this class of hormones. They chose *estrogen*, the brand name of the Parke-Davis and Company product. Parke-Davis graciously relinquished their trademark on Estrogen, as well as on another product called Estrone. I would give a lot to know what happened in that room. Estrogen and Estrone (the brand names) were a nod to the fact they could induce estrus in mammals and similar changes in women. The word *estrus* is from the Greek word *oistros*, which has a few meanings, including "sexual season," "gadfly,"

REPRODUCTIVE HORMONES: A HANDBOOK • 59

"sting," and "madness." With that in mind, though it would be challenging, I'm all for renaming estrogen.

Estrogen has many essential functions during the menstrual cycle, but it also has widespread effects throughout the body. Some of its key functions include:

- Triggering physical changes during puberty, such as breast development.
- Stimulating growth of the endometrium during the follicular phase.
- Changing cervical mucus so it becomes favorable to the presence of sperm.
- Helping the oocyte (egg) mature.
- Communicating with the brain to influence pulses of GnRH.
- Maintaining vaginal health by depositing storage sugar into the vaginal cells, supporting the vaginal microbiome, and increasing blood flow to the vagina.
- Stimulating waves of contractions in the muscle of the uterus that move fluid, and hence sperm, from the cervix up to the oviducts.
- Regulating temperature by quieting an area of the brain that communicates about heat.
- Influencing a myriad of other systems and activities, such as brain function, the immune system, blood clotting, and pain processing, to name a few.

Progesterone

The naming of progesterone was nowhere near as complex as that of estrogen. It was recognized early on that this hormone was vital for a successful pregnancy, so the name was derived from the Latin *pro gestum*. Progesterone is pro-gestation.

There are three sources of progesterone. Small amounts are produced by the developing follicle before ovulation and by the adrenal glands, although most of the progesterone in the adrenal gland is converted to cortisol (another steroid hormone) and into androgens (testosterone and similar hormones). Most progesterone is made by the corpus luteum in the luteal phase of the menstrual cycle. *Corpus luteum* means "yellow body," and if you were to cut an ovary in half and look at a corpus luteum, it would be easy to spot with the naked eye because the tissue is a striking yellowish orange, like a dark egg yolk, due to a large amount of lutein, which is yellow. The first time I saw one, the color was so saturated I thought I was looking at something fake. During the luteal phase, the corpus luteum produces so much progesterone—about 40 mg a day—that it's often seen as the gland that can produce the most hormone per gram of tissue, which is especially impressive considering it's a temporary structure that's about the size of a marble. The corpus luteum also produces estrogen.

We've already discussed the importance of progesterone regarding decidualization, but some of its other effects include:

- Stimulating breast tissue.
- Providing feedback to the brain about the status of the menstrual cycle.
- Relaxing muscles to stop the waves of uterine contractions triggered by estrogen.
- Converting estradiol to the less potent estrone.
- Promoting sleep.
- Elevating temperature (hence the rise in temperature post-ovulation).

Many of the troublesome symptoms during the menstrual cycle, such as mood changes and bloating, are believed to be due in part to progesterone.

Androgens

Androgens are the class of reproductive steroids that have traditionally been associated with male characteristics. They include the well-known testosterone, but also hormones that may be less familiar: dehydroepiandrosterone sulfate (DHEA-S), dehydroepiandrosterone (DHEA), androstenedione, and dihydrotestosterone. The word *androgen* comes from the Greek root *andros*, for "man." The name *testosterone* was coined in 1938, and the *Oxford English Dictionary* states that its origin is most likely from the Latin *testis*, for "witness," as in witness to virility. I get that this is supposed to be a very he-man-type sentiment, as in "I made fire" and "I make life," but honestly it makes me think more of a buffoonish cartoon character. Just as I'd be in favor of renaming estrogen, I'd be in favor of renaming testosterone. After all, it's entirely possible to have unproblematic names for hormones as long as sex (she writes in a stage whisper) isn't involved. For example, insulin (not a reproductive steroid) comes from the Latin word *insula*, meaning "island."

Androgens are produced in the ovaries, the adrenal glands, and other tissues that can convert certain hormones into testosterone. DHEA-S, DHEA, and androstenedione are primarily prohormones, meaning they don't play a big role themselves but exist primarily to be converted into estradiol, estrone, or testosterone. Testosterone has some effects on tissues, but it is also converted to dihydrotestosterone, which is much more potent. Testosterone can also be converted into estradiol.

The testosterone made by the ovaries is meant to act locally, so the concentration of testosterone in the follicle is much higher than the concentration in the blood. This makes studying testosterone a challenge because the amount that enters the blood from the ovaries is so low that it's difficult to measure. In addition, testosterone can be converted to estrogen, so we don't know in every case if testosterone is truly impacting the tissues or if it is testosterone that is being converted to estrogen that is producing the hormonal effect.

While it is true that testosterone plays an important role in many bodily functions, from building muscle and bone mass to balancing mood, and even in regulating the developing follicle and ovulation, the reality is that these functions are complicated, and testosterone is just one ingredient. For example, a study looked at a large group of women with a condition called primary ovarian insufficiency (POI), where the ovaries have stopped working before menopause. POI is associated with low levels of estrogen and testosterone, and many researchers believed some of its symptoms and health consequences were related to the lower levels of testosterone. In this study, women with POI were treated either with estrogen or with estrogen and testosterone to raise their testosterone levels to the typical range. Adding testosterone didn't improve well-being, quality of life, or mood when compared with just replacing estrogen. There were also no additional gains in bone density over what was achieved by estrogen alone. And another consideration: people with polycystic ovarian syndrome (PCOS) often have higher levels of testosterone, and especially higher levels of free, or active, testosterone, yet they do not report higher libido or muscle mass.

I think it's fair to say we don't know what we don't know about testosterone. What we do know is that while it's important, we must be careful not to make grand medical proclamations about testosterone and the reproductive cycle in the absence of robust data, especially given the amazing press that testosterone seems to get and the amount of money to be made in the libido industrial complex.

Prostaglandins

Prostaglandins are hormones released locally in tissue, often in response to injury. Prostaglandins aren't made in a gland and sent out into the bloodstream; rather, they are made on demand, like a hormone pop-up shop. Essentially every cell can make prostaglandins. Like reproductive hormones, they are also lipids, but they are made from arachidonic acid, not cholesterol. They are also unfortunately named because they were first identified in seminal fluid, and so their source was believed to be the prostate. SIGH! I must yet again insert an exasperated comment about how naming things because they were first found in men is hopelessly misogynistic. But if you have been doing medical research by looking primarily at men, what do you expect? It's a wonder the heart isn't called the andro because it was first studied in a man.

There are four main types of prostaglandins, and they help with many bodily functions, including blood clotting, triggering pain, generating a fever with an infection, and starting labor. As far as the menstrual cycle is concerned, prostaglandins are released from the follicle before ovulation and from the lining of the uterus during menstruation, and they also are active in the blood vessels that supply the endometrium. Some of their actions include:

- Triggering pain right before ovulation (aka mittelschmerz).
- Causing the uterus to contract, to stop bleeding with menstruation (hence they are a major factor in painful periods).
- Encouraging blood to clot in the blood vessels that supply the lining of the uterus, another way to stop menstrual bleeding.
- Playing a role in modulating hormone levels and the activity of hormones.

I've seen some naturopaths and functional medicine doctors post on Instagram about nonsteroidal anti-inflammatory drugs (NSAIDs), which inhibit prostaglandins, being "bad" for ovulation and a potential cause of infertility. While it's true that prostaglandins play a role in the menstrual cycle, there is no convincing data that links the use of these drugs with difficulty conceiving. There have even been studies to see if these drugs might improve outcomes with in vitro fertilization (IVF), although the studies are of low enough quality that a conclusion either way isn't possible. One study observed women over two menstrual cycles, and those who took NSAIDs in their follicular phase were actually *more* likely to ovulate than those who didn't. The researchers concluded their "use is likely not harmful to reproduction function."

It's always amazing to me how the people who fearmonger about modern medicine negatively affecting the menstrual cycle are usually promoting some type of unstudied supplement or botanical. Then again, fears about fertility are a big business. Also, these people seem to believe suffering is acceptable, and maybe even necessary, in the quest for mythical menstrual purity. While a fertility doctor might suggest stopping these medications for someone with infertility where no other reason can be identified, there is no data to suggest that anyone is harming their menstrual cycle by taking them.

Anti-mullerian Hormone

Anti-mullerian hormone, or AMH, is produced by the follicles, and it functions as part of the communication system that controls the primordial follicles waiting in the wings. The name *anti-mullerian hormone* is a bit of a mouthful, and it has nothing to do with the ovaries. AMH is so named because in a male fetus it inhibits the development of the uterus and upper vagina, which are known as the Müllerian system. Later it was determined that this hormone is also important in regulating the development of follicles; sadly, it was stuck with the prior, unfortunate name.

The ovary has a set number of follicles that must last over the reproductive span, approximately thirty-five to forty-five years, and a control mechanism is required so all the primordial follicles don't wake up at once and rush in and scream "PARTY!" During each cycle, only some primordial follicles will come out of hibernation and progress to the antral follicle stage so they can potentially be recruited by FSH, and while this process is complex and not fully understood, we do know that AMH is involved in regulating how primordial follicles enter the growing pool (the party prep phase) and how the follicles respond to FSH in each cycle. AMH is basically a bouncer extraordinaire, handing out the VIP tickets to the ovulation party and keeping an eye on everyone in line.

AMH is often called a marker of ovarian reserve, as the level reflects the number of follicles left that can theoretically ovulate—basically what you have left in the ovarian bank. For this reason, some people advertise AMH as a fertility test, but unfortunately this claim is misleading. If AMH levels could predict fertility, we doctors would be ordering that test, as it would be very useful! The reason we don't is because studies show it's not a fertility predictor, and a test that can't do what it claims to isn't helpful for anyone's fertility journey. In fact, it can be harmful. What if someone had an AMH test, was falsely assured that their fertility was "normal," put off getting pregnant, and was then infertile because of the delay? The opposite is also possible. I have seen people post online about stopping their hormonal contraception to check their fertility with this test, be falsely informed by the test that they had diminished fertility, and then have an unplanned pregnancy. There are real consequences here.

Knowing your AMH level can be useful in specific situations. For example, it can help predict success with certain therapies for infertility therapy, and for someone about to undergo cancer therapy and chemotherapy it may predict whether their menstrual cycle will return after these treatments, which can damage the follicles in reserve, potentially leading to premature ovarian insufficiency. Some researchers have wondered if AMH levels might also predict whether follicles can recover after prolonged testosterone therapy. This information would be helpful for those who are taking testosterone for transition and might want the option of stopping it at some point for pregnancy. More work is needed here. However, AMH levels are *not* a marker of someone's current or future fertility, and this kind of fertility testing isn't recommended by the experts at the American Society for Reproductive Medicine. The single best piece of information that can inform people about future fertility is their age.

Can You Balance Your Hormones?

There are two phrases from self-anointed hormone experts that are sure to elicit a cringe reflex from the evidence-based OB/GYN community. One is "hormone imbalance" and the corollary is "estrogen dominance." There are no research papers describing the symptoms and signs of these supposed conditions, meaning they are not medical conditions. At best, hormonal imbalance and estrogen dominance are bad analogies, but at worst, both terms are used by a menstrual rogues' gallery of functional medicine doctors, naturopaths, functional nutritionists, and "period coaches" to sell unindicated testing, concierge care, diets, and supplements.

"Oof," some of you may be thinking, "that's a lot of shade to throw at alternative providers." So this is a good time to discuss what qualifies as expertise. Functional medicine is not a recognized fellowship; therefore, it's a meaningless term. Naturopaths are not doctors; they receive significantly less training than medical or osteopathic doctors, and much of the training they do receive is not supported by evidence-based medicine. For example, most naturopaths are taught that homeopathy is real, but it's a scam. A health care provider believing in homeopathy is like a pilot believing in magic carpets. Do you want a pilot flying your plane who also believes that magic carpets can fly? In addition, much of naturopathic practice revolves around recommending unregulated and understudied supplements. As for functional nutritionists and period coaches, these are not protected terms, meaning you have no idea what training these individuals have, if they have any at all. I could start an online program for Dr. Gunter's certification in functional nutrition or period coaching, design a curriculum, charge $10,000 for completing it, and print out diplomas from my HP printer, and someone could do my training and call themselves a Dr. Gunter–trained period coach. But that won't happen because, well, I have ethics.

This is your health, and you want a real expert. If you needed your appendix out, would you want a doctor who is a board-certified surgeon, someone with recognized training, who has passed required exams, and is licensed? Or someone who did a non-recognized program and calls themself an organologist (to borrow an idea from the very funny comedian Dara Ó Briain)? A functional nutritionist and a period coach are the equivalent of an organologist.

Now back to the facts.

Estrogen makes the endometrium grow, and without enough progesterone to counteract or *balance* out that effect, irregular bleeding can develop. If this happens over a long period of time, it could result in cancer. Causes for insufficient progesterone can be irregular ovulation and obesity (as fatty tissue makes estrogen). Here, the diagnosis isn't a hormonal imbalance, but the word *imbalance* isn't a bad analogy to describe the effect of insufficient progesterone on the endometrium at the cellular level. However, its use has been corrupted far beyond this narrow meaning.

Reproductive hormones change normally throughout an ovulatory menstrual cycle, and while some people refer to the follicular phase as a time when estrogen dominates and the luteal phase as a time when progesterone dominates, this is a teaching tool, not a diagnosis. So what is meant by "hormone imbalance" and "estrogen dominance"? As these aren't recognized terms or a valid diagnosis, they can mean anything. It's possible they are used as an incorrect diagnosis for irregular ovulation, but in the world of functional providers, naturopaths, and period coaches, it seems that these phrases are also often related to estrogen metabolism and accumulation of excess estrogen and/or "harmful" estrogen.

Let's review estrogen metabolism. Estradiol and estrone are produced, do their jobs, and are then removed from the body, and the process of removal is estrogen metabolism. Removal is important; otherwise, hormones would accumulate. Estrogen metabolism is a complex biodynamic process that has lots of moving parts, but one main concept involves its conversion into other substances that can be removed more easily, either via the kidneys and urine or by being packaged by the liver and sent out through the bile duct into stool. (Basically, it's ending up in the toilet somehow.) There are two major ways that estrogens can be metabolized in the liver: one is hydroxylation (which means adding a hydroxy group) and the other is conjugation (which means adding a glucuronide or sulfate group). It's not important to know the details here, just that hydroxylation and conjugation happen in the liver and are different ways of packaging estrogens for removal.

Conjugation changes estrogens so they can leave the liver via the bile duct and enter the stool. Estrogen metabolites that enter the bowel cannot be reabsorbed. However, in the bowel, estrogen metabolites meet an enzyme called beta-glucuronidase, which can convert some metabolites back into active estrogen that can be reabsorbed into the bloodstream via a process called enterohepatic circulation. A healthy gut microbiome has lower levels of beta-glucuronidase, limiting the conversion of estrogen back into the active form and hence reducing reabsorption. Not all of the reactivated estrogen is reabsorbed—some sticks to the fiber in the stool, basically hitching a ride to the toilet. This is one hypothesis for how a high-fiber diet is associated with a lower risk of breast cancer, because it creates a healthier gut microbiome by limiting conversion back to activated estrogen.

The very real process of how estrogen is removed via the bowel has been twisted into a narrative of "estrogen imbalance" or "estrogen dominance." These terms are highly problematic because they have no legitimate medical definition. Some practitioners and lay practitioners use them to describe the idea that certain people absorb too much estrogen. Apparently, it's a fairly common belief among naturopaths that constipation causes estrogen to hang out in the bowel longer than it should, increasing its reabsorption into the bloodstream. This is untrue. The process of enterohepatic circulation is not affected by the frequency of bowel movements. It doesn't matter whether someone has three bowel movements a day or goes once every three days (the range of normal for bowel movement frequency). More bulk, regardless of timing, means more estrogen out. The important factors here are fiber creating a better microbiome and the estrogen sticking to the fiber.

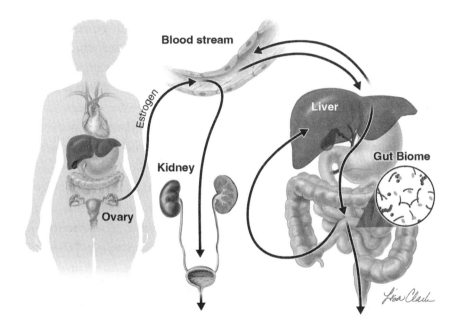

Figure 7• *Enterohepatic Circulation of Estrogen (Illustration by Lisa A. Clark, MA, CMI)*

There is even more complexity here because the body has many checks and balances. For example, one study tells us that when women eat a low-fiber diet and more estrogen is reabsorbed into the bloodstream, the amount of estrogen removed by the kidneys may increase to compensate. Some data suggests that fiber also decreases levels of follicle-stimulating hormone and luteinizing hormone, so it's highly likely there are complexities here that we don't yet understand. But as multiple studies link a high-fiber diet to lower risks of some cancers and diseases, the takeaway is that a high-fiber diet (meaning more than 25 g of fiber a day) and one with fiber from a variety of sources (meaning different legumes and vegetables) is probably best for both hormonal health and overall health. You won't see that promoted in heavy rotation in the naturopathic world, because it's not a message they can use to sell untested supplements. However, if you are looking to expand your fiber repertoire, my blog, *The Vajenda*, has a fantastic recipe for French lentils that is both high in fiber and delicious (and free).

The other way that estrogen can apparently be imbalanced or result in "estrogen dominance" revolves around cancer-causing metabolites made by the liver during the process of hydroxylation. When a chemical is metabolized for removal, it is often converted into intermediate chemicals, and sometimes these are harmful. For example, acetaldehyde is produced by the body when it metabolizes alcohol. Acetaldehyde is harmful, but it is quickly broken down into acetate, so exposure is brief. However, the more alcohol you drink, the greater your acetaldehyde exposure, and this is one of the ways that alcohol harms the body. Also, some people may be genetically more vulnerable to harm from acetaldehyde, or because of other illnesses may be at more risk of consequences from acetaldehyde exposure. Whether a metabolite causes harm for a particular person depends on many factors.

When it comes to estrogen metabolism, hydroxylation can occur by three different pathways, which for simplicity's sake I'll refer to as the 2, 4, and 16 pathways. Estrogen metabolites produced by the 4 and 16 pathways have been linked in some studies with cancer. The good science tells us this is very complex, and while estrogen metabolism is an important component in the genesis of some cancers, we don't have any definitive answers yet. Consequently, testing for metabolites outside of research studies is simply not useful until we do have a better understanding. Yet some functional providers and naturopaths recommend direct-to-consumer testing for estrogen metabolites, and they often call the metabolite produced by the 4 pathway "dirty estrogen." In addition to this testing being useless, the word *dirty* is a common way to scare women and sell products, as it ties into purity culture and binary statements that something is either good or bad, which are sadly effective marketing tropes.

Some functional providers also recommend MTHFR testing. MTHFR is the gene that produces the enzyme methylenetetrahydrofolate reductase. There are different variants of this gene, and yes, in our heads, we evidenced-based providers think of it as the "MoTHerF*ckeR gene" because of the acronym, but also because, despite the fact that it's a genetic variation with no health implications, it is used by quacks to fake an issue where none exists and sell unnecessary products. About 40 percent of people have an MTHFR variant, so a large percentage of people coming into their offices will "fail" this worthless test. MTHFR is possibly one of the most studied genes, so we have good information here, and the real experts at the American College of Medical Genetics and Genomics have recommended against testing for MTHFR variants since 2013.

Why do functional providers care about MTHFR and estrogen? Metabolism of estrogen via the 4 pathway involves an enzyme called catechol-O-methyl-transferase (COMT), which requires S-adenosylmethionine (SAMe), which is related to MTHFR. However, there is no need to learn any of these names, because none of it matters. MTHFR isn't associated with cancers or estrogen metabolism or really anything, which is why we call it a variant, like brown or blue eyes, and not a mutation, which implies disease.

Unnecessary testing for estrogen metabolites and/or MTHFR variants leads to recommendations for unstudied supplements to "correct" these metabolic pathways. I've seen people refuse to take hormonal medications that could help them, based on these worthless tests, and I've also heard from people who were eating carrot salads daily to help rid themselves of "dirty estrogen." "Dirty estrogen" ties into purity culture. No one ever says "dirty testosterone," ya know?

The only takeaway here is that estrogen can cause cancer by multiple mechanisms; this is well known, and there is no need for anyone to be tested for estrogen metabolites and to follow recommendations based on this testing. However, someone who isn't ovulating regularly may be at risk for endometrial cancer. For more on that, see page 231.

My Doctor Won't Test My Hormones—Help!

There are people with medical conditions who have their concerns ignored, and there is also inappropriate testing for hormones. Both of these statements can be true, and they are both reasons why I wrote this book, so people can learn about their symptoms and advocate for the right testing, while also learning what isn't helpful, as unindicated testing can often be harmful.

There is a plethora of direct-to-consumer tests for reproductive hormones, which makes it seem like medical providers should be doing more testing than they are, but a test that isn't needed can lead to false reassurance or take you down an expensive and unnecessary path. I know that blood tests can make some people feel as if their concerns are being taken seriously, but inappropriate testing is bad medicine. The answer to medical disenfranchisement is not unnecessary tests that provide an illusion of caring. And it's not just listening to people, because lots of functional quacks spend a lot of time with their patients. It is listening to people combined with practicing evidence-based medicine. And it's important to remember that direct-to-consumer hormone tests exist to benefit the company's shareholders, not you, the consumer.

Whether or not a reproductive hormone test is indicated depends on what question needs answering and whether this test can provide the answer. Testing levels of reproductive hormones can be very helpful in diagnosing causes of irregular periods and when periods seem to have stopped. They can also be useful when there is excessive hair growth in places where hair doesn't typically grow on women (for example, on the face and chest), and in the evaluation of infertility and planning infertility therapy. So relevant questions here might be "Why are my periods irregular?" or "Why do I have excess hair growth?" or "Why am I having difficulty getting pregnant?" If the menstrual cycle is regular, reproductive hormone tests don't need to be ordered as a baseline check, or as a periodic check, or because of a general feeling of unwellness. In general, a regular menstrual cycle is a good sign that reproductive hormones are within typical ranges.

Bottom Line

- There are three different types of estrogen, but estradiol is the significant one as far as the menstrual cycle is concerned.
- Progesterone is essential for preparing the lining of the uterus for implantation, in a process known as decidualization.
- Testosterone is an important hormone for reproductive health, but its role is complex and not yet fully understood.
- Anti-mullerian hormone levels reflect the number of follicles waiting in the wings, but they can't predict future fertility.
- "Hormone balancing" and "estrogen dominance" are fabricated terms and don't reflect fact-based medical care.

6

Menarche: Journey to the First Period

Many people think of the start of menstruation as the first period, and while it's true that's the first visible sign of the menstrual cycle, the story of menstruation—that is, everything leading up to the first period—begins in the way way back.

For those who don't know, that's a reference to the rear-facing last row of seats in a station wagon, cars you don't see much of anymore. I have glorious memories of sitting in the way way back with a friend in her mom's avocado-green station wagon with wood side paneling. Uncomfortable for adults, but a throne for kids. The way way back was a place to dish secrets, far from the prying ears of the adults in the front seat, and a space to see the wonders of the road you had just traveled.

Our way way back is what happens in the womb. Have you ever made anything out of modeling clay or playdough? Most of us have had the experience of taking clay and shaping it into one structure or another, sometimes adding another color, perhaps twisting the colors together, depending on the finished version we are imagining. Modeling clay is a good analogy for how the reproductive tract forms. An embryo is initially a single cell created by the joining of the ovum and the sperm. But that single cell divides, and then those two cells divide again, and so on. After a few weeks of dividing and developing, primitive tissues are created that are, for the purposes of our analogy, not unlike raw modeling clay. These primitive tissues receive instructions from genes that will transform them into organs. There are four groups of primitive cells (or four colors of modeling clay), each destined to become a different part of the reproductive tract. We all start out with the same four types of tissues, so each embryo retains the potential to develop a vagina, uterus, and ovaries or a penis, prostate, and testicles until the end of the seventh week of pregnancy (five weeks after conception).

These primitive tissues that we all have during our first few weeks as an embryo are:

- *Paramesonephric ducts*, also called the Müllerian system, which are destined to become the oviducts, the uterus, and the upper portion of the vagina.
- *Mesonephric ducts*, also known as the Wolffian system, which will become the epididymis, vas deferens, and seminal vesicles, classically thought of as male structures.
- *Primordial gonads*, which can develop into either ovaries or testicles.
- *Urogenital sinus*, which can develop into either the clitoris, lower vagina, and labia or the penis and scrotum.

If there is a Y chromosome, the primordial gonads are signaled to develop into testicles, which begin producing testosterone. It's testosterone that triggers tissues to transform into a penis, scrotum, and all the necessary accoutrements. In the absence of a Y chromosome, the tissues never receive this signaling, so the entire mesonephric system disappears and we are left with three types of tissue. The primordial gonads develop into ovaries, the paramesonephric ducts become the oviducts, uterus, and upper vagina, and the urogenital sinus transforms into the lower vagina, labia, and clitoris. So, yes, having a vagina, a uterus, and ovaries is the default, something that never ceases to charm me, as many origin stories, such as the ones from Greek mythology and several religions, involve a man being fashioned first.

The ovaries accumulate primordial follicles (immature eggs in hibernation) until a fetal age of twenty weeks. At this point, there are six to seven million primordial follicles. No more follicles can be made after this. From twenty weeks until birth, millions of primordial follicles disappear, and at birth approximately one million remain. Primordial follicles continue to reduce their overall number throughout childhood, and by the first menstrual cycle about three to five hundred thousand primordial follicles remain.

Some "fertility influencers" have claimed that ovaries keep making follicles into adulthood, the implication here being if your ovaries don't, then you should buy my supplement and we can unleash that power. There is no evidence at all that human ovaries can make follicles after birth. There was some research that suggested human ovaries might have what are called germline stem cells, cells with the capability of being coaxed into making new follicles of eggs. The bulk of the research suggests this is not the case. Some researchers have even used advanced technology to identify every single cell in a human ovary, and not found these stem cells.

The oviducts, uterus, and upper vagina develop from two paramesonephric ducts, one on either side of the body. Imagine these ducts as two ropes of clay on either side of a line. Through complex signaling, including genes that code for spatial orientation (if you've ever wondered how tissues know where to head and the final direction they should face, there are genes for that!), the lower halves of these clay ropes join, and this intersection will become the uterus and the top of the vagina; the two separate pieces at the top will develop into either oviduct. The developing uterus and upper vagina attach to the urogenital sinus (another lump of differently colored clay), which is destined to become the lower half of the vagina. As the fetal uterus and urogenital sinus grow, the cells inside disappear so the uterus and vagina are not solid at birth.

Some residual tissue at the vaginal opening becomes the hymen, which is simply a membranous fold that partially occludes the vaginal opening. The hymen is possibly the most offensively named of all the structures in the body, as it is named after the Greek god of marriage. However, the hymen has nothing to do with marriage or sex, and it is not possible to tell if someone has had penetrative vaginal sex by examining their hymen.

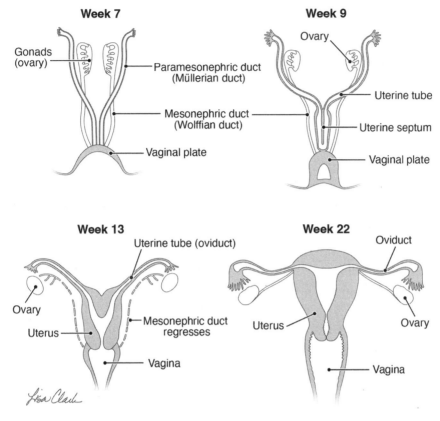

Figure 8 • *Formation of the Uterus, Ovaries, and Vagina (Illustration by Lisa A. Clark, MA, CMI)*

Besides the coolness of how the oviducts, uterus, and vagina form (I mean, genes that instruct your uterus and oviducts how to spatially orient themselves in your body? It sounds like the plot of a science fiction novel, except it is science fact and they are called homeobox genes), it can be useful information to know, because approximately 3 percent of people with a uterus, or who were embryologically meant to have a uterus, are born with abnormalities affecting the reproductive tract, and one of them might be you or someone you know.

At each point in the process there can be a misstep. Think of this as a complex IKEA project: if you get the instructions in the wrong order or a page is missing, the structure of the finished product might not be the same as the image shown on the box. The entire paramesonephric system can fail to develop, a condition known as Mayer-Rokitansky-Küster-Hauser syndrome, where no oviducts, uterus, or upper portion of the vagina are developed. Or one side may fail to develop, and while the vagina is normal, there is what's called a unicornuate uterus—a smaller-than-normal uterus, because there was less tissue to start with—and a single oviduct. There can be a problem with how the two paramesonephric ducts join, resulting in two uteruses that are fused together. Or, after the paramesonephric ducts join to form the uterus, if the middle doesn't disappear, a septum, or dividing piece of tissue, can remain. The signaling that causes the ovaries, uterus, and vagina to form can also be affected by chemicals known as endocrine disruptors, which act like hormones and can disrupt biological processes.

If the uterus has failed to develop, no bleeding will occur. If the vagina has not developed completely and is still blocked by tissue, menstruation may happen, but it is blocked from leaving the body and builds up inside the uterus and upper vagina. These are conditions to consider when a first menstrual period hasn't happened by sixteen years of age. Many of the conditions that affect how the uterus forms are associated with an increased risk of pregnancy complications. In addition, because the tissues destined to become the kidneys develop alongside the paramesonephric ducts, if there is an abnormality with the uterus, it is important to make sure there is no issue with the kidneys.

The Very First Period

The first time the uterus bleeds is not always with puberty; it may happen shortly after birth. It's not that one of the follicles in the growing pool accidentally ovulates. Rather, high levels of estrogen in the pregnant person's blood cause estrogen to cross the placenta and reach the fetus, where it can stimulate the endometrium to thicken, just as it would during a menstrual cycle. Progesterone also crosses the placenta, so the endometrium doesn't get too thick, but sometimes there is enough estrogen that with delivery, when the baby is separated from the placenta, withdrawing the source of progesterone, a small amount of bleeding occurs.

Interestingly, the progesterone in the placenta does not result in decidualization of the lining of the uterus, meaning it doesn't cause the changes that make implantation possible. During pregnancy, estrogen and progesterone aren't delivered sequentially, as they are during the menstrual cycle; rather, there is continuous exposure to both. Decidualization occurs only when estrogen comes first and primes the lining of the uterus and then progesterone follows—further proof that this phenomenon exists solely for implantation.

We know this information because of autopsies on infants who died at birth. It's important to acknowledge the generosity of parents who, in the crushing event of their newborn's death, allowed autopsy information to be used for research purposes. Autopsies are often done on stillbirths and neo-natal deaths in the hope that they might provide a clue to the cause of this ultimate tragedy, and at times that tissue is also used, with permission, for research. When we rightfully ask "Why don't we know that?" about the repro-ductive tract, it's often because there have been insufficient funds or interest, but even money and motivated researchers can't give us every puzzle piece. Sometimes it takes a great personal gift from a grieving parent to provide the information we need about human anatomy.

Menarche: The Start of Menses

Puberty is the combination of biological changes that leads to the physical transformation from child to adult. While the appearance of the first menstrual period, known medically as menarche, is a sign of puberty, and one that typi-cally occurs later in the process, I want to be clear that menstruation does not make one an adult. There is often much discourse about the first menstrual period being an ascension to womanhood, and in my opinion that is danger-ous. A twelve-year-old, the average age of the first period, is not an adult, and bleeding from the vagina does not magically change that fact.

This isn't a book about puberty, but there are some basics to cover to set the stage for the first period. The part of the hypothalamus with the chemical signaling to control ovulation wakes up, for lack of a better phrase. Exactly how this happens isn't fully known. But it's likely a combination of genetics (basically, we inherit a puberty clock of sorts), health, nutrition, and the envi-ronment, which includes stress and potential exposure to endocrine-disrupting chemicals. Interestingly, when this process first starts, the chemical signaling is primarily released during sleep.

There are three main physical events associated with puberty in girls:

- *Thelarche:* Breast development from the estrogen produced by the developing follicles. The initial signaling from the brain rouses the follicles to produce estrogen and raise levels of

> it, enough to trigger breast development but not enough to trigger ovulation.

- *Adrenarche:* The appearance of pubic hair and axillary (armpit) hair. This is under the control of hormones produced by the adrenal glands.
- *Menarche:* The first menstrual period. This is the last of the three main biological events. The average age of menarche in the United States is twelve, but the medically normal range is nine to fifteen years.

Looking at menarche among the Hadza, people in Tanzania who live a traditional hunter-gatherer lifestyle, the average age of the first menstrual period is approximately sixteen, which is likely close to the baseline for pre-industrialization. The age of menarche has decreased in the past century, and a major theory for why that might be revolves around nutrition. A critical body weight is necessary to trigger the GnRH pulses needed for the menstrual cycle (this threshold is believed to be around 45–47 kg/100–104 pounds), and we are now heavier sooner. Endocrine-disrupting chemicals may also play a role, and it may not always be about dose, meaning the amount of the exposure, but about timing at critical points in development, either as a fetus or as a child. Ultimately, many factors may be involved in lowering the age of menarche. I will summarize with a quote from Dr. Louise Greenspan, who is a pediatric endocrinologist and an expert on puberty, and who was my son Victor's doctor for his thyroid disorder, so clearly someone I trust! She wrote: "most studies have only been able to identify correlations with alterations in the timing of different pubertal milestones but . . . causality is difficult to glean from environmental epidemiology studies." Basically, it's complicated and we need to know more, though I appreciate that this answer may not be satisfying.

It is important to know that earlier periods are associated with some health conditions, most notably breast cancer, endometriosis, and chronic pain conditions. This isn't meant to scare you; rather, having information allows you to make informed choices. The increased risk of breast cancer is believed to be the result of a greater cumulative lifetime exposure to estrogen, but the mechanism for the increased risk of endometriosis and chronic pain is not well understood. It could be an impact of early or longer lifetime exposure to estrogens, or even early exposure to painful periods, as pain changes the nervous system in a way that increases pain.

Menarche starts when pulses of FSH and LH are sufficient to trigger the follicles that are entering the growing pool and are now at the final stage in their journey. Until this point, these follicles have disintegrated, but now, with FSH and LH, they can be induced to enter the menstrual cycle. The system may not initially be mature enough to get a follicle through to ovulation, so menstrual bleeding is often irregular during the first year after menarche. The average length of the menstrual cycle at this time is thirty-five days, but sixty to ninety days between periods isn't abnormal in the first year. During years two and three after the first period, cycles of twenty-one to forty-five days are normal. By age eighteen most teens have reached the typical cycle length of twenty-four to thirty-eighty days. Interestingly, the older a child is when they reach puberty, the longer it takes to establish ovulatory cycles.

Irregular menstruation in the first few years can be due to sporadic ovulation as well as anovulatory bleeding, meaning a follicle develops partially and produces estrogen, but not enough for ovulation, so there is no progesterone. The withdrawal of estrogen destabilizes the endometrium, and bleeding ensues.

Menstrual bleeding in the first one to two years can be problematic. Periods can often be heavy, which can be challenging to manage even for experienced bleeders, never mind an eleven-year-old in a bathroom stall at school. (Teens with heavy periods should be evaluated for a bleeding disorder. See page 215 for more on this topic.) The irregular nature of the bleeding can also make managing menstrual hygiene challenging. I was caught unawares several times as a teen, as were friends of mine, and we had an unwritten rule in school that if you saw someone with bloodstains on their paints, you walked up and offered a jacket to wrap around their waist or walked behind them as they went to the bathroom to clean up. Of course, no one should be embarrassed because they have leaked blood onto their clothes. It should be the equivalent of untied shoes: just something you might want to know about. But even when—because I do believe it is when—we get to a place where it's no big deal, there is still the issue of wet underwear and the hassle of washing out blood.

Regardless of whether their periods are heavy or light, or regular or irregular, many teens are bothered by them. While some of their discomfort might be related to shame imposed upon them by the patriarchy, for many it's simply practical. Who wants to be bothered with pads and tampons ever, let alone at age ten or eleven? And, of course, period diarrhea, premenstrual syndrome, and other unpleasantries don't help. Not all teens feel comfortable with tampons or menstrual cups or discs (not all adults do either), or with swimming in period underwear, so this can affect their ability to be on a swim team or go to the beach. Pads can chafe and may be uncomfortable, and not just during sports.

Not knowing when your period will start can also be stressful, whether you are twelve, twenty-two, or fifty-two. It was a nuisance to unexpectedly get my period on a transatlantic flight and be completely unprepared because I was fifty years old and thought I was menopausal (surprise! no); I had to rely on airline pads, which left me with a rash. If this had happened to me when I was fifteen, I would probably have been devastated.

In one study, approximately 70 percent of girls between the ages of fifteen and nineteen said they would prefer to have their periods less frequently than once a month. So it didn't surprise me at all when, a few years ago, I was writing a women's health column for the *New York Times* and one of the questions was from a mom whose teen was bothered by having a period. I recommended options such as period underwear for surprise gotchas; nonsteroidal anti-inflammatory drugs such as ibuprofen before the start of each period to reduce the amount of bleeding, as well as cramps and period diarrhea; and taking the birth control pill, which can regulate and reduce the volume of bleeding or even be taken in such a way that periods can be skipped altogether (all things you will read about in more detail in later chapters). I explained the risks of blood clots, which are very low but do exist. I wrote that by two years after the first period, most teens have stopped growing, but the younger someone is when they start bleeding, the longer they may continue to grow. I also explained that most of our current data indicates that the birth control pill with estrogen has no impact on height, but when a period starts very young, "a discussion about height with a pediatrician or pediatric and adolescent gynecologist may be in order."

I had sourced my recommendations from the latest literature and even consulted with a pediatric endocrinologist. Following the publication of the column, I was attacked online by a "natural health" contingent consisting of naturopaths, functional nutritionists, and period coaches who make a living telling people that they can solve any menstrual problem by taking unregulated supplements and eating different foods. It's an interesting overlap of the "natural" movement and the religious right that is rooted in purity culture, not empowerment. They said I was "promoting canceling teen periods with hormonal birth control." Apparently, it's a sin to empower teens and their parents with information; it's preferable for them to suffer in the name of purity. The amount of vitriol I received surprised even me (and I get a lot of hate online!).

Then again, a doctor telling people that they can improve their quality of life through science probably affects one's ability to sell completely useless menstrual detox products for "only" $39.99 a month, $29.99 with a subscription.

The desire to control your bleeding, either how often or how much, to improve your quality of life isn't a frivolous pursuit or an abomination. And *you* get to decide what "quality of life" means, because it is, after all, your life. Wanting to feel better just makes you human and that, my friend, is reason enough.

Bottom Line

- The ovaries, oviducts, uterus, and vagina develop in a fetus when there is no Y chromosome.
- All of the primordial follicles (immature eggs) have developed by twenty weeks of fetal life.
- The hymen is a membranous fold that has nothing to do with sexual activity or virginity.
- The average age of menarche is twelve. The age when menstruation starts is largely triggered by genetics and body weight, but environmental factors may also play a role.
- Irregular menses are common for the first year or two after the first period.

7

Menopause: The Afterparty

In the not-too-distant past (and sadly in some cases the present), girls were taught nothing about their periods. My own mother, born in 1933, had no idea that she would menstruate until one day in her early teens she woke up covered in blood. As her sister had recently been coughing up blood, which led to a diagnosis of tuberculosis and being sent to a sanitorium, my mother was terrified she too had a serious illness and would be sent away! Fortunately, there has been some headway when it comes to communicating about the start of menstruation, but what about the end? Not so much. Even today, many people face the end of menstruation with as little information as my mother had with her first period.

Why don't we talk about menopause? It has long been viewed as an expiration date for worth, which translates, not so loosely, to a loss of "breeder" status and "hotness" to the male gaze. In June 1986 (1986!), *Newsweek* ran a cover story that proclaimed a woman over forty had a greater chance of being killed by a terrorist than getting married. As if marriage to a man should be the goal of one's life. The piece was bunk, as the statistics were garbage, and it was eventually (and quietly) retracted twenty years later. But I was twenty years old when it came out, and it had an impact thanks to the dual messages of "You are nothing without a man" and "Your purpose is to make babies."

Basically, at forty your countdown to irrelevance was in high gear, and the only way to salvage that situation was with a man.

Before I started medical school, the only things I'd heard about menopause were tired jokes on television, maybe a raised eyebrow about not having to worry about getting pregnant, in an awful nudge-nudge-wink-wink kind of way, and a *Golden Girls* episode in 1986 where Blanche misses a period and thinks she is pregnant. Of course it's menopause, and so her joy at potentially raising a baby is replaced with the belief that she is now entering a phase of life that might as well be death's antechamber.

Who wants to discuss a sexless pre-death? Better to pretend it doesn't exist. Unfortunately, this cloak of shame means that many people with ovaries have no idea what to expect when they are no longer expecting a period. The consequence of the lack of education about menopause—and I'll put a lot of the blame on medicine that has dismissed generations of women—is a stunning 65 percent of women who feel unprepared for this phase of life.

What Is Menopause?

Menopause is the planned end of ovarian function, and it has occurred when someone is one year past their final period. Like puberty, it comes with many hormonal changes. In fact, the journey into menopause, known medically as the menopause transition, can be thought of as puberty in reverse.

From a fetal age of twenty weeks, the march of the primordial follicles, meaning recruitment from their hibernation, has been ongoing. This follicular attrition happens whether someone has had multiple pregnancies, took hormonal contraception that suppressed ovarian function, or was never pregnant or never took any hormones. Menopause happens when about a thousand primordial follicles remain. At this point, no more follicles are capable of ovulating. Production of estrogen by the follicles stops, but smaller amounts are still produced by other tissues, such as the brain, bone, and fat. Testosterone production doesn't drop with menopause, as the ovaries and the adrenal glands continue to produce it; rather, there is a gradual age-related decline in levels.

The language of menopause can be clunky, which only adds to the confusion. In medicine, we refer to everything after the final menstrual period as *postmenopause*, the time leading up to menopause as the *menopause transition*, and the actual date of the last menstruation as *menopause*—but obviously that's not something people can know at the time. To make things even more confusing, there are other terms that may be used. *Premenopause* is another name for the menopause transition, and *perimenopause* is the menopause transition plus the first year after the final menstrual period.

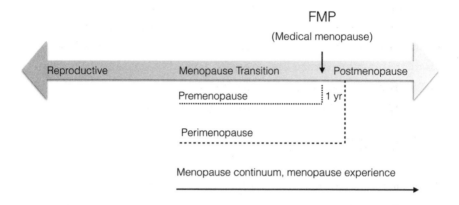

Figure 9 • *Phases of Menopause (Illustration by Dr. Jen Gunter)*

Medically, the years between puberty and the menopause transition are known as the reproductive phase, although I hate this term because it may as well say "breeding time." In addition, men do not have their hormonal status distilled down to stages of penile aging, yet the rate of penile dysfunction increases by 10 percent each decade.

To simplify things, I typically refer to menopause as the final period onward, and the menopause experience or continuum as the menopause transition onward.

The average age at the final period is fifty-one years, but the typical range is forty-five to fifty-five. If menopause happens between ages forty and forty-four it's considered early, and after fifty-five it's late. The menopause transition typically ranges from four to ten years, and the average age at onset is forty-six years. Typically, the earlier the onset of the menopause transition, the longer the transition tends to last. When ovarian function stops before age forty, the term is *primary ovarian insufficiency*. Surgical menopause occurs when both ovaries are removed before the final period.

Many people wonder if an earlier first period means an earlier menopause, and the answer is no. The loss of follicles doesn't start with the first period; it starts years before, at a fetal age of twenty weeks. Primordial follicles have been developing and disintegrating for long before the first period. The only difference with the first period is now there is FSH to catch some of those follicles and pull them into a menstrual cycle.

What about removing an ovary? Surely that affects menopause, as it cuts the supply of primordial follicles in half. The impact here varies with age. If an ovary is removed later in the reproductive years or during the menopause transition, the age of menopause will likely drop, as the number of primordial follicles that can enter the development stage is already at the lower end. However, if an ovary is removed earlier in life, when the number of primordial follicles is high, there seems to be a compensatory mechanism that helps to conserve primordial follicles, so the age of menopause is less likely to be affected.

Chaos Explained

Hormone levels stabilize after the final period, with low levels of estradiol and no progesterone. The dominant estrogen during this time is estrone. A small amount of estradiol is found in the blood, but this is hormone that has essentially spilled over from other tissues, such as bone and muscle, into the bloodstream.

However, things are quite different during the menopause transition. The time leading up to the final period is a bit of a hormonal potpourri, thanks to disordered ovulation. Remember, the normal menstrual cycle is a tightly regulated hormonal symphony, with estrogen arriving at the right time and in the right levels, and then the correct amount of progesterone making an entrance on cue. But everything changes with the menopause transition. I often think of the brain-brain-ovary connection during this time as bad management of an office full of people close to retirement. The workers are tired and might not always be performing at their peak, and the management is unable to motivate them or compensate for them. With that analogy in mind, here are some of the ways ovulation can change during the menopause transition:

- There are fewer waves of follicles, which shortens the follicular phase of the menstrual cycle.
- The dominant follicle takes longer to produce enough estrogen, which can lengthen the cycle.
- Follicles get recruited and estrogen is produced, but ovulation doesn't occur. Menstruation may be skipped or delayed.

- Double development occurs, in which one wave of follicles develops, a dominant follicle is selected, and everything appears to be progressing according to plan until a second follicle starts to develop. The original dominant follicle ovulates, but the late-to-the-game runner-up does not regress. Rather, it persists, and when the next cycle starts, it has a jump on the other follicles and is able to quickly produce enough estrogen to trigger ovulation sooner than expected. Estrogen levels in this second cycle are often higher than is typical.
- The corpus luteum malfunctions, which can result in a skipped period, a delayed period, a regular period, or spotting.
- No follicles are recruited. The cycle is skipped altogether, and no estrogen or progesterone is produced.

The menopause transition doesn't typically happen in an orderly fashion, and several of these phenomena can even occur together in one cycle. It really is hormonal chaos—estradiol levels may be low, normal, or even high, and progesterone levels may be low or normal. Cycles can be as usual or they can be shorter or longer. Even when they appear to be of normal length, the seemingly punctual bleeding may be from a cycle without ovulation. One thing that is certain is that hormone levels don't predict symptoms, so that's why we don't use them to guide therapy.

Hormonal chaos explains why the most common experience in the menopause transition is changes in bleeding. For approximately 40 percent of people, cycles are initially shorter, representing the change between the reproductive phase and the menopause transition. Then cycles may lengthen, initially by seven days or more (remember, a variation in cycle length of up to seven days from cycle to cycle is normal). When there are sixty days or more between periods, the final menstrual period is likely to occur within the next two to three years. However, menstrual changes don't always follow this pattern of slightly shorter, then longer cycles, then skipped periods. When you're in the menopause transition, the only thing to expect, hormone-wise, is the unexpected.

The hormonal chaos often also results in heavier and longer bleeding. During the reproductive years, the upper limit of "normal" for blood loss per cycle is 80 ml (2.7 ounces), because 90 percent of the time that is the experience for 90 percent of people. During the menopause transition, 90 percent of people have periods of up to 133 ml (4.5 ounces). Heavier bleeding is often the result of the varying levels of hormones, which can affect the process of building, destabilizing, and repairing the endometrium in a variety of ways. In addition, as we age, we accumulate medical conditions that can increase menstrual bleeding (see Chapter 16 for more). Obesity can also increase menstrual bleeding, and because rates of obesity increase with age, this may be another factor.

Hormonal chaos can also impact other conditions. For example, shorter cycles can worsen premenstrual syndrome, as it is typically the follicular phase that is shorter, and consequently more time is spent in the luteal phase, when PMS symptoms occur. Fluctuating hormone levels can also exacerbate menstrual migraines.

You don't need to learn all these ovulation permutations, although I hope you agree it's fascinating from a biological perspective—although perhaps less so while it's affecting you personally. When I went through my menopause transition, I had several episodes of soaking my clothes at incredibly inopportune times, such as right after takeoff on a transatlantic flight with the seatbelt light still on, sitting in an examination room discussing a patient's medical care, and while driving home. I did not marvel at the biological complexity of my body during any of these events. However, I knew the biological reasons why this was happening, so none of it scared me and I didn't feel broken.

Why Menopause?

There is a common and offensive trope that menopause is a disease of "ovarian failure" and women are simply now living long enough to experience it, hence exposing their biologically flawed ovaries. Those who espouse this must believe that women used to drop dead shortly after giving birth to their last child. No word from these folks on how the increasing rate of erectile dysfunction with age positions the penis as a paragon of aging perfection.

The concept of menopause as a disease isn't based on research; rather, it was a Big Pharma talking point from the 1960s, created to sell estrogen, which had become easy to mass-produce in an oral formulation. It's distressing to see doctors still using it today. And really, have they never heard of grandmothers and great-grandmothers? It's not as if the concept of elders emerged in the last century.

While it's true that before modern sanitation and medicine average life expectancy was much shorter, a lot of that was due to high rates of infant mortality. Historically, more women died in childbirth than do today, and of course more people died of conditions we can now readily treat. But many women lived to menopause. The Ancient Greeks were accurate about the expected age of menopause, and if everyone had been dying before age forty, they wouldn't have known it existed!

"Okay, that's all well and good," you are thinking. "Sure, menopause isn't a disease, but why does it exist?" Almost everything the body does is in support of reproduction, be it gestating a pregnancy, stopping menstruation in times of famine, or thinking creatively to find enough calories. Traits that don't contribute to the grand design of making the next generation tend to disappear. So how does menopause, a state where reproduction can't happen, benefit society?

Once the job of creating offspring is done, almost all mammals exit stage left, including chimpanzees, which have similar ovarian function to humans and are our closest living relatives. But humans keep on living. The question, therefore, isn't "Why do ovaries fail while women keep on living?" That's a concern for someone who thinks being alive after age fifty is a mistake for women and the natural order for men. The correct question is "Why do women keep on living even though the potential to directly pass along their genetics no longer exists?" How can they turn energy into offspring when they can no longer have offspring?

The answer may lie with grandmothers. Research tells us that, historically, grandmothers provided useful physical help so that their children were free to have more children, hence passing on the grandmother's genes. I like to call it "Genetics: the long game." There is supporting evidence for the grandmother hypothesis among killer whales, the only other species known to experience menopause that has been well studied. Like humans, female killer whales live in social groups and survive past their reproductive years. Grandmother killer whales share food with their grand-offspring and may be able to help the pod locate hunting grounds in times when food is scarce. When a grandmother killer whale dies, the likelihood that her grand-calf will die increases. If you want to read more about the data that backs up the grandmother hypothesis, please check out my book *The Menopause Manifesto*.

In the meantime, don't tolerate menopause being framed as the death of ovaries, a marker of irrelevance, and a loss of worth. Instead, know that it has been vital to humanity and has helped drive our evolution as a species.

How Will I Know It's Menopause?

The average age of starting the menopause transition is forty-six, but some women may notice menstrual irregularities a few years before, maybe even in their late thirties. If you are in your forties or early fifties and are experiencing irregular periods and/or other menopausal symptoms (we'll get to those shortly), then you are likely in the menopause transition. Checking reproductive hormones isn't necessary. It's the same as with puberty: if a growth spurt or a first period happened when it was expected, no one checked estrogen levels; you just kind of slid out of puberty the same way that you are sliding into menopause.

Furthermore, blood tests to determine menopause can be unreliable. Think back to the ovulatory patterns I just described—some cycles can even have higher levels of estrogen than normal. In fact, in the year before the final period, 23 percent of cycles can be associated with normal or higher levels of estrogen. If blood work is done and the tests are normal, giving a false reassurance that menopause is far off, it could still be one of the last ovulations, with the final period just one or two months away. Conversely, the blood work can look like menopause, with low estradiol and elevated FSH, and then ovulation can happen two months later and a normal cycle can restart. It's also important to know that we don't use blood levels to determine whether to manage menopause. If you are forty-nine and having hot flashes, we can treat them whether you are three years away from your final period or your final period was last year.

Distinguishing between the menopause transition and menopause is only essential, medically speaking, for a few reasons:

- *Risk of pregnancy:* People who don't want to get pregnant typically want to know when they no longer have to be concerned about it. Unfortunately, blood tests are not reliable here and are not recommended for this purpose. Before the age of fifty, the recommendation for stopping contraception is two years without a period; at fifty and older, it's one year without a period.
- *Evaluation of vaginal bleeding:* Any bleeding after the final period is *not* a menstrual period; it's abnormal uterine bleeding and needs to be investigated to ensure it is not a precancer or cancer. We don't use blood levels to determine this—if there is any suspicion that

someone is menopausal and bleeding, a doctor should do an ultrasound and/or take a sample of cells from the lining of the uterus.

- *Managing some hormonally responsive cancers:* With some breast cancers, it may be important to know if menopause has happened, as the therapies that are offered may change.

- *Someone is under age forty-five and has gone ninety days without a period:* This could be early menopause (age forty to forty-four) or primary ovarian insufficiency (under age forty), so blood work is indicated in this instance (see page 229 for more on POI). Similarly, for someone under forty-five who doesn't get a period, such as after a hysterectomy or endometrial ablation, or who had a hormonal IUD, persistent symptoms of menopause should prompt the same question: Is this early menopause or POI? In these cases, ovulation isn't suppressed, but the uterus can't be used as a barometer for the ovaries. Blood work may also be helpful here. It's important to know about early menopause and POI, as both are associated with an increased risk of osteoporosis, heart disease, and dementia, and because recommendations for menopausal hormone therapy, or MHT, are a little different than they are for those who start menopause at age forty-five or older. With POI, screening for other health conditions may also be needed.

What about people who are taking hormonal contraception with estrogen? They will not be expected to have significant symptoms; in fact, many have none. Estrogen-containing contraception (ECC) essentially replaces the hormonal chaos of the menopause transition, so estrogen levels never go up or down. The hormones in the pill, patch, or ring are also great for controlling bleeding, and estrogen protects bones.

Fertility and Age

Fertility starts to decrease years before the final period because of a reduction in the pool of follicles and a decline in the quality of the remaining eggs, which are more likely to have chromosomal abnormalities. We know age-related infertility is primarily related to the follicles, because people with age-related infertility can overcome that barrier with egg donation. Fertility starts to decrease in the thirties, the decrease is more significant at age thirty-five, and by age forty-five pregnancies without assisted reproduction are rare. This fits with the grandmother hypothesis, as our ancestral grandmothers could only help offload the stress of child-rearing if they weren't burdened with that task themselves. In cultures that don't practice contraception, pregnancies after age forty-one are uncommon. That doesn't mean people who don't want to be pregnant should give up contraception at age forty-one, as pregnancies absolutely can happen; it is simply information for those who are looking ahead and for whom being pregnant one day is important.

Evaluation and management of infertility are beyond the scope of this book, but for those who are interested in one day being pregnant, age is the most important predictor of fertility. For those hoping to freeze eggs, it is far more likely to be successful before age thirty-eight, and freezing more eggs increases the likelihood of success.

Symptoms and Health Concerns

Unfortunately, many medical practitioners still incorrectly believe that symptoms don't start until menopause, but many people have their worst symptoms before their final period. This misbelief can result in medical gaslighting, where someone is sitting in their health care provider's office talking about how they have been impacted by hot flashes or night sweats, and they are told, "That's not possible" or "It can't be that bad, you aren't even in menopause yet!" And of course the person is thinking, "WTF, are you in this body?" as they fan themselves.

When thinking about symptoms that could be related to the menopause transition, it is equally important not to blame your hormones for everything. Menopause doesn't happen in a vacuum. For example, if you are forty-five years old and having sleep disturbance, it could be related to the menopause transition or not—depression and sleep apnea can also affect sleep. The menopause transition can cause joint pain, but so can arthritis. While it's important to ask "Could this be menopause?" it's also important to ask "What else could this be besides menopause?"

You want to consider the emotional context as well. If you believe menopause is the end of your useful life, versus believing you are having some difficult symptoms that can be managed with modern medicine, and that after the hormonal rapids settle, things will improve, it changes your perspective. It is so important not to see menopause as a disease.

Some of the main symptoms of menopause, which can also occur in the menopause transition, include:

- Hot flashes
- Sleep disturbance
- Depression
- Anxiety
- Brain fog
- Palpitations
- Joint pain
- Weight gain around the middle
- Vaginal dryness
- Changes in sex drive

In addition, the risk of some medical conditions increases after the final period. They include:

- Bladder infections
- Dementia
- Heart disease
- Osteoporosis

That doesn't mean everyone with ovaries will develop these conditions, but it's a good idea to think about how you can modify your life to reduce your risk factors. Plus, knowing what to expect can help you advocate for the best care. If you want to learn more about all the changes that can happen during the menopause transition and menopause, about menopausal hormone therapy and other treatments, and how to get the best medical care and thrive, I suggest getting a copy of my book *The Menopause Manifesto*. There is simply too much on this topic to cover in one chapter.

The Upsides!

Too often we discuss only the negative aspects of menopause, but I'm here to tell you there are many positives. First, not having a period after having had one for thirty-five years is nice. I don't have hair on my legs or armpits anymore

(I'm someone who prefers not to have hair there, so for me this is a bonus). I also feel a clarity of thought, which other women report as well. During the menopause transition, there is brain remodeling. This is often viewed as negative because areas of the brain shrink, and who wants a smaller brain? However, other areas grow to compensate. One theory is that the shrinkage represents pruning of neurological pathways we no longer need: those involved with menstruation and pregnancy. The change in platform from reproducing capability to post-reproduction might be one of the causes of brain fog. It's a bit like updating the operating system on a computer. Just as your computer doesn't perform up to spec right before an update, so might your brain be a little glitchy during its remodeling. But afterward, things run smoother because you have a new operating system!

Treatment

Whenever I'm asked what is the one thing someone can do for a healthy menopause, I always say exercise. Look, I don't like that answer any more than anyone else, but the truth is, the cornerstone of a healthy menopause transition and menopause is exercise, meaning moving more, aerobic physical activity, and strength training. Exercise reduces the risk of dementia, heart disease, and osteoporosis. In addition, it improves balance, which reduces the risk of falls, so is important in fracture prevention. Exercise also helps preserve muscle mass and alleviates depression. It's hard to find a part of your body that exercise doesn't help.

Modern medicine can also play a role in treating the symptoms of menopause and preventing some of the medical aftereffects. There is a wide variety of options, which I cover in depth in *The Menopause Manifesto*. A full discussion of hormone therapy and other treatments is beyond our scope here, but it is important for you to know that therapies exist.

Be wary of medical practitioners who oversell estrogen as the fountain of youth, those who recommend hormone testing to guide therapy (it's not needed; we prescribe hormones based on symptoms, not levels), and those who recommend compounded hormones (special mixes of hormones made by compounding pharmacies), as they're not standard of care, are not as well studied or tested as standard pharmaceutical hormones, and have more risks.

Menopausal hormone therapy (MRT) may be recommended in the follow-ing situations:

- To treat hot flushes and night sweats.
- To help with mild depression early in the menopause transition.
- To prevent osteoporosis for those at high risk.
- To prevent cardiovascular disease and osteoporosis with POI and premature menopause.

We currently don't have good evidence to support MHT for the prevention of dementia or cardiovascular disease for those over age forty-five, and no medical professional society recommends it for these indications. MHT does not treat brain fog, and it does not affect the increase in fat around the middle that can occur with menopause (the exact reasons for this shift in the distri-bution of fat are unknown).

Vaginal estrogen, the hormone DHEA, and oral ospemifene are effective at treating vaginal dryness and pain with sex, and vaginal estrogen has also been shown to prevent urinary tract infections, which become more common in the years after the final period. The only people who need to have a detailed conversation with their health care provider about the safety of vaginal estro-gen and DHEA are those with breast cancer or endometrial cancer.

I'm Years from Menopause, So Why Should I Care?

Although menopause is typically not on anyone's mind until they are knee-deep in it, that isn't ideal. Think of menopause as a different and currently unfamiliar phase of life, and compare that to how you would think about a move to a different and unfamiliar town. If you were changing towns, you would probably look at houses and schools, restaurants or nightclubs, and maybe gyms before you moved. You would do so to be prepared. For example, if there was excellent public transportation in your new town and parking was expensive, you might sell your car before the move. Think of menopause the same way. If you know what to expect, you can be prepared and proactive. While menopause can be associated with bothersome symptoms and an increased risk of some health conditions, preparation allows you to be proactive.

It is rare to hear someone say, "Wow, I was so overprepared for my health concerns," but really, wouldn't that be great? If you know what kind of changes in menstruation might happen as you transition into menopause, and what they might signify when or if they happen to you, it will be less scary, and you will know whether you need to contact your health care provider.

In addition, approximately 1 percent of people experience POI, which can sometimes occur years or even decades before menopause is expected. Knowing about it can help you be proactive about a diagnosis and therapy if you are at risk for POI or notice symptoms of it (for more on POI, see page 229).

Bottom Line

- The average age of menopause, or the final menstrual period, is fifty-one, and the average age of onset of the menopause transition is forty-six.
- Fertility starts to decrease in the thirties, and by age forty-five, pregnancy without assisted reproduction is uncommon.
- There is no hormone test that can tell when menopause might occur; testing is indicated when menopause appears to be happening earlier than expected, meaning before age forty-five.
- There are treatment options for many symptoms and health concerns that arise during the menopause transition and menopause.
- The prevailing theory about why women live long past menopause is that grandmothers provided worth to society, increasing the reproductive capabilities of their own children (genetics: the long game).

Part 2

COMMON CONCERNS AND MENSTRUAL MAINTENANCE

8

The Pelvic Exam

When I was ten years old, I needed a nuclear medicine scan to check my kidneys. Between the Cold War and the overhyped fear of nuclear energy in the 1970s, I was terrified. I was going to be injected with radioactive material, and everyone seemed so calm about it! I envisioned toxic, neon-green nuclear sludge coursing through my veins, but I kept my fears to myself. They didn't have the capability to do this test in the children's hospital, so when I showed up at the adult hospital for the injection, the tech explained the test to me as I suspect he would have explained it to an adult. This did not soothe my fears about being injected with radioactive material, nor did the equipment that would perform the scan: car-sized metal machinery hanging rather precariously, to my ten-year-old eyes, from the ceiling. And I was supposed to lie beneath it? Moments later, they plopped me in a chair, swabbed my arm with alcohol, and injected me with the radioactive material. I stood up and fainted.

I'd had much more painful and scary tests before that scan, and none had caused me any emotional distress. But they had all been explained to me in a way that I understood, and probably most importantly, I hadn't been scared heading into any of them. The impact of this negative experience was profound. For years I felt woozy whenever I smelled an alcohol swab, and it was something I had to work hard to overcome.

Now let's consider a pelvic exam. As a gynecologist who has done thousands and thousands of pelvic exams over a more-than-thirty-year career, I see them as an essential tool for evaluating the health of the ovaries, uterus, vagina, and vulva. When I have one, it feels as familiar as brushing my teeth. But to someone who has never had one before, or who has been sexually assaulted, or who has pelvic pain or pain with sexual activity, or who has been traumatized previously by a pelvic exam, it might sound as scary as that nuclear medicine scan sounded to me. And the speculum? More like an instrument of torture than a piece of essential medical equipment.

The fear and dread around pelvic exams aren't surprising. These exams are rarely discussed in an accurate way outside of a medical office, so people often head into one with little or no knowledge, which is disempowering. Many medical providers rush patients and/or fail to explain the pelvic exam in ways that they can understand before it's happening, which is wrong. And waiting to explain the process until it is happening is equally unacceptable, because at that point your mind is preoccupied by what is happening to your body.

The consequences for individuals who fear pelvic exams or who find them painful are significant. The pain and trauma are problematic on their own, but they can also lead people to avoid needed exams and vital screening tests. I've spoken to numerous patients over the years who have skipped a needed pelvic exam and suffered medical consequences such as heavy bleeding and anemia or late detection of cervical cancer that could have been caught by cervical cancer screening.

And there is even more potential fallout due to poor communication about your specific pelvic examination. Not knowing exactly what happened can lead people to think they had a test, such as a cervical cancer screen, when they didn't. "Oh, I'm up to date on my Pap smears" is something I hear a lot, but then I can't locate any evidence of cervical cancer screening in the patient's medical record. What my patient means is they had a pelvic exam, perhaps in the emergency department or at a doctor's office, and they assumed they were checked for "everything." It wouldn't surprise me if some doctors even say "I checked for everything," but that usually means "Everything that is relevant to evaluate your health at this moment." A patient cannot be faulted for thinking that "everything" meant, well, everything, which would include cervical cancer screening!

What Is a Pelvic Exam?

A pelvic exam involves evaluation of the external and/or internal pelvic structures. External means the vulva and vaginal opening, and internal involves the vagina, cervix, uterus, oviducts, and ovaries. The exam may also include cervical cancer screening, insertion of an IUD, and/or investigation into symptoms such as pain, abnormal bleeding, or vaginal itching. The components of a pelvic exam can include some or all of the following:

- *Inspection of the vulva:* This evaluation typically involves separating the labia (lips) to look at the vestibule (the tissue that connects the vulva with the vagina).
- *Speculum exam:* The insertion of a speculum into the vagina (see below). This is used to evaluate the vagina and cervix, and to access the cervix for a procedure such as inserting an IUD.
- *Single finger exam:* The doctor inserts a single gloved finger into the vagina to check for any abnormalities and assess the degree of muscle spasm, a possible cause of pain with sex and pelvic pain.
- *Bimanual exam:* The doctor uses one or two fingers of a gloved hand inserted vaginally, with the other hand pressing on the lower abdomen. This exam evaluates the size and shape of the uterus and the oviducts and ovaries, which together are known as the adnexa (distinguishing what is oviduct and what is ovary by pressing with your hands isn't possible), and checks for any other pelvic masses. After a bimanual exam, some doctors might mention the angling of the uterus or say that the uterus is "tipped" (see page 104).
- *Rectovaginal exam:* The insertion of a gloved finger into the vagina and rectum at the same time to evaluate the tissue that divides the two. This exam can be useful in diagnosing potential cancers and pelvic floor prolapse.

The Speculum

A speculum is a tool that spreads or widens an orifice in the body to improve the quality of a medical exam. There are rectal speculums, ear speculums, nose speculums, and vaginal speculums. The speculum exam is reported as the most embarrassing and painful part of a pelvic exam, but as I'll discuss shortly, there's a lot that a good medical provider can do to reduce negative experiences.

The vaginal speculum we use in the office today is called a bivalve speculum. Its design is sometimes falsely attributed to Dr. J. Marion Sims, an awful doctor who tortured enslaved women in the United States with surgeries in an attempt to cure vaginal fistulas (connections between the vagina and bladder and/or the vagina and bowel). While Sims did invent a type of speculum, it's used in the operating room, not in the office for pelvic exams or cervical cancer screening. This speculum has been renamed the Lucy, after one of the women who suffered at his hands.

The bivalve speculum was invented in the nineteenth century by Marie Boivin, a French midwife who was called "one of the wisest midwives and the most truly medical woman of modern times." The reason we are still using it today is that it's well designed for its purpose. There are some issues with it, which I will discuss, but it was a revolutionary instrument for its day, and invented by a remarkable woman.

A bivalve speculum consists of two main parts, each with a bill and a handle that come together at a screw that acts like a hinge, so the speculum can be collapsed for insertion and then opened, pushing up against the bladder and down toward the rectum. Only the bills are inserted vaginally. The purpose of the speculum is to hold back or retract the vaginal walls to see the cervix, and it can be rotated so all the vaginal walls can be seen through the open sides.

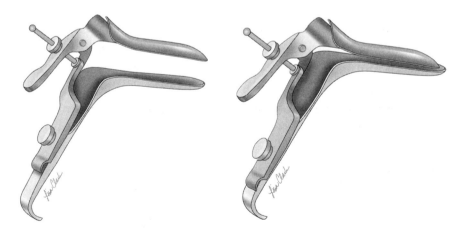

Figure 10 • *Speculum Open (Left) and Closed (Right) (Illustration by Lisa A. Clark, MA, CMI)*

Speculums come in different lengths and widths, and there are many minor variations in design, such as the shape of the bills or the handles. For example, a Pederson speculum is narrowest at the tip, so it's easier to insert, while a Graves speculum is wider at the tip. A Cusco speculum has handles that angle away so they don't touch the buttocks, and there is even a newer modification with two additional arms that push laterally. Speculums can be metal, silicone-coated metal, or plastic, and one newer speculum claims to be biodegradable. It's good to see companies trying to improve the design.

There are advantages and disadvantages to each type of speculum. Metal can be cold if not warmed prior to the exam, and the sound and/or feel of metal bothers some people. Metal has a lower carbon footprint, but there is cost involved in maintenance and cleaning after each use. Some people prefer the feel of plastic, but the handles click in a way that can bother others and, depending on the brand, unclicking them to reposition can sometimes be cumbersome and even painful. Silicone can feel better for some, but it can be harder to sterilize, and the silicone coating can break down, resulting in the added expense of replacing the speculum sooner.

Because we are all built differently, an office would ideally have access to a variety of speculums. However, it's important to acknowledge that, for reasons of cost and access to sterilization equipment, every choice simply may not be possible. Regardless of the type of speculum a medical provider decides to stock, speculums of different sizes should be available.

Some things that can help reduce pain with a speculum exam include:

- A provider who explains what is going to happen, meaning what parts of the pelvic exam are needed and why, and that the exam will be stopped if it is uncomfortable. This conversation should happen while the patient is still dressed. Absorbing information can be more challenging when you are naked and sticking to a plastic sheet that is making your bottom sweat. Also, in my experience, knowing that the exam will be halted if it's uncomfortable or triggering can help people feel in control.
- Raising the head of the bed about forty degrees. This allows you to have eye contact with your doctor and lets them see any signs of discomfort in your facial expressions. This position can also help relax the abdominal and pelvic muscles.

- Seeing or touching the speculum before the exam starts.
- Receiving good communication from your doctor during the exam so you know what is happening with each step. Your doctor should also seek affirmation before moving on to the next step. For example, after inspecting the vulva, they should ask if it is okay to proceed to the speculum exam. If not, the exam should be stopped.
- Trying alternative positions. The standard position for exams in the United States and Canada, called the lithotomy position, involves lying on the table with your feet in supports (often called stirrups, but I hate that term). Instead of supports, the feet can be placed on the corners of the bed (called the M position), and in one study this position was preferred by patients. Another option is to bring the feet together and let the knees flop out (often referred to as the frog-leg position). A speculum exam can even be done with the patient lying on one side. It is difficult to insert an IUD that way, but it can be used for cervical cancer screening or to collect a sample to evaluate for vaginal infection.
- Using the narrowest speculum. Some speculums, when collapsed, are about the width of a finger. Often these narrow speculums are adequate, but for other people they fail to push the vaginal walls apart sufficiently for the doctor to see what they need to. In that case, it may be necessary to move up to a bigger speculum.
- Self-insertion of the speculum, meaning the patient inserts it themselves and then the doctor repositions it if needed. In one study, there was a high degree of satisfaction with this method.
- If metal, a warmed speculum.
- Using a lubricant, which makes the speculum insertion easier and less painful. Lubricants do not affect the quality of cervical cancer screening or testing for STIs.
- If the feel of metal is bothersome and plastic or silicone isn't available, placing a condom over the metal speculum and cutting out the tip of the condom so there is minimal to no metal touching the vagina, but the doctor can still see the cervix.
- Taking time.
- Applying lidocaine, a topical numbing ointment or gel, at the vaginal opening to reduce pain from the speculum.

- For trans men and nonbinary people on testosterone, using vaginal estrogen for a few weeks before an exam, which can help reduce discomfort.
- If an exam is painful but needed, offering pain control and sedation by an anesthesiologist. This is an underutilized option. I have stopped exams and said, "I think we should regroup and talk about how we can do this for you in a non-painful way." I always emphasize that needing more pain control is not a sign of weakness or a fault; you simply need the pain control you need.

Most of my patients have previously had pain with exams, and many tell me their experience in my office is the first time they have had a non-painful pelvic exam. This is heartbreaking and unnecessary. But it also tells me that these measures can be very effective. In addition, if the first exam with me is not traumatizing, it increases the chance that we may be able to do a more thorough exam at the next visit.

There are some factors that increase the risk of an exam being painful: being under twenty-five; a history of sexual abuse; a history of pain with inserting tampons and/or penile vaginal sex; and previous pain with exams. Vulvodynia (a nerve pain condition of the vulva), vaginismus (spasm of the muscles that surround the vagina), endometriosis, some infections, and hormonal changes of menopause can also cause pain with pelvic exams.

Why Do I Have to Scoot Down the Table?

Many people think, "If I scoot down any farther, I'm going to be on the floor!" This maneuvering exists only with the lithotomy position, because when the leading edge of the buttocks is a little lower, it can make it easier to see the cervix with a speculum exam. The same effect can be created by placing your fists, a rolled-up towel, or a bedpan under the hips.

My Uterus Is Tipped—What Does That Mean?

Many people hear after a bimanual exam that their uterus is "tipped." This is something I wish health care providers would stop saying, as it is almost always uttered without context, leaving the patient wondering if it is good or bad. A "tipped uterus" is not a medical term, and confusingly, doctors may use it to mean one of two anatomical situations. Also, we are talking about uteruses, not cows in a field!

Vert means "to turn in a particular direction," so an introvert turns inward. With the uterus, it refers to the angle or spatial orientation in the pelvis. An anteverted uterus is angled forward, toward the bladder; this is the most common orientation (see Figure 11 below). A retroverted uterus angles backward, toward the rectum. If it's in the middle, we use the very non-medical-sounding term *mid-position*. Hold a hand up in front of you. If you tip your hand forward at the wrist, that is anteverted; if you move it so it's in a straight line with your wrist, that's mid-position; if you angle it backward at the wrist, that is retroverted.

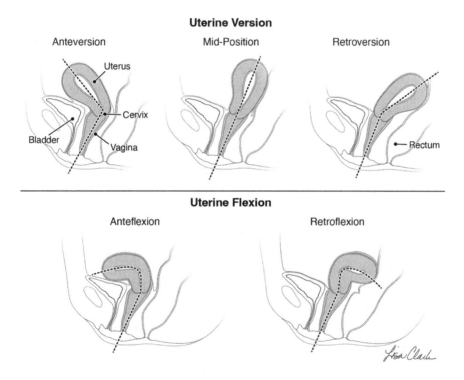

Figure 11 • *Positioning of the Uterus (Illustration by Lisa A. Clark, MA, CMI)*

Sometimes the body of the uterus is flexed upon itself, meaning its shape is no longer a gentle C but a very curved one, almost as if the uterus is folded. If it is flexed forward, this is called anteflexion. If it is flexed backward, pushing into the rectum, it is retroflexed.

While they may look extreme and uncomfortable, these variations in position are usually as meaningful as the shape of your nose, and they most definitely don't impact fertility (a common question). However, there are a few situations where the position of the uterus matters:

- *Finding the cervix:* Okay, the cervix can't really get lost, but when the uterus is anteflexed or retroflexed, the cervix can be angled in such a way that it is not visible in a straight line from the vaginal opening— meaning once the speculum is in, it may need to be repositioned to find the cervix, and this can sometimes make the pelvic exam uncomfortable. If you know your uterus is anteflexed or retroflexed, let your doctor know so they can insert the speculum in a way that makes it more likely they will find your cervix on the first attempt, reducing discomfort. I find it very helpful when someone says, "Hey, my last doctor told me that my cervix is angled weirdly."
- *Procedures such as an IUD insertion or an abortion:* The instruments we insert need to follow the direction of the inside of the uterus.
- *When it's a sign of a medical condition:* A uterus can be retroflexed just because that's how it's shaped, but it can also be because of scarring due to endometriosis, a previous infection, radiation (from cancer therapy, not an X-ray or CT scan), or a previous surgery. When a uterus is retroflexed because of scarring, it can be painful if it is pushed with a penis, fingers, or a sex toy; when there is no scarring, a retroflexed uterus typically moves and doesn't cause pain with penetrative sexual activities.
- *During pregnancy:* As the uterus enlarges, it lifts out of the pelvis so it has room to expand; this is best imagined as a balloon being blown up. With a retroflexed uterus, the top part can get trapped against the sacrum, which can be very painful. Fortunately, this is a very rare condition, affecting one in twenty thousand pregnancies, and there is treatment.

Do I Need a Regular Screening Pelvic Exam?

In medicine, a screening exam or test is something designed to identify a problem early to reduce negative health outcomes in a specific population. For example, screening for chlamydia is recommended for everyone with a cervix who is twenty-five years or younger, because studies show testing everyone in this age group is beneficial given the increased risk of chlamydia in the age group. Screening is also recommended for other people at higher risk, for example, someone with a new sexual partner. A screening exam or test should show that it has benefit for the population being tested.

Previous guidelines used to recommend an annual pelvic exam, but the reason was always nebulous, for example, "to make sure everything is okay" (not a reason) or to pick up ovarian cancer early. This was at a time when we also did annual Pap smears, so the pelvic exam was all folded into the same visit. Cervical cancer screening (CCS) has now changed radically, and annual exams for that reason are no longer necessary, so many people have rightly wondered if the annual pelvic exam (everything but the CCS) is still needed.

There is no study that shows an annual pelvic exam saves lives or identifies any health condition for people who don't have symptoms. Meaning, if someone doesn't have symptoms, the exam doesn't add anything health-wise, and it also is not a good test for identifying ovarian cancer. Guidelines vary from not recommending it at all to leaving the decision up to the doctor and patient, but no medical professional group in the United States, Canada, or the United Kingdom recommends an annual pelvic exam. Some health care providers claim they still choose to offer an annual pelvic exam because it reassures patients and can strengthen the bond between doctor and patient. I'm just going to say that the second part is creepy. And while it's true that some people say they're reassured by a pelvic exam, it is false reassurance, because we have no studies that show medical benefit from these exams.

If you have symptoms such as bloating, pelvic pain, or heavy periods, that's a completely different story; in that case, a pelvic exam is important. But then it isn't a screening exam; it's meant to investigate symptoms. An annual screening test for chlamydia for sexually active people under twenty-five can be accomplished with a speculum exam, but it can also just as easily be done with a urine test and skipping the exam. And as most labs are open after hours and on the weekends, a urine test is typically more convenient than a pelvic exam—and, of course, less traumatizing.

How Do Doctors Learn to Do Pelvic Exams?

At my medical school we worked with standardized patients, women who were paid to teach us to do pelvic exams. These women had specific training and had often worked with medical students for years. Before I ever touched a "real life" patient, I had done four pelvic exams where the patient herself guided me through how to insert the speculum and how to position it, and then afterward explained what I had done right and what I had done wrong. This experience was invaluable, and in my opinion it should be mandatory.

I've heard that there are medical schools where students are brought into an operating room to do pelvic exams on anesthetized patients without their consent. That is assault. A pelvic exam should be performed during surgery only if it will contribute to the surgery. For example, a pelvic exam before a hysterectomy can provide information that may be useful during the surgery, just as examining a knee might be helpful before knee surgery. But a pelvic exam will not contribute to gallbladder surgery or a knee replacement. In situations where the information from a pelvic exam may be useful, only the doctors and students who have met the patient and will be scrubbed into the surgery should be involved with the pre-procedure pelvic exam in the operating room. I wouldn't have the skill set I do today if it were not for all the patients who graciously allowed me to learn while caring for them, and that includes doing a pelvic exam before I assisted with surgery.

If a pelvic exam under anesthesia is part of the surgery, this should be discussed with you at a preoperative visit, and if any trainees might be involved this should be discussed and your consent obtained. Surgeons are in positions of great power, so asking for permission when you have fasted the night before and are nervous and about to be rolled into the operating room is not appropriate. And of course, you always have the right to limit these exams.

Cervical Cancer Screening

Cervical cancer screening includes the Pap smear, named after Dr. Georgios Papanikolaou, one of the two doctors who independently invented this method of CCS as well as testing for human papillomavirus (HPV). It's important to point out that the Pap smear isn't truly cervical cancer screening—it's screening for precancers, conditions that can be treated to prevent cancer. If cancer is suspected, different testing is required.

Almost all cervical cancers are due to HPV, which is why HPV testing has become a larger part of CCS. There are over two hundred types of HPV, but only thirteen of them can live in the tissues of the genital tract and are oncogenic, meaning they can cause cancer. The big guns here are HPV types 16 and 18, which cause approximately 75 percent of cervical cancers (HPV 16 alone causes 60 percent). The remainder are due to HPV types 31, 33, 35, 39, 45, 51, 52, 56, 58, 59, and 68. There are other cervical cancers that are not HPV-related, but they are rare and not easily identified with Pap smears, so switching to HPV testing doesn't mean we are missing these other rare cancers.

HPV infections are common. About 80 percent of women will have at least one in their lifetime, but not every HPV infection leads to cervical cancer. In fact, within two years of a positive test for HPV, the immune system will have cleared the virus 90 percent of the time. It's when the virus doesn't clear, something we call *viral persistence*, that it becomes a risk factor for cervical cancer. Before we knew about the key role of viral persistence, many women with mild changes to their cervix due to HPV—changes that would have cleared without medical intervention—were overtreated. Current guidelines balance the importance of detecting precancers when they can be treated with minimizing the risk of overtreating changes that will not become cancer.

CCS is important because cervical cancer is the fourth most common cancer among women worldwide and the second most common among women of reproductive age (fifteen to forty-four). Worldwide, 250,000 people die from cervical cancer every year. Health care disparities have a huge impact here: those who die from cervical cancer may not have access to the HPV vaccine or to appropriate CCS. In addition, trans and nonbinary people are less likely to get cervical cancer screening, almost certainly because of difficulties accessing care and how they are treated within the health care system.

The rates of cancer and precancer have decreased for those who have been vaccinated for HPV, but also for those who have not been vaccinated (although the decrease is less). This is due to herd immunity: because many people are vaccinated, there is less virus in circulation, which benefits the unvaccinated.

A Pap smear involves a light scraping of cells from the surface of the cervix and the cells are then evaluated under the microscope. With HPV testing, cells are collected from the cervix and analyzed by a machine. CCS can be a Pap smear, HPV testing, or a combination of the two. A speculum is required to see the cervix to collect a Pap smear, and while the current recommendation is to use a speculum for HPV testing, there is a lot of data that shows collecting a sample with just a brush inserted into the vagina is accurate. In addition, there is research showing that menstrual blood and urine specimens are also accurate for HPV testing, meaning one day (hopefully soon) we might be at the point where a urine sample could be all that is needed to test for cervical cancer screening, and so it's possible we may one day see HPV testing that doesn't require a speculum. Currently, for someone who cannot have a pelvic exam because of pain or fear, collection of an HPV sample from the vagina with the brush and no speculum might be an option to consider; another option is having sedation, if available and affordable, to reduce anxiety and pain.

Cervical cancer screening guidelines, meaning the type of testing and the frequency, are based on several factors, such as age, the type of screening, previous results, whether the patient is living with HIV, and the country where the patient lives. The age when screening starts varies from twenty-one to twenty-five. Overall, the bulk of the research currently favors HPV testing as the preferred screening option, but for those who are between twenty-one and twenty-four, a Pap smear is recommended. HPV infections are so common for people under twenty-five that using HPV testing for this age group may yield too many positives that ultimately are unlikely to be concerning.

Some people are concerned about going five years between cervical cancer screens with the HPV test, but it's important to remember that it takes years from acquiring the virus to develop a precancer. Spacing out testing helps to limit unnecessary procedures while catching most cancers. And also remember, the single best way to prevent cervical cancer is to get the HPV vaccine. For those whose partner has a penis, condoms also help reduce the rate of HPV infections. Smoking is another cofactor in cervical cancer, so quitting smoking is as good for your cervix as it is for your lungs.

Bottom Line

- A pelvic exam is an essential tool for gynecological health; unfortunately, for pain-sensitive people it is painful and traumatizing.
- A pelvic exam shouldn't be painful, and there are many ways to improve the experience.
- Pelvic exams should be performed only with consent, including in the operating room.
- Many doctors mention a tipped uterus, but it's not a concern except in certain specific situations. For most people, it's just the way you are built, like the shape of your nose or ears.
- Cervical cancer screening can be accomplished with HPV testing, Pap smears, or a combination of both. The guidelines may vary between countries for a variety of reasons.

9

Premenstrual Symptoms: PMS, PMDD, and Breast Pain

There is a wide range of bothersome physical and/or emotional symptoms that can appear in the luteal phase of the menstrual cycle and then disappear shortly after menstruation starts. Table 1 lists the most common ones, but some researchers report up to 150 different symptoms. By some estimates, up to 80 percent of people experience at least one of these symptoms, so it's fair to say they are part of the typical menstrual "experience." That doesn't mean they don't suck, or that I'm being dismissive about the distress they may cause. Rather, they are so widespread that they are almost as common as bleeding.

Table 1 • COMMON PHYSICAL AND EMOTIONAL SYMPTOMS OF PMS

COMMON PHYSICAL SYMPTOMS	COMMON EMOTIONAL SYMPTOMS
Breast pain	Anger
Bloating	Anxiety
Fatigue	Food cravings
Headache	Irritability
Hot flashes	Mood swings

COMMON PHYSICAL SYMPTOMS	COMMON EMOTIONAL SYMPTOMS
Joint pain	Sadness
Swelling in hands and legs	Social withdrawal

For most people, the symptoms don't have a major impact on their daily life. When two or more (at least one physical and one emotional) are present in the luteal phase of most cycles and they negatively affect quality of life, be it at work, at school, at home, or within relationships, the diagnosis is premenstrual syndrome, or PMS, which affects 12 to 20 percent of people who menstruate.

Premenstrual mood dysphoria, or PMDD, is a severe form of PMS that affects 3 to 5 percent of people. With PMDD, there is a greater focus on emotional symptoms, and for a diagnosis of PMDD, five symptoms from Table 2 must be present, with at least one from each column. The symptoms must be severe enough that they cause significant distress and have a significant impact on quality of life.

Table 2 • DIAGNOSIS OF PMDD

ONE OR MORE	ONE OR MORE
Significant mood swings, including increased sensitivity to rejection	Feeling overwhelmed or out of control
Significant irritability or anger, or increased conflict in relationships	Sleeping too much or insomnia
Significantly depressed mood, feelings of hopelessness, or self-deprecating thoughts	Physical symptoms such as breast tenderness, swelling, joint or muscle pain, feeling bloated, weight gain
Significant anxiety, tension, and/ or feelings of being on edge	Significant change in appetite in either direction
	Feeling lethargic, tiring easily, very low energy
	Difficulty concentrating
	Drop in interest in usual activities, such as work, social life, hobbies

The most important aspect in making the diagnosis of PMS or PMDD is the timing of when symptoms appear: they must be limited to the luteal phase, meaning they don't appear before ovulation. In addition, they must go away completely within four days after menstruation starts. The symptoms must also be present for most of the menstrual cycles in the previous twelve months.

The History of the Mad Menstrual Woman

It's hard to mine historical writings about women's health and find a diagnosis that we might now recognize as PMS. First, there is the problem of different disease models. Until the nineteenth century, Western medicine revolved around the four humors: black bile, yellow bile, phlegm, and blood. Illnesses were due to imbalances, and treatments were meant to correct these imbalances. Diagnoses made with humoral medicine can't be translated to scientific medicine; it's like working with two incompatible languages.

In addition, most illnesses were attributed in some way to the uterus (a disease model we thankfully abandoned), women were often viewed as weaker, and beliefs about menstruation were different. At one point menstruation was linked with vampirism and rabies, and for centuries menstrual blood was believed to be toxic. If your medical model literally treats menstrual blood as toxic waste, it's unlikely you will make much of swelling or mood swings right before menstruation—clearly, the toxins were building up!

To underscore the difficulties in identifying PMS or PMDD in historical medical writing, here is an example from a textbook that was published in the 1800s. Mary W. was diagnosed with "melancholia with suicidal tendencies" and a "nervous affliction" related to her periods. Mary also had a lot of gynecological symptoms, and she said she could bear all of them if it weren't for her "nervous state." Might Mary really have been suffering from PMS or PMDD? Poor Mary was given all manner of awful therapies, including douching vaginally with lead acetate, to treat the nervous state that was "clearly" related to her periods. And then, almost as an afterthought, we learn that Mary had sick children at home, had a drunken husband who spent all their money, was hemorrhaging regularly from her rectum, and was leaking large amounts of black blood and tissue from her vagina (I know!), not to mention that over the past months her abdomen had become so swollen that she looked seven months pregnant! All of this is mentioned in passing as if these details are completely unrelated to her emotional state. Untangling what were physical and emotional symptoms related to her menstruation, what was likely advanced cancer of the uterus or ovary, and what was a truly terrible home life just isn't possible. I think a lot about the Marys I've met from reading old textbooks.

The first mention in the medical literature of what we could today call PMS/PMDD was in a 1931 paper by Dr. Karen Horney called "Die Prämenstruellen Verstimmungen" (Premenstrual Tensions), where she wrote (according to a translation) that it is "remarkable that so little attention has been paid to the fact that disturbances occur not only during menstruation but even more frequently, though less obtrusively, in the days before the onset of menstrual flow." She described the symptoms as "varying degrees of tension, ranging from a feeling that everything is too much, a sense of listlessness or of being slowed down, and intensities of feelings of self-depreciation to the point of pronounced feelings of oppression and of being severely depressed."

Understanding the Cause

The specific reasons why people get PMS and PMDD are not well understood. Like many things in medicine, there are a lot of moving parts that result in PMS/PMDD. There is clearly a hormonal component, as PMD/PMDD doesn't occur before puberty, ebbs and flows with the menstrual cycle, disappears with menopause, and resolves temporarily during pregnancy. The theory is that it's not hormone levels per se, but rather the fluctuations in their levels, as during the luteal phase progesterone and to a lesser extent estrogen rise and then drop. Some research suggests that allopregnanolone, a metabolite of progesterone, may have a role in the symptoms. Certain people do appear to be exquisitely sensitive to progesterone from a mood standpoint.

Another theory revolves around serotonin, a neurotransmitter that is involved in regulation of mood and anxiety. Hormones impact serotonin levels, and there is data showing that women with PMS/PMDD have dysregulation in their serotonin system. There are also genetic and environmental factors that make some people more vulnerable than others. For example, smoking increases the risk of PMS/PMDD.

The hormonal changes in the luteal phase are complex. While progesterone appears to be an appetite stimulant, some studies suggest that estrogen may be an appetite suppressant and that a high progesterone level antagonizes this effect, essentially negating estrogen's ability to reduce appetite. Other hormones that affect appetite, including ghrelin and leptin, also vary throughout the menstrual cycle. While the exact mechanism isn't yet known, cumulatively the hormonal changes result in an increase in appetite and calorie intake in the luteal phase, as well as cravings for foods high in carbohydrate and fat. Estrogen and progesterone also interact with several neurotransmitters, such as serotonin, dopamine, and gamma-aminobutyric acid (GABA), which may explain many of the mood symptoms. Moreover, these hormones affect the renin-angiotensin-aldosterone system, a critical system that controls blood volumes and how blood vessels contract and relax. Changes in it could lead to bloating, swelling, and fatigue, and even cravings for salty food.

Ultimately, we understand some of the basic biology, and there are lots of plausible ways that hormonal fluctuations can interact with body systems to produce the myriad of symptoms, but we are not able to predict who will develop PMS/PMDD and who will not.

PMS/PMDD and "Perimenopausal Rage"

Some women describe both mood fluctuations and a varying range of moods during the menopause transition (colloquially called perimenopause). Whenever a woman tells me she feels "perimenopausal rage," I always want to rule out PMS/PMDD. I also think of PMS/PMDD when someone tells me they started hormone therapy in the menopause transition because of mood symptoms, such as feeling on edge, irritable, angry, or low, and instead of improving, they felt worse.

There are a few reasons for these mood changes. The first is that in the early stages of the menopause transition, the menstrual cycle shortens a little, always in the follicular phase (before ovulation). The length of the luteal phase, the time after ovulation, stays the same. PMS/PMDD symptoms appear only in the luteal phase, but if you spend less time in the follicular phase, you lose "good days"—meaning, percentage-wise, you spend more of your time with PMS/PMDD. If your cycle shortens by four days, that's four days of feeling good that you lose, which can make it harder to recover. And the early menopause transition can easily last five to seven years, so that is, unfortunately, a lot of time to deal with fewer good days. In addition, fluctuations in hormone levels are far more extreme during the menopause transition, which could worsen symptoms. Sleep disturbance, typical of the menopause transition, might also play a role: if you are tired all the time, your ability to cope with PMS/PMDD may decrease. Some people develop mild depression related to the menopause transition, which could also amplify PMS/PMDD.

Diagnosing PMS/PMDD

PMS/PMDD can be a confusing diagnosis to pinpoint, as medical conditions with similar symptoms can fluctuate with the menstrual cycle, including depression (up to 60 percent of people report a worsening of depression before the menstrual cycle), anxiety, irritable bowel syndrome, and fibromyalgia, to name a few. However, it is atypical for these conditions to flare only during the luteal phase and then completely resolve during the follicular phase.

Most research supports tracking symptoms over at least two menstrual cycles to help obtain a diagnosis, and there are a variety of ways to do so. You can use a pen and paper, mark up a calendar, or create a file to track what you are experiencing daily. Many menstrual tracking apps (see Chapter 11) allow you to track PMS/PMDD symptoms as well. There are also resources available through the International Association for Premenstrual Disorders (IAPMD). If you search for them online, you'll find a link to a free app for tracking symptoms, a medically vetted questionnaire for tracking symptoms, and lots of other resources.

Getting a diagnosis early is critical. Many people develop PMS/PMDD as adolescents and never receive treatment or even the validation of a diagnosis. Even just knowing what is happening can be liberating, because believing you are alone in having distressing and even disabling symptoms is an incredibly isolating and destructive experience.

Blood work for hormone levels isn't recommended in diagnosing PMS/PMDD, but most guidelines suggest a screening test for thyroid conditions. Screening for depression with a validated questionnaire is important as well. Vitamin D levels are the same for women with and without PMS/PMDD, so testing for vitamin D isn't necessary.

Managing PMS/PMDD

When it comes to managing PMS and PMDD, the guidelines regularly recommend exercise, but the data on its effectiveness is sparse. Look, we know exercise is good for health, and it has been shown to have a positive impact on mood, but whether it can specifically help PMS/PMDD isn't known. Another non-pharmaceutical strategy, with more evidence to support its use, is cognitive behavioral therapy (CBT). There is also some weak evidence supporting an increase in complex carbohydrates (think whole grains, legumes, vegetables) in the luteal phase, but then, like exercise, that's just a good health strategy overall. The two management therapies most supported by science are:

- *Selective serotonin reuptake inhibitors (SSRIs):* Antidepressant medications such as citalopram (Celexa), escitalopram (Lexapro), fluoxetine (Prozac), paroxetine (Paxil), and sertraline (Zoloft) work very quickly for PMS/PMDD and can be taken in one of three ways: daily; in the luteal phase only (starting with ovulation); or when symptoms start. The latter two options appeal to people who want to be on the medication only when they need to be. For example, if symptoms start five days before your menstrual period and last for two days after bleeding starts, you might be able to take an SSRI for just seven or eight days a month. People with more severe symptoms, or those with more unpredictable cycles or symptoms, may need a daily option, but it's nice that SSRIs offer this flexibility.
- *Estrogen-containing oral contraceptive pills:* It may seem counter-intuitive to take more hormones, but the pill stops ovulation and replaces the cyclic fluctuations with a steady state. The pill can be taken every day, meaning no placebo, so menstruation is skipped altogether. There is some evidence that the pill with drospirenone/estradiol, taken in such a way that the pill-free or placebo time is only four days (so twenty-four days of active pills), may be specifically useful, but the data is not that robust.

When SSRIs and estrogen-containing oral contraceptives are ineffective, another prescription medication to consider is a class of drugs called gonadotropin-releasing hormone (GnRH) agonists or antagonists (I'll call these GnRH medications). These medications interfere with the pulses of GnRH released by the hypothalamus and bring about a chemically induced, though temporary, menopause. Pausing the menstrual cycle in this way can help when PMDD is severe. When GnRH medications are stopped, the cycle starts up again (for more on these medications, see page 219). GnRH medications require monitoring as they can have long-term consequences, such as osteoporosis and cardiovascular disease, because as far as your body is concerned, it is in early menopause. The risks can be mitigated by adding back a small amount of estrogen and progesterone or progesterone-like hormone (this is called add-back therapy—original, I know). The dose of the hormones added back is less than the body makes (like the doses in menopausal hormone therapy) and provides a constant level with no fluctuations and doesn't trigger PMDD.

GnRH medications used to be available only by injection, so if people didn't like how they felt afterward, they were stuck waiting one or even three months (depending on the dose) for it to wear off. This idea was understandably scary for some people, but now there are oral forms available, which makes these medications easier to try and easier to stop if you don't like how they make you feel.

GnRH medications are also useful for people who are considering removing their ovaries because of PMDD. (In that situation, several other therapies should have been tried first.) These medications can give you a window into how you might feel without ovaries. When the ovaries are removed before age forty-five, we recommend menopausal hormone therapy until at least age fifty-one to lower the risks of osteoporosis, heart disease, and dementia, so trying out these hormones beforehand is useful as well. Basically, GnRH medications allow you to road-test the effects of surgery and the hormone therapy needed to mitigate the drop in estrogen in a reversible way, helping you make an informed decision about surgery.

Over-the-Counter Therapies

The Internet is filled with supplements and special diets that claim to cure PMS/PMDD, but most of them are poorly tested and/or make no sense, biologically speaking. The two with the best evidence are:

- *Calcium carbonate supplements:* Calcium affects many biological processes, and two studies suggest that calcium carbonate might be effective at managing PMS/PMDD, either 500 mg twice a day or 1,200 mg once a day (in the latter study they used Tums, an over-the-counter antacid—no expensive designer supplements needed).
- *Vitex agnus-castus:* Also known as chasteberry, *Vitex agnus-castus* binds with the dopamine D2 receptor, opioid receptor, and estrogen receptor beta. Multiple trials support the use of chasteberry for PMS/PMDD; however, the studies were recently evaluated in a meta-analysis and were all found to be low-quality. That said, there seems to be little harm in trying it. The dose is 20 to 40 mg a day.

There are a whole host of other botanical and "natural" products used for PMS/PMDD, such as vitamin B_6 (100 mg a day), oil of evening primrose, and acupuncture, but the data supporting their effectiveness is of even lower quality or they just don't work, and I don't recommend them.

Breast Changes and the Menstrual Cycle

I had a boyfriend who could reliably tell when my period was coming because of the change in my breast size. We would lie in bed, spooning, and one of my breasts would be cupped in his hand, and then out of nowhere he'd say, "Is your period coming?" This wasn't weird or creepy for me—it was highly entertaining, because he was always right, and he was very proud that he knew my breasts so well. Also, he wasn't the kind of man who was grossed out by sex during menstruation; the first time it came up, he said, "That's why they make navy-blue towels!"

To understand breast changes related to the menstrual cycle, it's helpful to know how hormones affect breast tissue. Breasts undergo hormonal changes each cycle, much as the endometrium does. Think of this as prep work for a theoretical pregnancy. Unlike what happens with menstruation, if no pregnancy occurs, the tissue changes in the breasts can reverse. One group of researchers performed MRI scans during different phases of the menstrual cycle and found that breast volume, or size (both the amount of tissue and the water content), was lowest right after menstruation (the early follicular phase). Around ovulation, increases in tissue size and water content were detected, and breast volume increased rapidly from days 16 to 25, with breast size reaching its maximum on day 25. On day 5 of the cycle, the amount of breast tissue is 30 percent lower than at the peak right before menses, and water content is almost 18 percent lower. Basically, there is a rapid increase in the amount of breast tissue and in the fluid in the tissues during the luteal phase. These changes are largely driven by estrogen, which causes breast ducts to grow, and progesterone, which increases the growth of the lobules (milk glands) as well as fluid retention.

We are limited in our ability to know all the changes in breast tissue based on the menstrual cycle, because it is unethical to biopsy breasts for such a study, even if there were volunteers, as biopsies can cause scarring that could later affect mammography and breast cancer screening for the participants. So we are restricted to studies where biopsies were done for other reasons or after death on autopsy, which might produce different results.

Cyclic mastalgia is breast pain that varies with the menstrual cycle. It is a diffuse pain that is hard to pinpoint and is often described as a generalized tenderness and/or a heavy sensation. It can be very uncomfortable and distressing for some people. Cyclic mastalgia occurs during the luteal phase, and while the exact cause is unknown, it could be from fluid retention, the growth of the breast tissue, or even a hormone-induced impact on pain signaling. As I mentioned earlier, with hormone-related changes, it often isn't the actual level of the hormones but rather the fluctuations that are responsible for the symptoms.

Treatment of cyclic breast pain revolves around ruling out causes that are more serious, including cancer (although breast cancer is rarely painful), and then finding therapies that reduce the discomfort. A biopsy is not needed, but if there is any concern about breast cancer, then appropriate screening and/ or testing is indicated. First-line therapies involve wearing a well-fitting, supportive bra and medications like acetaminophen (Tylenol or paracetamol) or nonsteroidal anti-inflammatory drugs (NSAIDs) such as ibuprofen (Advil, Motrin) or naproxen sodium (Aleve, Naprosyn). Starting these pain medications one to two days before ovulation, or before the pain typically starts if it is later in the cycle, can sometimes make them more helpful.

Many physicians recommend quitting smoking, and while the link between smoking and cyclic breast pain is controversial, smoking does raise the risk of breast cancer and numerous other health conditions, so there are many reasons to quit. A lot of people ask about caffeine and breast pain, but the data linking the two is weak at best. Oil of evening primrose and vitamin E are common over-the-counter medications for breast pain, but these likely have a placebo effect; there is no good data to support their use. There is some low-quality evidence supporting the use of *Vitex agnus-castus* (chasteberry) and *Matricaria chamomilla* (chamomile) for breast pain. Although more studies are needed, if you are interested in trying nonprescription medications, these are two to consider.

If cyclic breast pain doesn't respond to these measures, it is reasonable to consider a trial of birth control pills, skipping any placebo pills to eliminate the fluctuations in hormones. Other options include danazol and tamoxifen, which are medications that can block the effect of estrogen on breast tissue. They can have side effects, so a discussion of the risks and benefits is important, as with all medications.

Bottom Line

- PMS and PMDD are conditions with physical and/or emotional symptoms that impact quality of life. These symptoms develop during the luteal phase and resolve with menstruation.
- PMS affects 12 to 20 percent of women. PMDD, a more severe version, affects 3 to 5 percent.
- Hormonal fluctuations appear to be the trigger for PMS and PMDD, but the exact reasons why some people have these conditions and others don't are unknown.
- The most effective therapy for PMS/PMDD is SSRIs. Estrogen-containing birth control pills are another good option.
- There is a rapid increase in both breast tissue and fluid in the breast tissue during the luteal phase.

10

Beyond the Uterus: Hormones and Your Health

The menstrual cycle has wide-ranging effects beyond the uterus, ovaries, and vagina, affecting overall health and well-being. The immune system, nervous system, blood vessels, muscles, and gastrointestinal system can all be involved; in fact, there seems to be no nook or cranny of the body that can't at least theoretically be impacted. Some of these changes exist to favor the implantation of a potential pregnancy—for example, the small rise in temperature after ovulation. But the impact of hormonal fluctuations can also be collateral damage, meaning there can be a price to pay for the wiring (for lack of a better term) that is needed for a menstrual cycle and gestating a pregnancy. And the reverse can also be true. Many medical conditions can impact the menstrual cycle.

Your experience may not be reflected in these pages, as it's not possible to cover all the interactions between the body and the menstrual cycle in one chapter. If one medical condition is typically worse right before menstruation, yours might be the opposite. This doesn't invalidate your experience. Rather, given the vast number of hormone receptors throughout our bodies, the dynamic nature of hormone levels, individual genetics, and other medical conditions, along with environmental factors, there really is an endless number of potential permutations and combinations of interactions between the body and the menstrual cycle. How we feel, and the changes we experience during each cycle, is the sum of many parts.

Diet and Menstruation

Most studies suggest that the basal metabolic rate (how many calories you burn at your baseline) increases slightly during the luteal phase. This translates to burning about an extra 100 calories a day. We don't know whether this is due to the minor increase in temperature and other changes during the luteal phase or it represents the energy needed to build the endometrium. Either way, appetite and energy intake often increase in the luteal phase, and specific food cravings aren't uncommon. It's probably no surprise to anyone reading this that the food most commonly craved is chocolate. Perhaps there is a specific chemical in chocolate that fulfills a need, or maybe it's just the pleasure of it? There is also conflicting data about whether the menstrual cycle has a noticeable impact on when people gravitate toward eating more protein or more carbohydrates.

Is there a diet that can optimize the brain-brain-ovary connection and how the uterus responds? In other words, is there an ideal diet for menstruation? No, not as such, though that answer may infuriate the numerous coaches and naturopaths who are invested in recommending expensive services or books to supposedly "repair" periods.

Adequate calorie intake is essential for ovulation. This makes sense, as pregnancy and lactation are metabolically demanding, so a system that can reduce fertility when there are not enough calories to sustain a pregnancy is beneficial. It takes a significant drop in calories—about 30 percent—to interrupt the signaling from the brain that triggers follicles in the ovaries to develop. We know this because of studies where people had bariatric surgery and hormone levels were interrupted before there was a substantial amount of weight loss, meaning it was the impact of the calorie restriction that affected the system and not the loss of weight. In the long term, the impact of inadequate calories on hormones can be significant; for more on this, see Chapter 17.

But what about the best foods to eat? Are carbs bad? Is fat bad? Are there menstrual superfoods? If you spend any time on Instagram or TikTok, you wouldn't be faulted for thinking you need to eat raw carrot salads, avoid seed oils, avoid "grain carbohydrates," and eat only during a six-hour window each day for optimal menstrual health. Good news: that's all a load of garbage. Carrots are a fine vegetable, but if you prefer cauliflower, that's great. Canola oil is fine. Whole grains are part of a healthy diet. And the number of books and experts promoting intermittent fasting for menstrual health is inversely proportional to its value.

The idea that humans need a special or restrictive diet to optimize menstruation is simply not true. First, humans are fantastic omnivores. We have adapted to living in a multitude of climates with very different food sources, and fertility keeps trucking along. Also, if there were a single superfood or a few essential superfoods, what would happen if the weather affected that food? "Too hot for acai berries this season, sorry. That's it, folks. Fertility is canceled for the year. Fingers crossed that the crops recover." Reproduction can't afford to be a picky eater.

While it's true there is limited research on optimal diets for menstruation, we can look at studies that use natural fertility (conceiving without technological intervention) and pregnancy outcomes as a proxy. Here, the data tells us that the best diet is one that is low in saturated fat, high in a diverse number of vegetables, high in legumes, and high in fish. Basically, the same foods that are best for almost every health condition. It may not be sexy or sell coaching services, but the take-home message is to eat more protein from fish and plants, more plant foods in general, more whole grains, less meat, and less added sugar. You want a balanced diet so you'll get micronutrients such as calcium, iron, and vitamins. Because vitamin B_{12} is found only in animal products, vegans and some vegetarians will need a source of vitamin B_{12}, such as nutritional yeast or a vitamin B_{12} supplement.

Fiber is an important macronutrient. The average American diet includes about 15 g of fiber a day, but the recommendation is to eat 25–30 g or more per day, so people looking to optimize their health through diet should consider counting their fiber intake. I count fiber every day because it really is so important. Yes, it requires meal planning, but it's worth it. I often start the day with a high-fiber cereal, something with 10–13 g of fiber per serving, because then I'm nearly halfway to my daily fiber goal already. A high-fiber diet is associated with a lower risk of breast cancer, possibly because fiber is essential to the process that removes estrogen from the body. Other reasons to focus on fiber are to prevent constipation and hemorrhoids (incentive enough, really) and to lower the risk of colon cancer, heart disease, and many other medical conditions.

Along with claims about intermittent fasting, some people promote a keto diet to "optimize" hormones, or even a combination of both keto and intermittent fasting. There is no data to support their assertions. If you like either of those dietary approaches and they don't lead you to disordered eating, they are fine—they're just no menstrual miracle.

Some functional medicine doctors and functional nutritionists promote wearing a continuous glucose monitor to track or improve diet in pursuit of resolving menstrual issues. These devices are meant for people with diabetes, and although they are very useful for monitoring that disease, if you don't have diabetes, you will gain nothing by learning that your blood sugar normally goes up after eating a meal and then comes back down. A study among people who didn't have diabetes showed that 96 percent of the time their blood sugar levels were normal, and when they weren't, the likely reason was often a false reading. If you don't have diabetes, continuous glucose monitoring will not contribute to your menstrual health, but it will cost you a fair bit of money and could lead you to enjoy food less or even develop disordered eating.

It is important to know if you have diabetes or metabolic syndrome (a cluster of risk factors that increases the risk of cardiovascular disease, one of which is an elevated blood glucose level while fasting), as these conditions have implications for your heart health. You do not need a continuous glucose monitor for this purpose. There are a variety of different screening guidelines, but in general, every year for adults forty-five years or older, and anyone younger with risk factors for diabetes, is recommended. The test can be of fasting plasma glucose level, glucose tolerance (you drink 75 g of glucose and have your blood glucose tested two hours later), or HbA1c level, which reflects your average blood sugar over the past three months. Some risk factors that should prompt testing in people under the age of forty-five are a waist circumference of 89 cm (35 inches) or more, a diagnosis of polycystic ovarian syndrome, a history of gestational diabetes, high blood pressure, or a family history of diabetes.

Physical Fitness

Extreme athletics can have a negative impact on the menstrual cycle and this effect is discussed in Chapter 17, but what about the reverse—can the menstrual cycle affect athletic ability? Is there an ideal time to train? Is there a better phase of the menstrual cycle for cardio or lifting weights or should you even avoid those activities during certain times of the cycle? When considering these questions, it's important not to get tripped up by older, patriarchal messaging that women are less physically capable during menstruation. In 2019, Stephanie Rothstein Bruce won the USATF Half Marathon Championships in Pittsburgh with a time of 1:10:44 the day after her period started. According to *Runner's World*, that was a new personal best for her. We don't all need to be breaking personal bests on cycle day 2, but we do need to be careful how we think about limits.

But what about a workout geared toward maximizing the impact of the cyclic changes of estrogen and progesterone on things like flexibility and muscle recovery? Some adjustments are intuitive. For example, if for two days before your period you have severe breast pain, that might not be the best time for you to focus on upper body work or activities that make you bounce up and down (sports bras can provide only so much compression). If you have period diarrhea, you may not feel up to a long run outside where accessing a bathroom might be challenging. However, missing an arm workout or a distance run once a month because it's poorly timed with your menstrual cycle likely has fewer consequences for those of us who are not professional athletes.

According to Dr. Alyssa Olenick, who has a PhD in exercise physiology, the literature is mixed on how the menstrual cycle affects training. She told me there may be a slight decline in performance in "the last few days of the luteal phase or the first few days of the menstrual cycle." But the most important thing for non-elite athletes is "adequate nutrition and a good program," meaning something you can do and stick with. If you feel better during different phases of your cycle, go for it; if you don't, then don't. Dr. Olenick also told me, "It's perfectly safe and fine to lift and do cardio at any point" in your cycle. Basically, listen to your body. And you may need a few extra calories, 50–200, during your luteal phase to match the change in energy use. I recommend following Dr. Olenick on Instagram, as she has a lot of great content and often debunks disinformation about exercise and the menstrual cycle. You can find her at @doclyssfitness.

It could potentially provide a psychological advantage to believe that your training program is superior because you are incorporating exercises that have been specially tuned to your menstrual cycle. It is possible that elite athletes might see results with these programs; for them, a 1 percent change might be the difference between Olympic gold and tenth place. But for me (and most of you reading this book), with my ten-minute mile and my weight routine (of which I am quite proud, by the way), not so much. The theories are interesting, and maybe we will see more data on them. Meanwhile, if you feel that some workouts are better at certain times in your cycle, then adjust your routine to account for that. Listening to your body is always a good idea.

Emotional Stress

The topic of emotional stress requires the strictest science; otherwise, what we think we know can easily be contaminated by the stench of patriarchy. For example, during medical school, I often heard different variations of this medical truism: "The stress of an exam can make you skip a period." But the exam might easily be replaced with a breakup or international travel or a few nights of insomnia. This often felt like the "nervous woman" trope, meaning women are too high-strung and you, little lady, are too type A. Calm down and your cycles will get regular.

The interactions between stress and the menstrual cycle are complex. There is data to suggest that extreme stressors can suppress GnRH and pituitary hormones, potentially affecting the development of follicles and hence the menstrual cycle. But how much stress? Obviously, we must be able to tolerate some. Imagine the stress of being the first group of people ever exposed to −20°C (−4°F) and having to figure out how to live in that environment—and yet the brain and ovaries did not perform the biochemical equivalent of "Nope"!

Emotional and physical stressors are a large part of the human experience, so we must be able to withstand some without the ovaries packing up shop. But on the flip side, we know that high levels of stress increase the risk of a premature delivery and other poor pregnancy outcomes, meaning limiting pregnancy during times of high stress may be beneficial for optimizing reproductive success. The biological mechanisms for an impact on the menstrual cycle are certainly in place, as stress produces hormonal and inflammatory changes that can affect the hypothalamus.

So how much stress does it take to impact the menstrual cycle?

Answering this question is harder than you might think. First, it probably isn't ethical to expose people to massive amounts of stress to see who is negatively impacted. There are also historical and environmental factors, such as childhood trauma, that make some individuals more vulnerable to stress, and genetics may play a role. In addition, stressors are sometimes associated with food shortages, which can affect menstruation. And let's be real: during times of great stress, who is going to go to the trouble of recording their cycle and what they eat in real time? On the other hand, looking back at a time of stress, say, six months ago, is subject to recall bias and may not be accurate.

People who tracked their menstrual cycle via the app Natural Cycles before and after the start of the COVID-19 pandemic provided an opportunity for researchers to look at the effect on menstrual cycles of the stress of a global pandemic. The study compared the menstrual cycle experience of over eighteen thousand people, 45 percent of whom reported pandemic stress. There was no link between experiencing stress and menstrual cycle irregularity, not even for the subset of people who reported the most stress. Studies using data from menstrual apps are great because the data is recorded in real time, so there is no misremembering when you had your period, and large amounts of data can be collected. The downside is they may not reflect the general population. For example, in this study, users were more likely to be over thirty, White, and college-educated, so as a group they may have had other resources to cope with pandemic-related stress.

Menstrual cycle regularity might also not tell the full story. The Menstruation and Ovulation Study 2 (MOS2) followed 125 women ages nineteen to thirty-five with regular menstrual cycles during 2020 and 2021 (the first two years of the COVID pandemic). This study obtained more in-depth data than the Natural Cycles study, as there were questionnaires about how the women were living their lives, their basal temperature recordings, and even their hormone levels. In addition, researchers could compare these women with those in a similar, pre-pandemic study called the Menstruation and Ovulation Study (MOS). While the length of the menstrual cycle and menstrual flow were the same pre-pandemic and mid-pandemic, during the pandemic 63 percent of women had subtle changes in ovulation picked up only by the hormone testing, compared with 10 percent pre-pandemic. Unsurprisingly, those who recorded more stress, depression, anxiety, and sleep disturbances were more likely to have these subtle changes. The long-term implications of these hormonal disturbances that didn't change the menstrual cycle length or flow aren't yet known.

Another study evaluated the impact of COVID-19 on the menstrual cycle among health care workers, and it did find an association with menstrual irregularity, but that study asked people to remember their menstruation, so it may or may not be a true impact. It is also possible that health care workers had much greater levels of stress, especially at the start of the pandemic, when we had few good therapies for COVID-19, no vaccines, and trailers doubling as makeshift morgues in hospital parking lots.

What about stressful situations that are more personal than a pandemic? A study from the 1990s evaluated workplace stress and menstrual function. Its participants not only reported whether they felt stressed or not, but their menstrual cycle data was recorded in real time and urine samples were collected so ovulation could be determined. The findings? Workplace stress was associated with a shorter menstrual cycle—every twenty-one or twenty-two days—but not with an irregular or longer cycle. This result doesn't surprise me; anecdotally, I've witnessed a big impact from a toxic work environment. Sometimes I see people struggling with a medical condition despite maximal therapy, and when they visit me for a follow-up later, their recovery is simply amazing. When I ask, "What happened?" I often hear "I quit my toxic job." Several studies have also linked intimate partner violence with menstrual irregularities, and I have seen the same medical improvement after people leave harmful relationships.

The impact of stress on the menstrual cycle has been evaluated in the context of war, and the most common finding was periods stopping temporarily, but the conclusion was that it was related to malnutrition. One study found that women who had been able to flee a war zone early were less likely to experience irregularity during that time of stress than those who could not escape the conflict. Again, this relies on remembering cycles, which is prone to recall bias.

Exposure to toxic stress as a child can have profound physical effects later. These adverse childhood experiences (ACEs) are is something we are actively learning more about. ACEs include traumatic childhood events such as sexual abuse, physical abuse, witnessing intimate partner violence, and parental substance abuse. Researchers believe that chronic activation of the stress response system in childhood produces lasting changes in the brain. There is data that links exposure to four or more ACEs with increased rates of heart disease and diabetes, and some research also links multiple childhood ACES with a higher rate of skipped periods, infertility, and earlier menopause. It's possible that people who have experienced ACEs might be more vulnerable later in life to the impacts of stress on the menstrual cycle, basically lowering the threshold at which stress might have an effect.

Depression is linked with menstrual cycle irregularities, possibly due to changes in neurotransmitters or inflammation; in situations of high stress, people who develop depression or have underlying depression may be more vulnerable to cycle irregularity.

The take-home message here is that stress does have an impact on the menstrual cycle, but a noticeable effect usually requires big stressors or stress that persists. We are all unique and may have different thresholds before stress affects our cycle.

Sleep

Some women report disturbed sleep at the end of their luteal phase or during menstruation, and there are chemical reasons for this. Estrogen and progesterone receptors in certain areas of the brain are involved with sleep, and progesterone can be sedating. In addition, surges of luteinizing hormone from the brain are linked with sleep at certain times of the menstrual cycle and during puberty. It's important to keep in mind that there are cycle-related factors other than hormonal fluctuations that may impact sleep. For example, if you are extremely bloated from PMS, you have terrible menstrual cramps, or your breasts are painfully tender, your sleep may suffer that night.

The studies on sleep and the menstrual cycle are small (it isn't easy to get funds and enough people to sleep in a sleep lab every other night for their entire menstrual cycle so changes can be monitored), but there may be small changes in some of the phases of sleep architecture over the course of the menstrual cycle. For example, there is a decrease in REM sleep (the stage where your eyes are darting around) during the luteal phase. Some data suggests that sleep apnea may be worse during the late luteal phase, so if you are getting tested for this condition, menstrual cycle timing might be something to discuss with your health care provider. And as people get closer to menopause, there is a trend toward waking up more at night, which is often driven by hot flashes.

In objective studies where women who report poor sleep during menstruation are hooked up to equipment that monitors sleep, no change in sleep quality is detected. We don't always accurately assess our sleep quality, which may be one reason for the discrepancy. It's also possible that people feel fatigued or not themselves because of premenstrual symptoms and blame their fatigue on lack of sleep, when it is really driven by hormonal fluctuations. I know if I feel unwell, I often wonder if it is due to a poor night's sleep, but frequently there are other factors.

What about the impact of disrupted sleep on the menstrual cycle? People who consistently sleep less than six hours a night are more likely to have abnormally short or long menstrual cycles, and teens who get five hours of sleep a night or less are more likely to have irregular cycles. People who work night shifts, which are associated with disrupted sleep, have a slightly (about 15 percent) higher risk of shorter or longer menstrual cycles.

Bowel Issues

As discussed in the introduction, menstrual diarrhea is a thing. It affects about 12 percent of people who menstruate and is likely due to prostaglandins. It can be treated with NSAIDs or hormonal contraception. Conversely, some people report constipation, often in the early luteal phase, right after ovulation. The theory here is that high levels of progesterone slow the bowel, as progesterone can act like a muscle relaxant. There are so many potential permutations and combinations of hormonal changes, coupled with each person's individual genetics.

People with irritable bowel syndrome (about 12 percent of the population) often report a worsening of their symptoms, such as abdominal pain and bloating, or worsening of their bowel patterns (constipation or diarrhea) with menstruation. One study measured the sensitivity of the rectum to pressure in different phases of the menstrual cycle for those with IBS and those without (this is done with a balloon inserted rectally) and found that during menstruation, people with IBS had a significant increase in sensitivity, meaning they felt more pain than at other times of the menstrual cycle. This finding suggests that the hormonal changes associated with menstruation might amplify pain signals for those with IBS.

Headaches

Fluctuations in estrogen levels can trigger menstrual migraines, meaning headaches that occur within two days before or two days after the first day of bleeding. These are slightly different from menstrually related migraines, which occur in proximity with menstruation but can also happen at any other time during the cycle, not exclusively in conjunction with bleeding. Whether these are two distinct medical conditions or one condition on a spectrum isn't known. With menstrually related migraines, the headaches must be temporarily linked with menstruation two out of every three cycles. Menstrual and menstrually related migraines are frequently reported as more severe than migraines that have no association with the menstrual cycle. This is another excuse for women to be falsely labeled as weak or hysterical.

Women are about three times more likely than men to develop migraines, so biology clearly has a role. The fact that a woman's risk of developing migraines starts to increase with the first period and decreases with menopause indicates that estrogen plays a key role in this phenomenon. There are a variety of mechanisms by which estrogen can trigger migraines, as it modulates pain pathways, amplifying pain signals (essentially turning up the pain volume), and may also affect blood vessels in the brain. The prevailing theory is that it isn't hormone levels themselves that are the trigger, but rather the fluctuations. This hypothesis is supported by the fact that estrogen-containing birth control pills, which prevent fluctuations in estrogen levels, can be an effective therapy for menstrual migraines.

One important factor with migraines is whether they're associated with auras, as this can affect the choices for therapy. Auras are neurological symptoms, such as zigzag lines, flashing lights, or extreme dizziness, that can accompany migraines. It is believed they represent spasms in the blood vessels in the brain; importantly, they are associated with an increased risk of stroke. For this reason, someone with auras should not use estrogen-containing contraception (ECC), as it raises their risk of stroke by six- to sevenfold.

In addition to all the standard therapies for migraines, people with menstrual migraines or menstrually associated migraines without aura can try ECC (the pill, the ring, or the patch). These medications provide a consistent level of estrogen, especially when taken continuously, with no placebo week, preventing the fluctuations that trigger migraines. For someone with auras, the birth control pill without estrogen is an option and will prevent big fluctuations in estrogen; however, there is some estrogen production and hence withdrawal each cycle. Whether it is enough to trigger migraines isn't known. It would not be wrong to give it a try for two to three cycles to see whether it works for you. For someone who is suffering with menstrual migraines and who has auras, and for whom nonhormonal medications have failed, it may be acceptable to try ECC after a full discussion of the risks. A consultation with a headache specialist is indicated in this situation.

Immune System

Pregnancy requires widespread changes to the immune system. Parts of it must be suppressed to permit a fetus to grow, but parts of it must be active to help control the invasion of the placenta. Overall, for people with ovaries, the balance is toward immune system overactivity. Consequently, women have a higher rate of autoimmune diseases, such as systemic lupus erythematosus (SLE), rheumatoid arthritis, and multiple sclerosis (MS). The risk of auto-immune conditions is three times higher for women; for MS, it is fifteen times higher. However, women have a lower risk of cancer than men. Basically, the immune system has more opportunity to attack itself, which we see in both the increase in autoimmune diseases and the destruction of early cancer cells.

Some of the immune system vigilance is hardwired into the X chromo-somes, but some is due to the significant impact of estrogen. Estrogen stimulates the immune system, whereas progesterone and androgens (such as testosterone) are inhibitory. Consequently, there is a jump in autoimmune conditions around puberty, and many people report worsening of these con-ditions at certain phases of the menstrual cycle. In addition, there are reports of trans women developing autoimmune conditions when they start taking estrogen during their transition. This information should not be used to advocate against transitioning—by that logic, we should give everyone with two X chromosomes puberty blockers to prevent the increase in autoimmune conditions with puberty. But the link is important for trans people to know about, so they can advocate for testing should they develop symptoms that might be suggestive of autoimmune conditions. More long-term data is needed.

Many medical conditions are in turn associated with irregular menstrual cycles, greater risk of infertility, and primary ovarian insufficiency. For example, almost 50 percent of women with SLE have less frequent periods than expected.

There is mounting evidence that the human immune system has become hypervigilant over the past hundred or so years because it is no longer occu-pied with the infectious burden of intestinal parasites and other infections. Remember, it evolved to protect us tens of thousands of years ago, when our bodies were exposed to much greater immune challenges. One of the great advances of the past few hundred years is that more and more people are living parasite-free lives. But those who have an immune system that is more easily revved up—meaning those who menstruate—may be paying a greater price.

Epilepsy

People with epilepsy are more likely to report irregular menstrual cycles. The main theory is that abnormal electrical activity in the brain affects the release of gonadotropin-releasing hormone (GnRH). Knowing this connection, it's still important to rule out other causes of irregular menstrual bleeding. In addition, some medications used for epilepsy can affect hormonal contraception and cause irregular bleeding, and can also potentially impact their effectiveness at preventing pregnancy, so it's especially important to tell the doctor prescribing medications for your epilepsy about your method of contraception. The medical provider prescribing your contraception should also know about your medications for epilepsy.

I Think I Notice Menstrual Cycle Fluctuations . . . What Now?

There are many symptoms that can vary with the menstrual cycle. If you wonder whether that's happening to you, consider tracking your symptoms with a calendar over at least three cycles. Discuss the variations in symptoms with your health care provider. This may be your gynecologist, but it could be another doctor. For example, if you have diabetes and your blood sugar is higher in one part of your cycle, you want to discuss that with your endocrinologist; if it's a change in bowel function, talk to your gastroenterologist.

If you pinpoint a menstrual cycle fluctuation in a condition, you may need to increase and decrease the therapy for that condition over the different phases of your cycle (if possible). Another potential option is a trial of eliminating ovulation with hormonal contraception. If the chosen method doesn't work, you can always stop, but you probably need at least a three-cycle trial to assess the contraception's efficacy on your symptoms.

Here's an example I see often: vulvar and/or vaginal itching that is worse right and during before menstruation. It could be related to changes in hormones, which can in turn impact itch or colonization with yeast; changes in inflammatory chemicals; or there may be other hormonal or nonhormonal explanations. For instance, the friction of menstrual pads might be the issue. One option in this situation is to preemptively increase the topical medication for treating itch a day or two before itching is expected to start, which often helps reduce or eliminate the flare. Another is to try continuous birth control pills, taken in such a way that there is no menstruation.

Bottom Line

- Hormonal fluctuations can produce widespread effects in the body, and changes in functioning or flares of medical conditions can be related to the changing hormones of the menstrual cycle.
- A healthy diet for the body is a healthy diet for menstruation. There is no diet to "optimize" hormones.
- Workplace stress, food scarcity, ACEs, and the stress of intimate partner violence can affect the menstrual cycle.
- Menstrual migraines and menstrually related migraines are believed to be due to the drop in estrogen at the end of the luteal phase.
- Having two X chromosomes and being exposed to estrogen both increase the risk of developing autoimmune conditions.

11

Menstrual Tracking

In the last few years, along with the creation of an app for just about everything, there has been what feels like an explosion of people tracking their
cycles with menstrual apps, and not for just a few cycles. These apps have
over 500 million downloads and more than 50 million users worldwide,
and even the newest version of the Apple Watch heavily promotes the menstrual tracking component. The popularity is undeniable. The availability
of these products suggests that menstruation is being taken seriously as a
biological process deserving of attention and care, but it's also part of a bigger
pattern of individuals gathering personal health data (how they sleep,
what they eat, how many steps they take, etc.) to improve functioning, a
phenomenon referred to as "the quantified self." It's important to remember,
though, that part of the reason for this menstrual app explosion is that there
is money to be made.

At their core, menstrual apps are high-tech versions of the cards we used
to hand out in the office with three calendar months and space to document
days of bleeding or spotting—when I trained, doctors often had branded
ones made up for their practice. Many apps allow the user to track other
menstrual-related symptoms, such as headache or bloating. Some also provide an algorithm and allow for input of biometric data, like temperature or
hormone levels in the urine, to predict fertile days; hence, some people use
them as tools for fertility awareness, either as contraception or as a way to know

their most fertile time, to increase their chance of conception. Here we'll cover the use of menstrual tracking apps in general. See Chapter 29 for their use as contraception.

The Benefits of Menstrual Tracking

Cycle tracking is of value for people with menstrual concerns. If you think your periods have been coming closer together or are spacing out, or are irregular, or are heavy, or you are having symptoms that you think might be related to menstruation, such as headaches or menstrual cramps, then three cycles of data will almost certainly help you communicate what's happening to your health care provider.

Here are a few examples:

- Sumara sits in my office with her phone. She has been feeling bloated and moody. When we discussed these symptoms several months ago, I asked her to track them for three cycles to see if they fluctuated in relation to menstruation. We look at the data, and it seems clear that her symptoms start around day 20 or 21 each month, about a week after she ovulates, and they resolve by the second day of bleeding. This information helps us determine that Sumara has premenstrual syndrome and allows us to decide on the best evidence-based therapy (see Chapter 9 for more on PMS).
- Jane's periods have been irregular, but on her first visit she couldn't remember the pattern—asking people to tuck away ninety or so days of bleeding data in their brain, to be recalled on a moment's notice when their OB/GYN wants it, isn't practical. But now that she has three months of menstrual data to share from her period tracker, it seems that she is bleeding every twenty-six to twenty-eight days, meaning her cycle is regular, but she's also bleeding for one or two days randomly mid-cycle (irregular spotting). This helps me come up with a better plan for investigating her abnormal bleeding pattern.
- Yumi has vulvar itching, and it has only partially improved with topical steroids. She isn't sure if it's related to her menstrual cycle or not. Hormonal fluctuations can affect how itchy some people feel, but the friction of menstrual pads can also be a factor, and

Yumi wears pads. I suggested she track her cycle for one or two cycles so we could see if her itch starts before her flow or once she starts wearing pads. With the data in hand, it's clear that her itch starts before her flow. We discuss using hormonal contraception in a continuous way, so she doesn't get a period, and that is the missing piece to her itch puzzle.

If you don't have any medical concerns, your cycle seems regular to you, and you are not interested in knowing when you are most fertile, then these apps are unlikely to be medically helpful. Medical concerns aside, though, some people like the idea of having a historical record of their cycle or being more aware of their cycle, for a variety of reasons, from making sure they have menstrual products on hand to booking a vacation that doesn't coincide with menstruation, to being able to look at the data from an app and think, "Oh, that's why I'm feeling crummy: my period is due tomorrow." For some, this kind of cycle awareness is reassuring and even empowering. For others, however, it may be anxiety-provoking over-monitoring. Data from sleep trackers shows that those apps can lead to both anxiety and hypervigilance about sleep—which, paradoxically, can negatively affect sleep. We don't have much data about the negative effects of cycle tracking, but one study tells us that, when their period comes at a different time than the app predicts, some people blame their body for the difference when it's often the app that has calculated incorrectly, meaning some apps may actually make you less in tune with your body.

Privacy Concerns: The Dark Side of Fertility Apps

Whether an app advertises that it can be used to track symptoms and bleeding to maximize chances of pregnancy or as a form of contraception, the business model is almost always the same: selling your private data. Just as for a pharmaceutical company, *you* are the source of income. While some apps are subscription-based, meaning you pay to download and use them, selling data is typically more profitable than charging $5 a month. And paying for an app doesn't necessarily mean it isn't also selling your data.

I remind my kids and myself of this all the time: no free app is free, and with an app that monitors health, especially one that tracks your period, that data is a level up, from a privacy perspective.

It's true that apps' collecting and sharing data can be helpful. There are excellent research papers that look at large volumes of data, some which I have used as references in writing this book. It's not otherwise possible to get so much information about so many menstrual cycles from so many people. Many users are pleased to contribute in this way, but the key is knowing in advance how your data might be used. If privacy matters to you (and we'll discuss why it might) but participating in research does too, then you might want to learn whether you can opt out of data collection for profit but into data collection for research.

The money in apps comes from selling your information to data brokers, who use your data to create user profiles—for example, "high earning, period tracking, gym user" or "student, period tracking, vegan." There is a frightening report from Apple called "A Day in the Life of Your Data," and it's well worth a read. Many apps don't just collect data about what you might have liked or looked at, they also troll through your device. Here is an excerpt from the Apple report that follows a fictitious father and daughter going to the playground and describes what happens to their data along the way:

> Later, at the playground, John and Emma take a selfie. They play with a photo filter app, settling on adding bunny ears to the photo. The filtering app, however, is able to access all the photos on the device and the attached metadata, rather than only the playground selfie. John posts the picture on a social media app. The app links John's current online activity to a trove of data collected by other apps, such as his demographic information and purchasing habits, using an email address, a phone number or an advertising identifier.

Data brokers know where you live, what you like to eat, where you like to go. And when menstrual data is added to that treasure trove, they know when you may or may not be pregnant. One result might be annoying advertisements for an unstudied and unregulated herbal supplement that falsely claims the ability to regulate hormone levels, and these ads might follow you from Facebook to the next article you read online to Instagram. But it can be a lot more sinister, because it's not that challenging to figure out from the raw data who belongs to what information profile. Apparently, given fifteen pieces of deidentified data, almost 99.98 percent of people can be identified. The Catholic news outlet The Pillar reported that they used "commercially available records of app signal data" from a data vendor to show that a priest had used Grindr and visited gay bars, which lead to his resignation from an executive position. It's abhorrent that data could be used in this way, and this should serve as a cautionary tale about the amount and the specifics of personal data that is available for sale.

Menstrual data could potentially be sold to law enforcement, and in the United States, this is a real concern now that many states are designating life as beginning at fertilization and making abortion illegal. Should you be in one of those states and have a clandestine abortion—or even if you have a miscarriage but someone thinks you had a clandestine abortion—data from your app could be subpoenaed to build a case against you. If you visited a clinic that does abortions or a pharmacy or a store that sells herbs, that data can all be retrieved. Remember, lots of apps track your location, whether it's obvious (a weather app or Google Maps) or not so obvious (many others). This isn't a theoretical dystopian future. In 2022 Vice reported that a company called SafeGraph was gathering data that indicated whether a user had visited Planned Parenthood. The cost of a week's worth of data for visits to the more than six hundred Planned Parenthood locations in the United States? Just over $160.

I can think of other ways period tracking data could be used against people. In many places it's illegal to ask someone if they are pregnant at a job interview, but data purchased from an app could provide that information or make it clear that someone is trying to conceive, if they've visited fertility clinics.

If privacy is a concern for you, here are some questions to ask about any menstrual tracking app you are considering:

- *Does the app use third-party trackers?* This allows the collection and sharing of potentially sensitive data. The privacy policy should tell you if the app tracks data and how they share it, but these documents can be long and confusing, policies can change, and an option for opting out of data sharing isn't always easy. In addition, consumers have previously been misled by these policies. Case in point, Flo Health promised to keep data private. Yet, they have settled allegations with the U.S. Federal Trade Commission for sharing "sensitive health data from millions of users of its Flo Period & Ovulation Tracker app with marketing and analytics firms" and "did not limit how third parties could use this health data." I encourage anyone who uses these apps to read more about privacy. Good sources are Consumer Reports, Mozilla, and The Norwegian

Consumer Council (just put one of their names and "period tracking apps" into your browser).

- *Is the app based in Europe?* Digital privacy protection laws are stronger there, but that doesn't stop an app from selling data. However, when it comes to a subpoena from a government looking to charge you with a clandestine abortion, the app's being based in another country may offer you more protection.
- *Does your data stay on the phone or go to the cloud?* Data that stays on your phone may be safer, although if law enforcement gets your phone and can open your app, they can get to the data. In 2022 *Consumer Reports* recommended the apps Drip, Euki, and Periodical as the safest from a privacy perspective, because at the time of their reporting, all the data stayed on your phone. In addition, none of these three apps track data.

The Other Dark Side of Apps: The Info That Comes Along for the Ride

Many apps provide health information embedded in the app or on their websites, and there is a wide variation in accuracy. In one study, almost half of the apps provided information about how the day of conception could impact the sex of the baby (reader, you may be shocked to learn that the day of ejaculation doesn't affect whether a sperm with an X chromosome or one with a Y chromosome is the one to run the gauntlet). I've read medical disinformation on several websites that support period tracking apps, and I've also read good information. But how does the consumer tell the difference between bad and good information when an app they trust presents both as equal? Once you've decided to trust an app with your health data, especially one to help you get or avoid being pregnant, you are probably more likely to believe the information it provides. After all, we know that when an app incorrectly predicts the date of the next period, many people blame their bodies rather than questioning the accuracy of the app.

For example, on menstrual apps or their associated Instagram accounts, I found claims that there is a post-pill polycystic ovarian syndrome (there isn't) and that hypothalamic amenorrhea can be treated with the herbal medicine ashwagandha (no quality data to support this), and that "seed cycling" might be a valid thing to try. "Seed cycling"—eating different types of seeds at different points in your menstrual cycle to "optimize" your cycle— is best described as a spell rejected from a second-rate magic compendium. And that raises another issue. When I read disinformation on a site that supports a menstrual app, it makes me wonder . . . if pseudoscience creeps into their content, does it also creep into the algorithms they use to predict fertility?

It's best to think of a menstrual app in the same way you think about a pharmaceutical company. Just use the product and then get your health information from unbiased sources that aren't invested in your choosing one specific product. After all, you wouldn't get medical information about gynecological conditions from the makers of a birth control pill. And be wary of content written or checked by naturopaths; I would personally double-check that information.

Some apps offer religious information, or barely veiled religious information, so that might also be a consideration for some people.

How Well Do Apps Work?

When choosing an app, consider why you want to track your cycles. For example, do you want an app that can tell you your fertile window, to help prevent pregnancy, or one that makes it easy to look back and see whether your period really has been irregular? If you are interested in finding your fertile window, either to maximize or to minimize your chance of conception, the performance of the app matters a lot more than if you are simply collecting data. Apps that specifically offer themselves as contraception by supplementing an existing fertility awareness method are addressed in Chapter 29.

How well do these apps do at predicting the start of the next cycle and/or the fertile window? As it turns out, many perform very poorly. Even worse, because their calculations are often proprietary, rigorous evaluation is challenging. Researchers can assess their performance only by looking at the tools and information they provide, by creating fictional patients or by entering historical data from real people into the app to see how well it does.

One 2016 study, published in the *Journal of the American Board of Family Medicine*, found that twenty-four of thirty apps incorrectly predicted the window of fertility—that's an appalling 72 percent failure rate. Another paper found that the apps studied incorrectly predicted the onset of the next cycle about 20 percent of the time.

One group of researchers created menstrual profiles for five fictional women and entered data over six cycles into ten period tracking apps. The apps all did well for the fictional patient with a regular twenty-eight-day cycle, but for the more irregular cycles, they frequently predicted ovulation earlier than expected. Another study looked at twenty free websites and thirty-three apps that claimed to be able to predict the fertile window to maximize the chance of conception; overall, the websites and apps correctly identified only 75 percent of the fertile days. Yet another study showed that 22 percent of apps had inaccuracies in content, the tools they used to predict the menstrual cycle, or both.

To sum up, if you are depending on an app as a predictive tool, choosing a quality app may be harder than you think. And if your period comes on a day other than the one your app predicted, there's a decent chance that the app was incorrect.

Bottom Line

- Menstrual tracking apps have become a big business.
- When you have a menstrual or a menstrual-related concern, tracking your cycles for three months can be helpful, but the only real benefit apps offer over a pen and paper is convenience.
- Data from apps, including menstrual data, can be purchased from brokers, which could have serious ramifications for some people.
- Some apps promote medical misinformation and even disinformation, so look at your app as a tool, not as a source of health information.
- Many apps have performance issues. If your period comes at a different time than the app predicted, there is a good chance the app is incorrect.

12

The History and Safety of Menstrual Products

Before we go any further, let's get on the same page regarding terminology. They are not "feminine hygiene" products because:

- Needing them is not a sign of being feminine; it's a sign that you need something to catch blood.
- They're not hygiene products because menstruating is not unhygienic.

They are menstrual products. And they're essential. And please, to any store that sells menstrual products: if you are still labeling them "feminine hygiene," spend the money for a new sign. Really. It will be a small cost for you, and people who menstruate will almost certainly look more favorably upon your store, which I imagine might be good for business—never mind that it's the right thing to do.

The enduring stigma surrounding menstrual products is something to behold, and not a good something! I'm amazed that even now, in the time of COVID, people will keep a box of tissues on their desk and think nothing of someone walking by, grabbing one, and blowing their nose. Snot is coming out onto the tissue in public. Sure, we can't usually see it, but we know it's there, and snot and the respiratory droplets that come with it can spread illness. ICK! Yet somehow this behavior is socially acceptable, while at the same time people often feel they need to perform magic tricks to hide a pad or tampon while walking to the restroom to take care of "business."

Without menstrual products, children, teens, and adults who menstruate are forced to socially isolate during menstruation, or risk going out and soaking their clothes. Period-related social isolation can affect schooling, the ability to support oneself financially, and even health. Access to menstrual products is, unfortunately, not universal, and period poverty—not being able to afford the needed menstrual products—is a real concern worldwide. In one survey, 60 percent of people said they needed to budget to afford menstrual products.

Menstrual products are also a big business. In the United States alone, the industry generates $3 billion per year. (You'd think with that kind of buying power, secrecy would be a thing of the past. But, hey, patriarchy.) It's absurd that 50 percent of the population should pay to menstruate while 100 percent of the population benefits from menstruation. To make it even worse, in many U.S. states, and in many other countries, menstrual products are taxed. Why should capitalism get all that sweet menstrual cash? The government wants in on the action.

And what action it is! Until recently, some states and countries taxed menstrual products as luxury items, on par with alcohol and tobacco, as if not bleeding onto your clothes was a luxury. In New York State, the revenue from taxing menstrual products was an estimated $14 million a year before the state stopped enforcing the law. Yes, $14 million was generated by half the population—the half more likely to live in poverty. The tax, and the cost of menstrual products overall, is a disproportionate extra burden for those who are struggling financially.

In the U.K., the average cost of menstrual products is about £10 (about US$12.50) per month. In the United States, the average is $13.25 a month; over a typical menstrual lifetime, that amounts to $6,360. Many people need that $13.25 a month for other expenses. Given the income inequality between women and men, if, instead of paying for menstrual products starting at age twelve, teens had been able to put that money each month into a U.S. Treasury account that generated 2 percent a year, they would have about $9,955 in that account at the age of fifty-two, the average age of menopause. If they found a corporate bond fund (slightly riskier) that generated 4 percent, they would have $15,872, and if they invested it in the S&P 500, which generates about 7.45 percent growth (on average over the last twenty years), they would have $38,482.

If anyone doesn't think that's a big deal, then I propose we start taxing those who *don't* menstruate each month, starting at the age of twelve, to level the playing field. The months where payment is late or missed will result in random spraying of red fluid on the seat of their pants to demonstrate the impact, inconvenience, and embarrassment of not having access to menstrual products because of the expense. And, of course, the added hassle and expense of laundry and dry cleaning should also be experienced.

Or, you know, we could just abolish menstrual taxes and then work to make products free.

Not all countries have a menstrual product tax. Kenya was the first to abolish a tax on menstrual products, in 2004. There is now no menstrual product tax in many countries, including Canada, Mauritius, Colombia, India, Rwanda, the Republic of Ireland, and the United Kingdom.

In the United States, menstrual products are at least now covered under flexible spending accounts (FSAs) and health savings accounts (HSAs), where you can set aside pre-tax money for medical expenses. Until we get to the point of free products, I believe schools, government buildings, and all office buildings should provide free menstrual products, just as they have free toilet paper and soap. Those who disagree apparently think people are going to run around stockpiling menstrual products, yet they never raise the same argument about toilet paper.

If you want to do your bit to fight against the system that forces people who menstruate to feel shame and pay more for the very biological machinery that gave you life, please call your local representatives and insist on changing the law if you have a tax in your area. Also push for legislation to make menstrual products available without cost in government buildings and all schools, and consider putting menstrual products out in the open in the bathroom in your home.

The History of Menstrual Products

What did people use before menstrual products were available commercially? The truth is, we know very little about this, likely because it didn't interest the men who documented most of world history. Or perhaps they didn't mention menstrual products because of modesty or because menstrual blood was linked with disease and, hence, was a topic to be avoided. Even texts written by midwives before the 1800s make no mention of how women managed menstruation. Given how detailed some of these texts are about diseases and body parts—for example, describing the length of a typical "man's yard" (aka penis)—it's unlikely that modesty was the reason. I wonder if they just assumed everyone knew what to do. The midwives didn't explain how to wipe after going to the bathroom either, so maybe the mechanics of menstrual care was considered common knowledge.

Even when women did write about their personal affairs, the practical management of menstruation is conspicuously absent. They used euphemisms in some cases, such as feeling "sick" or "poorly," that may have meant they were menstruating, but scholars can't be sure. In her book *Menstruation and the Female Body in Early Modern England*, Sara Read writes that housewifery manuals in the 1600s and 1700s included information on how to clean one's ears and nose, but nothing about menstruation. Dr. Laura Klosterman Kidd, in her graduate thesis "Menstrual Technology in the United States, 1854 to 1921," researched letters from pioneering women who migrated west across America, which were detailed enough to tell other women what they should pack, down to their underwear, but included no lists of menstrual provisions. Dr. Kidd also evaluated many diaries and went so far as to plot them out to see if being "sick" or "poorly" cropped up in a frequency that might suggest menstruation, but she wasn't able to come up with a connection. Such is the culture of silence. Women did not feel free to write about menstruation even in their own personal journals.

I've often wondered how early humans coped with menstruation. We can't know what our ancestors did ten thousand years ago, but we do have some information from the Hadza, a Tanzanian ethnic group who live a hunter-gatherer way of life and so don't use commercial menstrual products. Hadza girls and women use cloth and skins as reusable pads, washing themselves and the pads with soap they make from the seeds of the baobab tree. Interestingly, the length of their menstrual bleeding is less than we experience in "modern society"—two to three days—and the majority describe it as light (although the definition of *light* wasn't possible to parse out in the study). A shorter duration and lighter flow suggest that in pre-agricultural times menstruation might have been easier to handle without the aid of modern menstrual products because there was less blood.

There are reports in many cultures of ancestral women using internal products, such as cloths or grasses or even fabric wrapped around a stick, inserted vaginally as DIY tampons, but the accuracy of the reports isn't known. I spent some time going down Internet rabbit holes trying to validate some of the claims and never found a true academic reference. Were these products purely for menstruation, or were they being used medicinally? For example, the Ancient Greeks wrote about vaginal tampons made from wool soaked in fat, but there is no proof they were used like tampons as we now know them; they seem to have been medicinal.

We tend to "appeal to ancient wisdom"—in other words, to romanticize what people did or perhaps *might have done* in ancient times—in the belief that our elders knew best. If they inserted a stick wrapped in moss into the vagina, is that a practice we should resurrect? While I am fascinated by how our ancestors coped with menstruation, just because something was used historically does not mean it was safe, or even that it worked well.

Pre-1900, before menstruation was understood in the context of hormones and the endometrium, there seems to have been a cross-cultural belief that it was important for the blood to come out of the vagina, either because it was polluted and needed to be expelled for health reasons, or because it was significant for religious or cultural reasons. Sara Read points out that in England in the 1600s, sex workers used sponges inserted vaginally to absorb blood so they could keep working while menstruating, but otherwise this doesn't seem to have been common practice, meaning this was likely a risk these sex workers were obliged to take to make money to survive. It's unlikely that internal vaginal products for menstruation were common. Women used what they had on hand, tying or pinning bits of animal skin, rags, knitted sections of wool, or remnants of garments between their legs—the origin of the euphemisms "rag" and "clout." I imagine boundless creativity came into play here. Many cultures advised women to rest, so being confined to a bedroom or a hut, with no household tasks to do, might have limited soiling. However, women may also simply have bled onto their legs and clothes.

When undergarments such as shifts became fashionable, they likely served to absorb blood. One of the only descriptions of this use comes from the 1733 trial of Sarah Malcolm in England. Malcolm, a laundress, was accused of murdering three women: her eighty-year-old employer and two other servants. Her employer had been robbed and the two servants killed as a cover-up. One of the victims, Ann Price, had her neck slashed, and the other two women had been strangled. Blood on Malcolm's clothing was considered evidence of her guilt; however, Malcolm explained it was menstrual blood. In her own words:

> If it is supposed that I kill'd her with my Cloaths on, my Apron indeed
> might be bloody, but how should the Blood come upon my Shift?
> If I did it in my Shift, how should my apron be bloody, or the back
> part of my Shift? And whether I did it dress'd or undress'd, why was
> not the Neck and Sleeves of my Shift bloody as well as the lower Parts?

Malcolm claimed she was a lookout for the robbery and had no idea that the people she accused of committing the crime were going to commit murder. There was other evidence of her guilt besides blood on her clothing (she had some of the stolen articles in her possession), and ultimately she was convicted and hanged. Whether she committed murder or simply acted as the lookout is unknown. The people she accused were never tried. The case is a fascinating bit of history, though: one of the few times a woman spoke about how she managed menstruation was when she was defending her life in court.

The Dawn of Modern Menstrual Products

The first commercially produced disposable pads appeared in the late 1800s in the United States. They were named Lister's pads, a nod to Dr. Joseph Lister, who was a pioneer in surgery and introduced the concept of sterilizing surgical equipment, among other important discoveries, hence tying in the product with cleanliness and sterility. Disposable pads also appeared in the United Kingdom (Southalls' Sanitary Towels) and Germany (Hartmann's). The absorbent material was gauze, cotton wool (think cotton balls), or wood wool, which is made by breaking down wood strips with acid (it was commonly used in surgical dressings and is quite absorbent). The appearance of these pads coincides with the medical interest in hygiene, thanks to emerging knowledge about germs and the movement toward antiseptic techniques. Despite their price, disposable pads found a market in the United Kingdom and Germany, but according to *Under Wraps: A History of Menstrual Hygiene Technology*, by Sharra L. Vostral, Lister's pads did not sell well in the United

States, perhaps because they were expensive and weren't that much of an improvement on what women could fashion at home.

In the 1920s, women were working outside the home in greater numbers, and the idea that they should rest during menstruation, a long-standing medical belief, was falling by the wayside. The idea of a disposable menstrual product became more appealing. Into this modern era stepped Kimberly-Clark, with "Kotex," a portmanteau of *cotton-like texture*. Kotex was originally made from cellucotton, a wood pulp fiber that was used in surgical dressings, and the product was introduced with a savvy marketing campaign about hygiene in women's magazines. The pads were held in place by pins or menstrual belts, and the basic design did not change significantly, except perhaps for choice of absorbent material, until the 1970s.

The early forerunners of the menstrual cup and disc were made of oilskin or even noncorrosive metal (ouch!). These devices were quite large, because the doctors of the day believed women bled 120–300 ml (4–10 ounces) during menstruation (we now consider 90 ml/3 ounces to be excessive). Fortunately, they never went to market! Looking at the patents, I imagine they would have been *quite* uncomfortable. The first true menstrual cup in the United States was the Tassette, which was invented in 1937 by Leona Chalmers, an American actress. It was made of rubber, and the advertising focused on its discreet nature and the benefit of not needing cumbersome pins or belts. The Second World War brought a shortage of rubber, so production of the Tassette stopped. After the war, it was reintroduced with a marketing blitz, which included giving free samples to nurses in the hopes that a word-of-mouth campaign from trusted sources would be successful, but it never took off in a way that made it profitable.

The first tampons were produced in 1931: Wix, by Frederick Richardson, and Tampax, by Earle Cleveland Haas, who was an osteopathic physician (apparently his wife was extremely gracious in trying out his designs). As Sharra Vostral writes in *Under Wraps*, Dr. Haas's motivation was that he "just got tired of seeing women wearing those damn rags" and was trying to give them a better option. The name Tampax is a portmanteau of *tampon* and *pack*. Haas's design was unique in that the stitching allowed for the tampon to expand lengthwise, and it included a disposable plunger or applicator. In many ways, it was very similar to what we use today. The applicator was meant to prevent the need to touch the tampon prior to insertion, though fears about that posing an infection risk were, of course, unfounded. After all, it's not as if penises, fingers, and tongues are sterile, and they are inserted into vaginas. But I'm sure along the way there have been those who felt the applicator was a sensible precaution: putting fingers close to the vagina to insert a tampon might lead to mass masturbation, and hence the downfall of the patriarchy.

Kotex introduced a tampon shortly thereafter called Fibs. No, really. As in "Can I have a pack of Fibs?" Fibs was short for *fibers*, but it also played into the fact that the period was hidden and suggested that women were fibbing, possibly contributing to its failure to catch on.

The Truth about Toxic Shock Syndrome

Menstrual toxic shock syndrome, or mTSS, is a severe illness that results when the immune system responds in an aggressive and dangerous way to a toxin called TSST-1, which is made by the bacterium *Staphylococcus aureus*. Though it's often linked with tampons, the contraceptive sponge, diaphragms, and menstrual cups are also associated with mTSS. These products are used by fewer people, which creates the illusion that they are less risky; in reality, it's just that we have less data because they aren't as popular. The truth is, we don't know their risk relative to tampons.

Toxic shock syndrome can also happen when the toxin enters the blood through the skin in other ways—for example, after surgery or a burn. Both menstrual and non-menstrual TSS are serious illnesses, but fortunately they are rare. Menstrual TSS affects approximately 0.5 in 100,000 people per year, which is about the same rate as non-menstrual TSS. For women under twenty-four, the risk of mTSS is slightly higher, though still less than 2 per 100,000. Menstrual TSS occurs within four days of a period and causes fever, a dramatic drop in blood pressure, a rash that eventually peels, and even organ failure. Many people are sick enough to need intensive care, and sadly, even with aggressive modern medicine, some people die.

Proponents of "purity culture" frequently use the specter of mTSS to scare people away from vaginal menstrual products, especially tampons, so many people are surprised to learn about its rarity. I have heard more than once from people who were terrified of tampons because of mTSS and were stunned when they heard the true numbers. The risk of death from using tampons is 0.02 per 1000,000 people a year—less than the risk of dying from being struck by lightning (0.1/100,000), and much less than the risk of being killed as a pedestrian by a car (1.7/100,000 per year in the United States), yet we don't tell people they shouldn't go for walks because of lightning or cars.

Menstrual TSS was first described in 1979, and its appearance is linked with the introduction of a new tampon by Procter & Gamble called Rely. Before Rely, tampons were all cotton, cotton-rayon, or a cotton-viscose blend, and they expanded lengthwise (meaning up and down the vaginal canal). Rely had two key differences: the absorbent material was polyester foam cubes and chips with carboxymethylcellulose (a gelling agent), with a mesh covering (like a tea bag), and it expanded widthwise as well as lengthwise. The tagline was "It even absorbs the worry." I remember using one back in the day, and that sucker was so large, getting it out was like birthing a peach—a little shocking for a fourteen-year-old.

New material, greater absorbency, and a different direction of expansion meant Rely was a radical departure from previous tampon designs. Nowadays, such design changes would require studies before the U.S. Food and Drug Administration (FDA) would allow it to hit the shelves, but Rely was introduced before the FDA changed those rules. Rely was aggressively marketed, and by the late 1970s it was used by about 25 percent of American women. To compete, other tampon manufacturers added polyacrylate, a super-absorbent polymer, to their tampons to increase absorbency. And boom, mTSS was seemingly everywhere. I was a fourteen-year-old using tampons when mTSS hit the news, and to say my friends and I panicked would be to vastly underestimate the impact of these stories. Rely was pulled from the U.S. market in 1980 and cases of mTSS started to drop. Polyacrylate was removed from tampons in 1985.

Initial theories were that mTSS was all about tampon absorbency, but now we know more. *Staphylococcus aureus* is a colonizer, meaning that having it in your vagina, in your nose, and on your skin is normal and not harmful under typical circumstances—"typical" meaning you are otherwise healthy and your skin doesn't get broken, which would allow the bacteria to enter the bloodstream. About 10 percent of women of menstrual age carry *S. aureus* in their vagina, whether they use tampons or not. But it's not just having *S. aureus* that matters; you must have a strain that makes TSST-1, and only 1 percent of women carry a TSST-1-producing strain. And then the TSST-1 must get into the bloodstream, and finally, the body must mount that exaggerated immune response. But most people are protected from this response, as 60 percent of women have antibodies that can neutralize the toxin. Basically, your body has a built-in mTSS obstacle course, and it works well most of the time.

So how do vaginal products change this equation and set up a situation where mTSS can develop? First, they introduce air as they are inserted in the vagina. The oxygen and carbon dioxide impact the vaginal microbiome, favoring the growth of S. aureus and TSST-1. These products can also cause microtrauma with insertion and removal, creating a portal for TSST-1 to enter the blood. Vaginal menstrual products may also provide a place for the bacteria to grow—for example, the fibers of the tampon—and menstrual cups can potentially introduce biofilms, complex structures of bacterial colonies, which can further disrupt the vaginal microbiome.

Does absorbency play a role at all? The longer a product is inside the vagina, the more time there is for bacteria to grow and produce the toxin, and more absorbent products are typically worn longer. Using a tampon that is more absorbent than needed might also play a role, as some data shows that the greatest area of TSST-1 production on tampons is in the dry spots (interestingly, menstrual blood suppresses the growth of TSST-1-producing bacteria). It seems that absorbency is a proxy for other factors associated with TSST-1 production.

There is no evidence to support the claim that organic tampons are lower risk for mTSS. What about all-cotton tampons versus those with rayon? Although older studies indicated that cotton might produce a less-TSST-1-favorable environment than rayon, newer research that better replicates the vaginal microbiome suggests that cotton-only tampons might produce a *more* favorable environment for TSST-1. There isn't enough data for a conclusive answer either way, so until we know more, just use what you like and can afford.

Unsurprisingly, I see lots of "conventional tampons are toxic shock syndrome death sticks" on social media accounts, but I have never seen one of these influencers discuss the risks of TSS from abscesses related to skin injury from pubic hair removal. Then again, there is no organic razor to sell, or at least not yet (insert eye roll).

The bottom line is that mTSS is serious but fortunately very rare, especially considering that two-thirds of women in the United States use tampons at some point in their menstrual life. It's important to know about mTSS in the same way it's important to know about lightning strikes. Once informed, people may make different decisions based on the information about the risks and benefits of tampons or menstrual cups, and that's okay. With that in mind, here are some practical tips about menstrual product safety and TSS:

- Use the lowest-absorbency tampon that gets the job done. For people whose flow starts off quite heavy and who then have several days of light flow, a box filled with a range of absorbencies is ideal. Avoid using a large or a super plus on lighter days; this will also help reduce the microtrauma that can occur with insertion and removal into a drier vagina.
- Don't sweat cotton versus rayon; use an affordable tampon that fits your body the best.
- Change your tampon every six to eight hours (unless it soaks through more quickly). More frequent changes will introduce more oxygen and carbon dioxide and may increase trauma with insertion; less frequent changes give bacteria more time to grow.
- Don't assume menstrual cups and discs are safer, or less safe, than tampons. TSST-1-producing *S. aureus* can grow on cups, and there is some evidence that larger cups might increase risk (due to either a bigger surface area for toxin production or more air with insertion), so aim for the smallest cup or disc that suits your needs. If you can afford a larger cup for heavier days and a smaller one for lighter days, that might be an option.
- With menstrual cups, there is a concern that just rinsing between uses may not remove *S. aureus* or TSST-1. One option is to boil cups between insertions, meaning you need to have two. This is admittedly not sufficiently studied.

Menstrual Product Safety

The data on toxic shock syndrome makes it clear that regulation of menstrual products is important, but regulation varies from country to country. In the United States menstrual products are regulated as medical devices, and this is controlled by the FDA. They are registered and given clearance for marketing; they aren't approved like pharmaceuticals. A registered product is subject to manufacturing oversight, meaning the FDA can evaluate what's happening in a factory. Registration also means that complaints and adverse events must be tracked, and if there are issues, the FDA will ask the company to stop manufacturing and/or distributing the product.

Unscented and scented pads using materials previously cleared by the FDA are considered Class I devices. The manufacturer registers the product and it goes to market. Class II devices, which have a higher risk, include any product made with a material not previously cleared for use, or any device inserted vaginally. Safety studies are required when any new component or design is introduced. If everything looks good, the FDA registers the device and it can be sold. If it isn't registered, the product can't go to market. The exception is menstrual cups; they can hit the shelves without waiting for a go-ahead, but they must still submit the paperwork for registration.

The FDA doesn't require that ingredients in menstrual products be listed on the package or be available to the public via the FDA; recently, New York became the first state to require that information on packaging. Some brands listed their ingredients several years before this law went into effect, but on its own, the name of a chemical used in manufacturing doesn't tell you much, safety-wise. Formaldehyde is a concerning chemical that is associated with health risks, but our bodies make formaldehyde, and it's also found naturally in apples. Imagine if I listed the ingredients for a recipe with no information about amount—it makes a difference if there is ⅛ teaspoon, 1 tablespoon, or 1 cup of chili powder in a recipe! The dose of some chemicals is too low to have a meaningful effect; others might be concerning if they accumulate over time; and for others, no dose is considered safe. In addition, the application matters: was the chemical used in manufacturing but no residues remain, or is it found in the final product? And if it is found in the final product, is it bound tightly, meaning there is no chance it can get from the product onto the skin or into the vagina, or is there a risk it could leach out and pose a health hazard? Ingredient lists themselves aren't that useful, and while transparency is important, the ingredients need to be interpreted appropriately.

It has long been insinuated that so-called conventional pads and tampons are more likely to contain harmful chemicals, either from manufacturing or from pesticide residues, than so-called organic ones. There has never been a peer-reviewed study in the medical literature to back up this claim. Nevertheless, the mythology generates fear and is a convenient way for organic producers to charge more to bring you a supposedly "purer" product. In some cases, organic menstrual products cost twice as much as non-organic ones. Now consider how many people experience period poverty. I personally think it's a disgusting marketing tactic to scare people into paying more for a product that has never been shown to be superior.

The FDA "recommends that products should be free" of pesticide residues, and if there are any residues, they need to be reported to the FDA, as does the method used for detection. I haven't been able to find any pad or tampon manufacturer that specifically lists the residues in their products, but many say "pesticide-free," which is a marketing term and is not based on lab testing. Literally no testing or proof is required to slap a "pesticide-free" label on a box of tampons, so I personally consider it worthless. And "organic" doesn't mean pesticide-free; it means the company uses pesticides that are certified as organic, but that doesn't tell you how well they have been tested.

What about chemicals that might find their way into menstrual products in the manufacturing process? One group of chemicals that is a concern in personal care products is phthalates, which are endocrine-disrupting chemicals. Phthalates are often referred to as "plasticizers," as they make plastics more durable, but they're found in many things (shampoo, nail polish, perfumes, and shower curtains are but a short list) and so unfortunately find their way into us. Most people have detectable levels of phthalates. There is concern that exposure to phthalates during pregnancy may be harmful to a developing fetus, and they may have other negative impacts on hormones, but the full nature of the risk they pose isn't known. Indoor dust and food are big sources of phthalate exposure. Food may be contaminated by phthalates in the packaging or in the gloves worn by food handlers.

Phthalates are found in many personal care products, so it's unsurprising that they have been identified in menstrual pads, liners, and tampons, as well as "feminine hygiene" washes, wipes, douches, and sprays. How these chemicals get into pads, liners, and tampons isn't known, but there are several steps in manufacturing that could potentially be a source—for example, the process by which the adhesive or the top sheet that controls moisture is stuck onto the pad. Organic pads, liners, and tampons have not tested any better here than conventional products. One study tells us that people who use douches are at higher risk of having more phthalates in their system (a concern that only adds to the list of reasons why douches are harmful), but using tampons doesn't appear to be a risk factor for high levels, so that is reassuring. A study on diapers indicated that the quantity of phthalate transferred was very low (ranging from 0.00006 to 2.3 percent), meaning very little came off the diapers, so theoretically the risk of exposure would be low. Although we don't know how well phthalates are absorbed from menstrual products, they are likely a minor source of exposure compared with food and other routes. Admittedly, more work is needed here.

Another concerning group of chemicals is volatile organic compounds (VOCs), which include formaldehyde, benzene, ethylene glycol, methylene chloride, tetrachloroethylene, toluene, and 1,3-butadiene. Some can cause skin irritation and some have been linked with cancer, adverse reproductive outcomes, and poorer health outcomes in general. VOCs can be released into the air we breathe by paints, cleaning supplies, personal care products, air fresheners, forest fires, cigarette smoke, and even cooking, to name just a few examples.

A few studies have looked at VOCs and menstrual products. One from the United States found that while all products tested had some type of toxic VOC, the amount was quite low, and that tampons and most pads are associated with "cancer and non-cancer risks that fall below health protective guidelines," meaning they do not appear concerning. Sprays and powders were associated with more exposure to potentially cancer-causing chemicals. Another study, from Korea, evaluated menstrual products and also found that, although VOCs were in all the products, if they assumed 100 percent of the chemicals would be absorbed (which is unlikely), the weight of the person using the products was 43 kg (95 pounds)—to approximate the size of a twelve- or thirteen-year-old; smaller bodies incur a greater risk, as the amount absorbed leads to higher concentrations when there is less body mass to dilute it—and the products were used at a rate of ninety panty liners a month (or three a day) or twenty-one heavy menstrual pads a month (seven a day for seven days), the amount of VOCs found posed no risk.

Another study looked at VOCs in the blood of tampon and pad users and found no fluctuation based on the timing of the menstrual cycle. This may be the most important piece of data, because if VOCs were being absorbed from menstrual products, we'd expect to see fluctuations when they were used. In this study, the group who used tampons had higher levels of two chemicals overall: 2-butanone and methyl isobutyl ketone. While these chemicals may be used in tampon manufacturing, they are also found in other things; for example, 2-butanone is in tomatoes, tea, and white clover, and methyl isobutyl ketone is in coffee. Their presence doesn't prove causation, as the tampon users may have been exposed in other ways.

We should know more about what's in menstrual products, and our governments should set acceptable levels of exposure, but as of early 2023, there is no data that suggests any cause for alarm. While it may be scary to read about potentially harmful chemicals, and admittedly the area is under-researched and more quality studies are needed, here are some points to consider:

- Menstrual products have not been linked to cancers, early menopause, infertility, or any health concern connected with exposure to toxic or endocrine-disrupting chemicals.
- Phthalates and VOCs are found in many things, so focusing on menstrual products diverts attention from sources that are known health risks. The manufacturing we depend on often results in the use or release of potentially harmful chemicals, and the biggest exposure risks are likely from food, water, air, and soil. Current data suggests that exposure from menstrual products, if it exists at all, is far less than from other sources. Medically, the best course of action is to reduce the known, higher-risk exposures in your life, especially from nonessential products.
- "Feminine washes," douches, powders, wipes, sprays, and scented menstrual products should be avoided, as there is data linking them with exposure to phthalates and VOCs. Also, these products have no health benefit, douches have been linked with an increased risk of pelvic and vaginal infections, and wipes, sprays, and scented products can be irritating. Essential oils are included in this category, as both regular and "natural" essential oils have been found to release potentially hazardous VOCs. There is no requirement for essential oils to disclose their ingredients on their labels, so what you might be exposed to is truly unknown.
- Some brands have their cotton and rayon fibers tested for harmful residues by OEKO-TEX, an independent certification body for testing textiles. When a product receives a Standard 100 credential and seal (which you can usually find on the product's website), it means the fibers have been tested and are within the safety limits for over a hundred harmful substances. The testing doesn't include every potentially harmful substance, but it certainly adds another safety check.

The Safety of New Menstrual Devices

The legacy of the Rely tampon is a reminder of what happens when a new product aims to disrupt menstrual technology without first doing the important benchwork in the lab. A radically different menstrual product is helpful only if those differences are safe. And that means studies, preferably those published in peer-reviewed journals. Because of the rarity of menstrual toxic shock syndrome, even with Rely it took hundreds of thousands of women using the product before a concerning pattern appeared, so it's essential to study any new technology in lab conditions that approximate the vagina.

Keep this in mind the next time you see a start-up entering the menstrual product business. Companies can absolutely come up with helpful new technologies, but the burden of proof is on them. For example, if a company claims that its CBD-infused tampons can ease menstrual cramps, look for published studies on the impact of CBD on the vaginal microbiome, and specifically on the production of TSST-1. If these studies don't exist, the company is literally gambling with the health of its consumers. When people wonder why some of these products are not available in the United States, it is because the companies have not submitted data to the FDA.

Bottom Line

- Before the late 1800s, women primarily used skins, scraps of fabric, and other absorbent material as homemade pads, or they went without and bled on themselves and/or their clothes.
- Menstrual toxic shock syndrome is a serious but rare condition that was first associated with extraordinarily absorbent tampons that are no longer on the market. It still occurs at a rate of 0.5/100,000, and it can be caused by tampons, menstrual cups and discs, or even contraceptive sponges.
- There is no credible evidence that organic products are safer from a toxic shock syndrome standpoint, or that they are more likely to be free of potentially concerning chemicals.
- The FDA doesn't require that manufacturers of menstrual products release testing results for residues, and terms like "pesticide-free" on the label are meaningless. Consumers looking for additional peace of mind may want to choose products that have sought independent certification from OEKO-TEX.
- While chemicals such as phthalates and VOCs have been found in many menstrual products, based on what we know, there is currently no cause for concern.

13

Modern Menstrual Products

Today we have many options for menstrual products, which is great because one-size-fits-all just doesn't cut it.

There are many factors to consider when choosing a menstrual product, such as heaviness of flow, how long you need to use the product each cycle, desire and ability to use a vaginal product, the activities you want to do while menstruating, the environmental impact of the product, cost, and of course basic comfort. Some people may also need to take into account religious or cultural considerations. And what you like or need may change over time.

Studies suggest that what people find most distressing about heavy periods is when blood leaks onto their clothes, which is understandable, so having a product that can do the job is of paramount importance. But ultimately, a lot of the decision comes down to personal preference.

Disposable Menstrual Pads

Disposable pads are perhaps the most popular choice. There is very little learning curve, although it may take some experimenting to find one that fits in the way you need. Personally, I found I leaked off the back of my pad, so when extra-long pads came out, that was a game changer for me. I always wondered if it was due to my height, my heavy flow, or a combination of the two. But it could have just been the unique shape of my body.

Pads have several components. First is the absorbent filling, which looks like cotton but can be any one of or a combination of cotton, cellulose, rayon, and polyester. Some pads also have a core of gel or foam, which significantly increases absorbency. The gel or foam absorbs blood a little more slowly than the other filling but locks it in. There is also a top sheet that lets blood pass through while preventing it from wicking back onto the skin; it may be perforated to allow some air flow. Keeping the skin dry is important, to reduce irritation. The top sheet may be cotton or a synthetic fabric like polypropylene or polyethylene. In general, synthetics are better at preventing moisture leakage back onto the skin. Some pads have an emollient in the top sheet. Pads also have a waterproof back sheet, typically made of plastic, to keep the blood from leaking through. An adhesive similar to craft glue sticks the pad to underwear, replacing menstrual belts (if you don't know what menstrual belts are, consider yourself lucky).

Pads are typically very well tolerated, and we have no studies to say one is better than another. Touch and feel are very personal; you like what you like, and what irritates you may not bother someone else. Some people with skin conditions, vulvar itching, or vulvar pain (such as vulvodynia, a nerve pain condition of the vulva) tell me they find disposable pads more irritating, so if you find them irritating, it might be worth seeing your doctor to be evaluated for these conditions. And people with sensitive skin might find that one brand is better for them, just as some might prefer a particular brand of shampoo and conditioner.

Some disposable pads are compostable, which can also impact purchasing decisions.

Some manufacturers add fragrance to their pads, but to me the not so subtle implication is that you have an odor when on your period; I mean, why else would you need a pad that smells like the farts of woodland elves? But perpetuating ideas about menstrual odor aside, there are medical issues with these products, especially those that use essential oils (which is a way to add fragrance without directly saying there is added fragrance). Essential oils have the "natural" halo, meaning products that use them are assumed to have a health benefit—or at least to be safe. But that is not always the case. The most urgent issue, in a use-this-product-get-that-problem kind of way, is irritation from either contact dermatitis or an allergic reaction. Essential oils can irritate the skin, especially the vulva, which is more susceptible to irritants, but they appear to be in the top sheet with some of these pads. Someone once left a comment on my Instagram calling one brand "spicy pads" because of the resulting skin irritation from wearing them, and that is how I now describe them in the office. (Thank you to whomever that was, by the way.) If a pad is making your skin feel warm or tingling, that is not a beneficial effect, it's a sign of irritation. Essential oils also release potentially hazardous volatile organic compounds (VOCs) such as acetone, acetaldehyde, and toluene (and there appears to be no difference between regular and natural essential oils when it comes to hazardous VOCs).

The advantage of pads is that they aren't inserted vaginally and there is no risk of toxic shock syndrome. The disadvantages are that some find them uncomfortable or irritating, and they aren't helpful for swimming and may be uncomfortable for other sports. They can also shift, although wings or other side adhesives can help reduce that issue (but damn, it does hurt when your pubic hair gets caught in the adhesive).

Pads may have a small but measurable impact on skin temperature and surface moisture, but it doesn't seem to be clinically relevant; wearing panty liners regularly won't cause yeast infections, changes in vaginal pH, or other health concerns aside from possible irritation from the mechanical rubbing of the pad.

Reusable Menstrual Pads

These are exactly what you think, a modernized version of menstrual cloths. They are typically made of cotton, flannel, or fleece. Some reusable pads are fabric only; some have removable inserts; others have plastic backing. They generally fasten around the crotch of underwear with a snap or Velcro. A variety of pads can be purchased online, many with fun fabrics, but there are also sewing patterns available online for those who choose to make their own.

Women have been using cloth in this way for thousands of years, and the only major issue is the risk of irritation, either from the friction of the pads or from wetness against the skin. You also need to wash them, which could be a hardship for some. There are no studies comparing cloth with disposable pads, but using diapers as a proxy (understanding that urine and feces aren't blood, but wet is wet), disposable diapers tend to be associated with less bacteria on the skin and fewer irritation issues.

The big differences between cloth and disposable pads are:

- *The feel of the pad:* Cloth is softer. People with pain conditions or skin conditions that affect the vulva may especially prefer the feel of washable pads.
- *Sustainability:* Cloth is a winner here.
- *Absorbency:* No washable pad can match the ability of a disposable pad to prevent wetness from touching the skin, or the absorbency of a pad with a gel or foam core.
- *Convenience:* If you soak a disposable pad while away from home, you just toss it and use another one. If you soak your reusable pad while away from home, you need a bag to take it home to launder, or it isn't reusable.

Period Underwear

Just as it sounds, period underwear is underwear that absorbs blood—basically a hybrid of underwear and reusable pads. The absorbent part is made of layers of synthetic microfibers or merino wool, and some have a polyurethane (plastic) component to help with leaks. There are many brands on the market in the United States, and they come in a variety of absorbencies and styles (boy shorts, bikini, high-waisted, etc.). The *New York Times*'s Wirecutter does a good job reviewing period underwear, and I highly recommend searching on "Wirecutter period underwear" to get their latest take on the available brands, how they perform in real-world situations, their price, and how "diaper-like" they look and feel. In June 2022, Thinx Hi-Waist was their number one pick, but there were lots of great options for different budgets and needs. Some brands also make period underwear that is suitable for swimming.

The upside of period underwear is they don't have the bulk of pads and you can be ready if you think your period might be starting but aren't sure. Some people find them less irritating than pads, and they are a great option if you don't want to carry around menstrual products or don't like other menstrual products (if you have a super-soaker period, pay attention to the recommended absorbency). Period underwear may be especially comforting for teens with irregular cycles, because sitting in class when you are thirteen and realizing that you have just soaked through your clothes onto the chair is the worst. I'm fifty-seven and I still remember it clearly, even though it was forty-three years ago. I was in eighth grade English class and we were reading

The Red Pony (I know, right?) by John Steinbeck. I called my period "the red pony" for years afterward.

The downside of period underwear is the expense. Most are in the $30 to $50 range, although there are some less expensive options. How many pairs you will need depends on how heavy your flow is and how often you want to wash them. But it could set you back $40 to $150 for three to four pairs, depending on the brand you need, and that is a big upfront cost for many people.

You may need to change period underwear over the course of a day if it becomes soaked, which is a bit of a hassle if you are in a public restroom. However, there are some with a side entry, which means you don't need to take off everything from the waist down in a public bathroom stall. (I'm thinking mostly about the grossness of the floor here.)

There have been reports online that claim period underwear contains perfluoroalkyl and polyfluoroalkyl substances (PFAS), which are VOCs. And with scary headlines like "Report: 65% of Period Underwear Tested Likely Contaminated with PFAS Chemicals," you can see why people are concerned. But there's a lot of misinformation here, and straight-up chemical phobia. PFAS are used in many things because they have useful properties. For example, they make things waterproof and greaseproof, they can be fire-retardant, and they reduce friction. It's hard to find an industry untouched by PFAS. Paint, guitar strings, carpet, ski wax, cosmetics, shampoo, sunscreen, and water-resistant clothing only scratch the surface.

We don't know all the health ramifications of the more than nine thousand PFAS, but some are associated with thyroid disease, increased cholesterol levels, kidney cancer, suppression of the immune system, and low birth weight among fetuses exposed during pregnancy. There is also weaker evidence linking some PFAS with breast cancer, early-onset puberty, and certain pregnancy complications, such as high blood pressure. Interestingly, people who menstruate tend to have lower levels of PFAS in their blood, because some PFAS are removed with menstrual blood.

PFAS are known as "forever" chemicals because they enter our world but don't degrade, so they accumulate. They are found in the air, water, and soil around the world, even in the Arctic and Antarctic. In addition, they are in many things that we touch. So PFAS aren't just "forever" chemicals but also "everywhere" chemicals.

Most experts agree the biggest risk is from exposure during the manufacturing of PFAS or pollution from manufacturing (the basis of the movie

Dark Waters), where the water you drink, the showers you take, and the local food you buy all have higher than average levels of PFAS. People who work in industries that use products with PFAS, such as firefighters, carpet installers, and food industry workers, are also at higher risk. But ultimately everyone is exposed, because PFAS enter the environment as pollution from factories, they off-gas from products, and foods can become contaminated from packaging or from the gloves of people handling the food.

Regarding period underwear, several people have sent it to be tested and found PFAS, and this culminated in a class action lawsuit against the brand Thinx, which was settled. The lawsuit was about advertising, not the safety of the product. But if there are PFAS in period underwear, what does that mean? The PFAS may be there on purpose, or fabric can become contaminated, just as everything else can, or it might contain chemicals that later break down to PFAS. The textiles expert I contacted thought if PFAS were in period underwear, they were likely there on purpose, to strengthen the fabric and allow for water repellency. It is also possible manufacturers didn't know PFAS were in the fabric they sourced.

Can the PFAS from period underwear get into your body? The expert I spoke with said it was unlikely. If the PFAS were there on purpose, he felt they were likely well bound to the fabric. However, there is some data to suggest that some PFAS are removed with washing; the biggest risk here seems to be PFAS entering the water supply, not personal risk to the person using the product. Graham Peaslee, the University of Notre Dame professor whose lab initially identified PFAS in Thinx, when a reporter sent in her underwear to be evaluated, told Wirecutter, "Simply put, if you've already washed your period underwear a few times, you've probably washed the PFAS out, and now they're poisoning everything downstream instead of you."

An important takeaway here is that PFAS in all clothing, not just period underwear, are understudied, but the little data we have suggests that if PFAS transfer from clothing to people, it's a minor contribution to the body burden—less than 5 percent of what we get from other sources, like drinking water and food. Truthfully, though, we don't really know.

Might my running tights or yoga pants have PFAS? It doesn't matter how sweaty I get, they seem to barely get wet, and when I travel and wash them out in the sink, they dry incredibly quickly. They cover a much larger surface area than underwear. Sweating and increased blood flow to the skin could theoretically increase absorption, yet this potential issue doesn't seem to interest people as much. When the only scary headlines are about period products, it supports my belief that fearmongering, not safety, is the real goal, because it's scary vagina stories that make copy.

According to the National Academies of Sciences, Engineering, and Medicine, "It is difficult to provide clear advice on how to reduce exposure to per- and polyfluoroalkyl substances (PFAS) because there are many potential exposure sources." Based on the limited information we have on the risks of PFAS in fabric, individual exposure from clothing is probably not a significant source. Obviously, there are unknowns and asterisks here, but there is no indication that people should panic. And while the vulva is more absorbent than other areas, most things placed on the vulva don't absorb 100 percent. Overall, the biggest issue with PFAS in period underwear is likely the global contribution from manufacturing, washing, and disposal (it eventually ends up in landfill). That's not an insignificant issue, but it is less panic-inducing.

One of the biggest sources of PFAS exposure is drinking water, so focusing on period underwear and not water could lead people to overlook a major thing that poses a known health concern.

Some companies are posting testing results for PFAS on their websites, and I've seen websites that post independent testing, but they also contain some incorrect information about other chemicals, so I can't recommend them. This kind of third-party testing doesn't give the full picture because it's not peer-reviewed. Products with OEKO-TEX Standard 100 certification (discussed in the previous chapter, see page 159) have been tested for some PFAS, but not for all.

Tampons

The standard tampon design consists of two basic components: the pledget, which is the absorbent part, and the string. Modern tampons expand mostly lengthwise, which helps to reduce pain and potentially microtrauma with removal. In the United States, the wrapping and applicator are considered part of the tampon, and all components must be submitted to the FDA for clearance before marketing. Tampons with applicators—telescoping cardboard or plastic to push the tampon up into the vagina—are more common in North America; applicator-free tampons are more common elsewhere.

Cardboard applicators were part of the original design that became Tampax; they were supposedly for cleanliness and protection from infection, but the disposable applicator also increased the price and hence the profits. There is no infection risk identified with inserting a tampon with a finger versus an applicator. Although people typically get more blood on their hands with an applicator-free tampon, regardless of the method you choose, you still need to wash your hands afterward, so from a cleanliness standpoint, an applicator doesn't offer that much of an advantage. Tampons inserted with an applicator tend to sit a little deeper in the vagina, which some people may prefer and others might not. Basically, an applicator is a personal choice. However, once a tampon is inserted, you shouldn't feel it.

The pledget is made of either cotton or rayon, or a blend of the two. Rayon, a fiber made from wood pulp, is more absorbent than cotton. Tampon absorbency is standardized by the FDA, and the amount of blood each tampon can hold is listed in Table 3. (For reference, 1 g of blood is approximately equal to 1 ml.) Absorbency is tested in a device called a Syngina, which, it pains me to tell you, is a portmanteau of *synthetic* and *vagina*. I'm not sure why that word bothers me so much, but it does. I suspect devices used to test other products don't get coy names like Synthoheart or Synthectum (synthetic rectum). Can't we just call it a tampon tester?

Table 3 • THE AMOUNT OF BLOOD A TAMPON CAN ABSORB

ABSORBENCY LEVEL	AMOUNT OF BLOOD
Slender/light	<6 g
Regular	6-9 g
Super	9-12 g
Super plus	12-15 g
Ultra	15-18 g

Some people might look at Table 3 with skepticism, because 15 g (15 ml, or 0.5 ounce) is a lot of blood. But the amount of liquid a tampon can hold in the lab may be different from what it can hold in a vagina without leaking. One study looked at Tampax to establish real-life absorbency, and completely soaked regular, super, and super plus tampons all came in below or at the lower range of absorbency listed on the label.

Tampon designs follow one of three basic configurations as they expand. They all expand lengthwise, but some retain their cylindrical shape, some open more like a flower (or an upside-down Ms. Pac-Man), and others spread out side to side, a bit like a stingray. This latest design, the stingray shape, is based on modeling of vaginas by MRI, which was part of the design process for the Tampax Pearl. The vagina is collapsed front to back when it is empty, so the idea was that the most comfortable design, and one that would best reduce leakage, would fit that shape. In their 2022 review of tampons, Wirecutter recommended the Tampax Pearl as number one for comfort and protection among tampons with applicators, and the o.b. tampon for an applicator-free option.

Here are some other tampon tips:

- Choose a tampon with the lowest absorbency to match your needs and change it every six to eight hours unless it's about to leak through. Leaks aside, this optimal time frame is about the real but very rare menstrual toxic shock syndrome (see page 152 for more).
- Don't wear tampons for penetrative sex, but they are fine to wear during oral sex.
- Try not to forget about an inserted tampon. It happens, even to gynecologists. The scenario is usually that you thought you'd removed it and didn't. When a tampon is left inside the vagina, bacteria can overgrow, resulting in a foul-smelling discharge. If you realize you've left a tampon in for too long, remove it, and it's probably wise to see your health care provider for an exam.

What about first-time insertions? I remember trying to insert my first tampon. I couldn't ask my mother for advice, as she had made it clear that tampons were evil, and asking her about anything related to menstruation was just not worth it. I was thirteen years old and it was summer, and I wanted to go swimming. It was not an option to miss out because of my period (summers in Winnipeg are short). I hadn't been sexually active and had bought into the myth of "THE HYMEN," meaning I thought there was a barely penetrable tight band inside my vagina. I envisioned one of those paper circus hoops that a dog or tiger jumps through, leaving the edges of the paper in shreds. I knew very little about my body but was highly motivated to go swimming. So I read the instructions that came in the box, and as nothing was mentioned about a penis needing to go in the vagina first, I decided I was good to go. It took two tries. I remember sitting on the toilet afterward thinking how I (and many of my friends) had built this up to be a thing and it wasn't. I think this moment started my awakening about paying attention to what I was being told about my body and realizing it might not fit with reality.

When considering your first tampon insertion (or menstrual cup/disc insertion, for that matter), remember that the hymen is not a freshness seal but simply vaginal tissue. It is more rigid in infants, and its likely biological purpose in the first few years is to protect the vagina from urine, feces, and dirt. By the time someone starts menstruating, the remnants of the hymen are typically as stretchy as the rest of the vagina. The hymen doesn't break, because vaginal tissue doesn't break. A physical exam cannot reliably tell whether someone who is menstruating has been sexually active with a penis or whether they have inserted a tampon or menstrual cup. There is no such thing as a virginity check. I appreciate that there are disgusting doctors who offer one, but they are either ignorant about anatomy or profiting from fears about the hymen.

It's true that sometimes the vagina can feel tight when trying to insert a tampon, but that is rarely because of the hymen. The most likely reason is that the pelvic floor muscles that wrap around the vagina have tightened, creating a smaller vaginal opening and resulting in increased friction and pain with inserting the tampon.

Most people insert tampons while either sitting on a toilet seat or standing with one foot on the toilet seat (or something of similar height). If you go with sitting on the toilet, raising your feet on a stool can open the pelvic floor muscles and make insertion easier. Another option, if that feels weird or stressful, is to lie on the bed (on a towel if needed), put your heels together, and let your knees flop open.

Here are some other points and strategies to consider for first-time insertion:

- Put some lubricant on the tampon.
- If you feel uncertain, try inserting a finger into your vagina first so you have an idea of its direction.
- Try a tampon with a plastic inserter, as they are smoother, which some people find easier.
- If you feel like you are hitting a wall, that is usually the pelvic floor muscles. Taking three or four slow, deep breaths in through the nose and out through the mouth can sometimes help relax these muscles.
- Sometimes the pelvic floor muscles are so tight the tampon can't be inserted at all. If you have tried a few times and had no success, see

your doctor or nurse practitioner. Typically it's muscle spasm, and there are treatments available, such as working with a pelvic floor physical therapist. But there are some rare conditions where the hymen is rigid or larger than expected, so it's wise to be evaluated for them.

- Once the tampon is in, you shouldn't feel it. If you do, it's typically because it's too low in the vagina or because of pelvic floor muscle spasm. If the tampon is uncomfortable, remove it. If it wasn't too painful, you can try again, but if discomfort persists, it's a good idea to see a doctor and perhaps a pelvic floor physical therapist for diagnosis and treatment.

Reusable Menstrual Cups and Discs

Many people who want to reduce their carbon footprint are turning to reusable menstrual cups or discs as a more environmentally friendly option, and many choose these options because they prefer how they perform or feel. Reusable menstrual cups and discs are made of silicone, latex, or a thermoplastic elastomer, a polymer made from rubber that is generally considered safe for those with a latex allergy (though people with a latex allergy should always follow the advice on the package and ask their own doctor). Cups and discs sit in the vagina and collect blood. Discs sit higher than cups (see Figure 11), more like a diaphragm, and some people find discs more comfortable for this reason, but others find cups more comfortable.

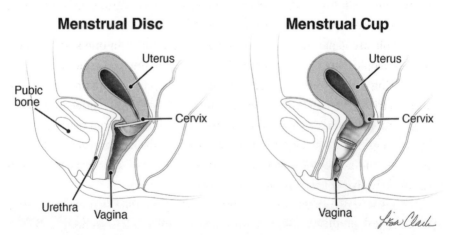

Figure 12 • *Placement of Menstrual Discs and Cups (Illustration by Lisa A. Clark, MA, CMI)*

Cups have a stem or a pull tab for removal and come in a range of firmness, which affects ease of insertion and removal, blood collection performance, and comfort. For example, soft cups open more slowly once inserted, so leaks might be more common, but they may be more comfortable, especially for those with bad menstrual cramps. For some people, cramps can come from contractions of a muscle layer around the vagina, which could increase with the pressure from a firm cup. The size of the cup and length of the stem or pull tab also vary. For people with a lower cervix—meaning you can easily feel your cervix by inserting an index finger in your vagina—it may take a few cups to find one that fits you the best and is comfortable.

There are a lot of cups on the market, so how do you choose? Wirecutter has a great in-depth piece on cup choices, including what makes a good starter cup. Period Nirvana (periodnirvana.com) is another excellent resource, and Kim Rosas, who runs Period Nirvana, also has an excellent Instagram profile with great videos and tips and tricks. Many sites have questionnaires to help match you to the cup of your dreams, but there are no studies evaluating their accuracy. Some cup manufacturers make recommendations based on previous pregnancies or age, but your age doesn't affect the size of your vagina, so I never understood what that was all about. In one study, women were provided with the same size cup and there was no difference in how it performed based on age or pregnancy history.

There are different techniques for folding the cup to make insertion easier, but ultimately, it just needs to go in your vagina and feel comfortable. This is where the flexibility, ranging from soft to medium to hard, comes into play, because some cups are easier to compress for insertion than others.

People are generally very satisfied with their cups. In one study, 91 percent of people who tried a menstrual cup as part of the study said they would keep using cups, and in another study comparing cups with tampons, where women tried each for three cycles and then switched, cups tended to be rated higher for performance and comfort. In general, it takes about two menstrual cycles to get comfortable with insertion and removal. Removal should happen over a toilet so the blood can be dumped. In general, they can be left in for up to twelve hours, but there is no good data here.

Menstrual discs are a newer addition to the reusable product market, and they are very similar to diaphragms that are used for contraception, but with a deeper bowl so blood can collect. They sit higher in the vagina than cups, positioned behind the cervix in an area called the posterior fornix, angling forward so the front sits above the pubic bone (like a diaphragm). Because they are inserted deeper in the vagina and need a little positioning, they can be harder for some people to insert, and it may take more tries to get comfortable using them. Some discs have a pull tab or a notch for your finger, and some people may find these easier to remove than the simple round discs that are removed by hooking the rim with your finger. Regardless of approach, there is often some spill with removal, so sitting over the toilet or removing the disc in the shower are both good options. Discs can also "autodump," which means when you are going to the bathroom, the shift in your position may cause them to leak into the toilet. If this happens, you may wish to check the disc position and correct as needed.

One advantage of discs over all other menstrual products is they can be used during penetrative intercourse; remember, discs are modeled after diaphragms, which are specifically meant to be worn during sex. A menstrual cup is not an option for penetrative intercourse, as it sits lower and blocks the vagina, and many also have a stem, which would be painful for a penis encountering it.

I asked Kim Rosas of Period Nirvana for some advice on using a menstrual disc during sex, and she suggested the following:

> If you have a heavy period, emptying your disc before sex is a good "just in case" practice. And here's another tip—the vaginal canal lengthens with arousal. Wait at least two hours after your romp to remove the disc, otherwise, you might find it harder to reach than you expected. If for any reason the disc is still hard to access, you can squat to make it easier to reach. A gentle push is ok to do in addition to a squat if it's still not accessible. Your muscles can help disengage the disc from behind your pubic bone, thus making the front rim easier to reach.

There are very few safety studies on menstrual cups and discs; certainly there are no large studies by the manufacturers. That doesn't mean they are unsafe, but cups and discs are often glossed over in the discussion about the risks of menstrual products, especially menstrual toxic shock syndrome (mTSS), as if tampons are riskier and the tampon companies are "hiding something." No one seems to say that about cup or disc manufacturers. I personally think it's because cups and discs are viewed as a greener source, so they benefit from the "natural" halo. I don't mean to imply that cups or discs are risky, but simply to raise questions about why specifically conventional tampon manufacturers are considered evil.

Cups are associated with mTSS, so it should be assumed that discs are too, especially since mTSS has been linked with diaphragms, but the actual incidence rate for cups and discs isn't known. It seems unlikely that it is higher than for tampons, though the air inserted with a cup or disc may be a risk factor.

Disposable Menstrual Discs

These devices have a firm ring with a clear, flexible pouch for collecting blood. Like a reusable disc, they sit high in the vagina, tucked behind the cervix in the back and the pubic bone in the front, and may require a little more skill to insert and remove than a menstrual cup. As with reusable discs, you can have penetrative sex, which may reduce mess. They may also be a good option for people who like reusable cups and/or discs and want to keep a backup on hand if their period starts earlier than expected, or for situations where access to water for cleaning is limited.

The main products in the United States are Softdisc, Flex Disc, and Flex Plant + Disc. According to their websites, these products are made of "medical grade polymers," a description that makes me roll my eyes because it doesn't tell me anything useful; polymers are just large molecules made up of repeating units of smaller molecules. Silicone, Teflon, wool, and DNA are all polymers and obviously these molecules are all very different! In a published study with Softdisc the material is described as a "proprietary blend of soft biocompatible polymer compounds in conformance with the United States Pharmacopoeia XIX Class VI criteria for plastics."

Flex has what I consider to be some problematic information on their website. They list toxic shock syndrome and the potential for leaks as a "con" for tampons, and as these are not listed as a con for discs, the implication, I suppose, is that these issues aren't a concern for discs. There is no data that assures us that menstrual discs are free from the risk of mTSS as there are cases associated with diaphragms, and disposable discs can absolutely leak (I have personal experience here). Flex also makes this claim on their website: "Tampons expand as they absorb, putting pressure on your vaginal walls. They're relatively rigid and unable to move with your body when your uterus contracts. Plus, they block the vaginal canal, trapping a little bubble of oxygen internally." But tampons don't put any meaningful pressure on the vaginal walls (it's not as if they are being pumped up like a balloon). As for the statement about tampons being "unable to move with your body when your uterus contracts," I have no idea what that means, and I am both an expert in period cramps and in the vagina. Vaginal menstrual products don't move to catch blood like someone running to catch leaks in the roof during a rainstorm with a single bucket. And as we reviewed in the previous chapter, air is inserted vaginally with tampons, cups, and discs. Additionally, there is no quality, peer-reviewed data that tells us menstrual discs are superior for people with menstrual cramps.

Can You Accidentally Remove an IUD with a Tampon, Menstrual Cup, or Disc?

This is a valid question. After all, the IUD string extends into the vagina and is typically long enough to feel when a finger is inserted vaginally. So it is plausible that the string could be inadvertently grasped or become entangled with a tampon, cup, or disc and pulled out with removal.

To answer this question, we must know the baseline risk of an IUD coming out on its own, known medically as expulsion. That risk is highest in the first year after insertion, and it happens to 3 to 10 percent of people with a copper IUD and 4 to 6 percent with a levonorgestrel IUD. Factors associated with expulsion are never having been pregnant; heavy and/or painful periods; being younger than twenty years old; having the IUD inserted immediately after delivery or a second-trimester abortion; and previously having had an IUD expulsion.

There have been reports of inadvertent IUD removal. One paper describes seven women who pulled out or dislodged their IUD (partial expulsion) while removing a cup, but this doesn't tell us how common it is, only that it's been described. A close friend who is also an OB/GYN accidentally pulled out her IUD while removing a tampon in a bathroom stall at an outdoor music concert. Alcohol was involved, so she freely admits that her judgment about what she was pulling, or how hard, may have been impaired.

Two studies gathered data from women who expelled IUDs, but they don't tell us whether the IUD came out at the same time as a menstrual product, making it hard to determine cause and effect. And frustratingly, the results conflict. One study revealed no difference in expulsion rate, but we don't know if internal menstrual products were used in the first six weeks after the IUD was inserted; the other study, which gathered data for longer, found the expulsion rate was 7.7 percent for those who used pads, 10.1 percent for those who used tampons, and 18.6 percent for those who used menstrual cups. The difference for menstrual cups was statistically significant, which suggests this result might be accurate. However, it still doesn't prove cause and effect, or that the expulsion rate is 18.6 percent among cup users. Menstrual cup users who had previously experienced IUD expulsions may have been more likely to sign up for the study, or menstrual cup users may be more likely to have other factors that increase the risk of expulsion.

It's certainly possible that the use of internal menstrual products could create a higher risk of accidental IUD removal, but there isn't enough known about the subject to give a formal recommendation about avoiding tampons, menstrual cups, or menstrual discs with an IUD. It's probably a good idea for those who use internal menstrual products to check their IUD string once after each period for the first year after insertion, and sporadically thereafter. And be mindful of the effects of alcohol or other substances that might affect your judgment about how hard you are pulling or what you are pulling.

If you inadvertently pull your IUD out, it doesn't necessarily mean you can't try again with another IUD and keep using your preferred menstrual product; however, it might be a good idea to cut the IUD string shorter so the risk of inadvertent removal is lower. Because this may impact the ease of IUD removal, it requires a discussion of the pros and cons with your medical provider.

Polyester Foam Products

Menstrual sponges made from the same polyester foam as the Rely tampon and the contraceptive sponge are available in some countries. We don't know how much the polyester foam contributes to the risk of mTSS, and I wasn't able to find any studies on mTSS with these products. This kind of foam is not only highly absorbent but also traps air, so additional air (and hence oxygen and carbon dioxide) might be introduced vaginally with menstrual sponges, though how much is unknown. Personally, I'm hesitant to recommend a product made from the same material as the Rely tampon, given the lack of safety data about the growth of TSST-1 and TSST-1-producing bacteria on these products.

Bottom Line

- There are many choices for menstrual products, and they all have advantages and disadvantages. What one person might find valuable in a certain product, another might find concerning.
- Menstrual pads are the most-used product. The biggest drawbacks are their bulkiness, the risk of leaking around the sides (wings help with this), interference with the ability to participate in some sports, and external irritation.
- Period underwear is a fine choice. Based on current knowledge, the concern about harmful chemicals is hype.
- The design of the Tampax Pearl was based on models of the vagina. Among tampons with applicators, it rates the highest for comfort and ability to do the job.
- Reusable menstrual cups and discs are becoming more popular, and they are great options for many people. It's possible they could increase the risk of dislodging an IUD during removal, but how often this occurs is unknown.

14

Menstrual Product Myths

Scaring people about menstrual products seems to have become its own cottage industry, probably because both purity culture and chemophobia (irrational fear of chemicals) sell papers, get page clicks, and generate views and likes. The way tampons especially are disparaged on social media—and even at times in the traditional media—you'd think they were toxic death sticks or incendiary devices. I suspect menstrual cups and discs get less negativity because they have a smaller market share, so are less likely to get page clicks for negative content. For now, anyway. Cups and most discs are also reusable, so they may also benefit from the "natural health" halo. But whatever the reason, certainly no menstrual product has been immune from these attacks. At times it seems like the groups involved won't be happy until everyone is bleeding onto their clothes.

There are no studies linking tampons, cups, or discs with any serious health condition outside of the very rare toxic shock syndrome, yet myths about these products persist, with some common themes: chemicals are evil; ancient wisdom is powerful; following a specific ritual (usually giving something up) will help you achieve better health; natural is best; and companies that make "natural" products are benevolent (and almost always held to a much lower standard).

The emphasis on "natural" is one of the most malignant concepts in menstrual mythology, as *natural* also means "not interfered with." Sit and let that wash over you. The implication is that menstrual products interfere with the vagina, removing its purity, its virginity, its perfection. "Natural" is deeply intertwined with purity culture, and that may be why this mythology speaks to us: most of us, to some degree or another, have been affected by purity culture. After all, we've been steeping in it for centuries.

Menstrual charlatans promote the idea that heavy periods, pelvic pain, painful periods, and cancer are caused by menstrual products, and insinuate that these products could harm future fertility. Because these conditions are biologically complex, and in the case of painful or heavy periods often go unaddressed, people who aren't bound by the truth can easily step in and make false claims that sound reasonable. Putting something in the vagina means a potentially harmful synthetic substance is closer to its target, right? It's easy to see how people reach this conclusion; after all, that's how menstrual toxic shock syndrome started.

Many of these myths are like Halley's Comet—they come around and around again with regularity. I've been watching this transpire since the late 1980s, and I've seen many of the same myths recycled, coming back each time with a different, scarier story. So let's tackle the oldies but definitely not goodies, as well as the nasty newcomers.

Do Tampons Affect Virginity?

This is probably the original tampon myth, the false idea that inserting a tampon before penetrative intercourse with a penis damages the hymen, hence destroying "virginity." I use quotation marks for "virginity" because it is a social construct and has nothing to do with the hymen. The fear of vaginal products affecting virginity appears to be a modern concept, because historically, many medications were used vaginally with no such concerns being raised.

Myths about tampons and virginity are tall tales designed to frighten women into thinking their worth is related to men's ignorance about the vagina.

Can Tampons Cause Painful Periods?

Possibly, but not in the way people think. Tampons, menstrual cups, and menstrual discs don't affect the chemicals that cause painful periods, but their physical presence could increase the muscle spasms (uncoordinated contractions in the musculature of the vagina) that can be part of painful periods. The spasms could also make the products difficult to position correctly, which could increase pain. If tampons, cups, or discs increase your period pain, see your provider and a pelvic floor physical therapist to be evaluated for spasm in the muscles of the pelvic floor.

Can Menstrual Blood Flow Be Controlled Without Products?

Free bleeding is the term for shunning menstrual products and simply bleeding into clothing. It's often seen as an act of rejecting the patriarchal shame associated with menstruation. But *free bleeding* can also be used to express the false idea that the egress of blood from the vagina can be controlled. Yes, "Just control yourself and bleed when you're sitting on the toilet" does sound like something an ignorant male politician might say in response to a request for the government to subsidize menstrual products, but apparently this claim is made by some people who menstruate. The idea is that the muscles that wrap around the vagina can be contracted to control the flow of blood.

Physiologically, this is preposterous. The pelvic floor muscles cannot contract enough to make a watertight seal for hours at a time. Think about briefly clenching your muscles to stop your stream of urine. Now imagine holding that clench, but tighter, while you walk, drive a car, and sit down for supper. How would these muscles stay tightly contracted while you sleep? There were times when I was in my menopause transition when my period would start out of the blue and I knew I was going to bleed everywhere. Even though I knew clenching my pelvic floor wouldn't help, I did it out of desperation, to try to stop the blood from leaking onto my chair or my car seat. Of course, it never helped.

If controlling bleeding were possible, don't you think people other than some influencers on Instagram would have figured it out? Wouldn't our ancestors have practiced it and taught it to their daughters? Considering all the people who have menstruated since the beginning of time, why would it be worthwhile to teach them how to control their urine, but not their menstrual blood, if such a thing were possible?

I think we all know the answer.

Attempting to contract the pelvic floor to hold in menstrual blood, besides being impossible, could lead to muscle spasm (a result of excessive clenching), which could cause pelvic pain or pain with vaginal sex. The other harm here is the mistaken worship of all things "natural" and the implication that voluntarily controlling your menstrual blood is unlocking the final level of being a RealWoman™.

Can a Menstrual Cup Cause My Uterus to Fall Out?

There is no evidence to support this theory. Pelvic organ prolapse is a condition where the tissues and muscles of the pelvic floor are no longer able to support the pelvic organs (meaning one or more of the uterus, bladder, urethra, and rectum). It can lead to these organs and the vagina itself descending. Sometimes a bulge can be felt at the vaginal opening; less commonly, tissues may hang out of the vaginal opening. Think of the vagina as a sock with a tennis ball sewn to the toe end on the outside of the sock. Now imagine inserting your hand into the sock and, from the inside, pulling down at the toe where the tennis ball is sewn. The part that telescopes inside the sock is the prolapsing vaginal tissue, and the tennis ball that you can feel but not see represents the organ that is dropping down. Pelvic organ prolapse is related to many factors, including genes that control the resilience of collagen (a protein that strengthens tissue and provides elasticity), injury during childbirth, medical conditions that affect connective tissue, obesity, constipation, and frequent straining.

The origin of the concern appears to be worry about bearing down, if needed, to help bring a cup or disc into reach for removal, as is recommended by some manufacturers. While it's true that repetitive straining is a risk factor for prolapse, only a brief bearing down is needed to remove a cup or disc. OB/GYNs often ask people to bear down in the office to see if a prolapse is visible, and we tell people they can bear down to help with removal of a pessary, a vaginal device that treats prolapse. Cups and discs are like pessaries in many ways, and as pessaries treat prolapse and don't cause it, the temporary bearing down for removal isn't a concern.

Is it possible that some people are straining, like with constipation, when they remove their cup? Sure, but they're using either the wrong size cup or disc or an incorrect technique for removal.

Is There Asbestos in Tampons?

NO. In capitals for emphasis! This myth has been around since I was in medical training. I can imagine the back cover of the novel: "EvilCorp has been secretly putting asbestos in tampons to increase menstrual bleeding and hence sell more tampons. Jennifer, a plucky young med student, uncovers the incriminating documents while writing a paper on occupational exposure to asbestos, putting herself and those she loves in danger." And voilà, we have a bestselling legal thriller. I'll call it *The Tampon Brief*. (Sigh.)

Asbestos is associated with health risks. It can cause cancer, but only after long-term exposure via inhalation, and no one is breathing in nonexistent tampon asbestos through their vagina. As with almost all of these conspiracy theories, there has never been a fiber of proof (or logic): no lab analysis showing asbestos in tampons, no incriminating documents marked "Top Secret." Someone, somewhere, made this up. It's likely a mix of garden-variety purity culture, the toxic shock syndrome fears of the late 1970s, and the increased awareness around the same time about the health risks of chronic exposure to asbestos.

Do Tampons Increase Menstrual Flow?

This myth seems to have two origin stories. In one, it's offered as proof for the asbestos myth just discussed. In the other, it's related to the incorrect belief that tampons create suction that draws blood out of the uterus. Remember, there is no blood sloshing around in the uterus, waiting to come out, and tampons don't create suction in the vagina. There is no biologically plausible way that tampons can increase flow.

Modern menstrual pads are very absorbent, especially those with gel cores. A heavy-day pad holds significantly more blood than a super plus tampon. A super plus tampon should hold about 12–15 ml (0.4–0.5 ounce) of blood, but there is no standard absorbency for pads, so I did a little home experiment to compare the two. After fifteen minutes in 15 ml of water, a super plus tampon was completely saturated, and I imagine it might leak or overflow if it were that wet in the vagina. I then poured 15 ml of water onto a heavy-day pad with a gel core and it was nowhere near capacity. Obviously, this isn't a scientifically rigorous test, but if you switch from pads to tampons and expect they will perform the same, you could easily conclude that your bleeding is heavier with the tampons. By nature of their design, and their reduced absorbency compared to pads, tampons are more likely to be prone to catastrophic leaks (I used to call these critical tampon events, or CTEs).

Are There Dioxins in Tampons?

A lot less than in your food! According to the World Health Organization (WHO), "Dioxins are a group of chemically-related compounds that are persistent environmental pollutants (POPs)." They can cause cancer, damage the immune system, and harm the reproductive system. They are hard for our bodies to break down and get rid of, so they can accumulate. Unfortunately, they're everywhere. Most of our exposure comes from food, mainly from meat, dairy, fish, and shellfish, because dioxins also accumulate in animals. The higher an animal is on the food chain, the more likely it is to contain dioxins.

As far as non-food exposure goes, dioxins are primarily a by-product of manufacturing, but they are also released into the environment from forest fires and volcanoes. They entered the tampon story because older methods of bleaching cotton and producing rayon created dioxins through the use of elemental chlorine. Bleaching methods have since changed, but there are still traces of dioxins in both tampons and pads—but not because of the manufacturing process. Rather, dioxins are in the raw material, be it cotton or wood pulp, because of pollution of the soil where the material was grown. And yes, that includes 100 percent organic cotton. In fact, in one study, an organic tampon had the greatest amount of dioxins.

However, most tampons have undetectable amounts of dioxins, and when detected, they are less than 0.2 percent of the allowable monthly intake. According to one group of researchers, the dioxin exposure from tampons is 13,000 to 240,000 times less than the dioxins we are exposed to by diet. For perspective, disposable diapers have the same traces of dioxins, but that doesn't seem to get any attention, probably because purity culture isn't involved.

Do Tampons or Menstrual Cups Cause Endometriosis?

This myth predates the Internet. In fact, at some point pre-MoveOn.org, there was even a petition to the FDA to get menstrual cups banned because of a false belief about an association with endometriosis.

There are two hypotheses here. One is based on the theory that endometriosis is caused by retrograde menstruation, meaning some menstrual blood essentially flows upstream and spills out the oviducts into the pelvis (for more on this, see page 268). There's just one major flaw with this hypothesis (and imagine me drawing out the *a* in *major* so it's about five seconds long). Neither tampons nor menstrual cups plug the cervix, so they can't create enough pressure to send more blood than usual backflowing out the oviducts. In other words, they don't contribute to retrograde menstruation. The second hypothesis was generated by unfounded fears about dioxins or endocrine-disrupting chemicals in tampons, as high levels of dioxins are related to an increased risk of endometriosis in studies with animals. However, as discussed above, tampons don't have dioxins in any concerning quantity.

A few studies have looked at risk factors for endometriosis and specifically asked participants about tampon use, and no clear link has been identified. In fact, one study found a lower risk of endometriosis among tampon users. No, this doesn't mean that tampons prevent endometriosis. There are several common-sense explanations for this result. First, if someone has terrible menstrual pain, they might be less inclined to insert a tampon, because everything hurts. Second, people with endometriosis are more likely to have pelvic floor muscle spasms, a condition where inserting tampons can be painful. So people with endometriosis are already less likely to use tampons than those who don't have endometriosis. It's also important to remember that most people with endometriosis experience symptoms early in their menstrual years. In fact, some have pain with their periods within the first year or two of menstruation. For this to be caused by chemicals in tampons, they would have to have started using tampons before their first period. Finally, if chemicals in tampons caused endometriosis, the risk of the condition would rise with age because of cumulative exposure over the years, but that isn't the typical pattern.

Is There Roundup in Tampons?

Glyphosate is an ingredient in some herbicides, most notably Roundup, so it may be used in farming the cotton plants destined for tampon glory (I, for one, appreciated cotton's dedication to this important service for thirty-five or so years). There is a myth that cotton in tampons is dangerous because it contains glyphosate, and this seems to have been started by a video of a presentation at a media event that was amplified by those who profit from, you guessed it, organic tampons. Like the origin stories of many of these myths, it is like a bad game of telephone based on unverified claims. But because most people don't have a good working knowledge of herbicides or agriculture, and because the WHO lists glyphosate as a possible carcinogen, and because it gets so much bad press (usually from those who profit from the bad press), it's easy to see why those of us who aren't experts in plant science could be frightened.

I'm most definitely not in Monsanto's pocket (they're the manufacturer of Roundup); however, there is a lot of science that disagrees with the WHO's conclusion. For starters, here's what the U.S. Environmental Protection Agency has to say: "There are no risks of concern to human health when glyphosate is used in accordance with its current label" and "Glyphosate is unlikely to be a human carcinogen." In addition, glyphosate works in plants via the shikimate pathway, but mammals don't have that pathway, so we humans can't metabolize it. Also, glyphosate isn't absorbed well across skin or mucosa such as the vagina. Glyphosate is also applied to the crops early in development, before the cotton fibers form. In addition, the amount that is applied is minute.

No one railing against co-called conventional tampons has ever provided legitimate evidence of a legitimate scientific concern with glyphosate. Regardless, several government agencies in Europe have evaluated tampons and found no evidence of glyphosate or its metabolite aminomethylphosphonic acid above the achievable limit of detection. If there are any residues present, they're in the parts per billion and not something that can be found with state-of-the-art testing. (I went down a deep glyphosate cotton rabbit hole.)

Wild claims with no backing science are a common tactic among those who promulgate these fears, and it's shameful. The onus is on the people making the claim to provide their point, but based on the information I've just provided, it's clear why they haven't. They have no case.

Is the Titanium Dioxide in Tampons Toxic?

In the summer of 2022, a TikTok video that went viral created panic about a brand of organic tampons containing the "dangerous" chemical titanium dioxide! How was that allowed? The story snowballed, with various people reciting the most common myths about tampons: "This must be why they make me bleed more" or "This might have caused the precancer on my cervix." Of course, "banned in Europe" only added to the hype. Unscrupulous health influencers (who really should be labeled "vectors of disinformation") amplified these unfounded fears, as did some in the media. I was even asked by a reporter how an organic product could have chemicals.

Le sigh. Everything is a chemical, and "organic" has nothing to do with titanium dioxide, which is not a pesticide. In fact, titanium dioxide, or TiO_2, is a naturally occurring mineral and a common ingredient in many products because it has whitening and reflective properties. It's used in toothpaste and some food, and to whiten the strings of tampons. It's also a major ingredient of some sunscreens. The fact that toothpaste use is not associated with oral cancers or other health concerns should have alerted the original alarmist to the fact that the risks could hardly be greater with a tampon string. With toothpaste, it's literally being rubbed into your gums! On a tampon string, the TiO_2 would have to dissolve into the vaginal discharge and then find its way to the mucosa to be absorbed.

One of the issues with TiO_2, which has been used for almost a hundred years in manufacturing, is that many products contain nanoparticles of it, meaning they're much smaller than the width of a human hair. Theoretically, this could change the way TiO_2 might act in the body, so there have been studies specifically looking at these nanoparticles and safety.

It's true that TiO_2 was banned in the European Union. They did so because recent studies showed that when rats were fed massive amounts of TiO_2 for several months, they might theoretically develop some bowel issues. Interestingly, the EU panel didn't identify any actual health concerns to prompt the ban. Health Canada reviewed the same data and concluded there was no evidence of cancer risk in animal studies with food-grade TiO_2, no changes to DNA in animal studies (something that could signify a cancer risk), and "no adverse effects in animal studies on reproduction, development, immune, gastrointestinal or nervous systems, or general health when rats were exposed from pre-conception to adulthood."

The International Agency for Research on Cancer (IARC) does classify TiO_2 as a Group 2B carcinogen, meaning "possibly carcinogenic to humans," but that applies specifically to inhalation. Though you might hear advice to let your vagina "breathe" by not wearing underwear, inhalation isn't a method by which a chemical can get from the outside world through the vagina and into your body.

But I get it, these viral claims are scary, and the first piece of information you receive about something can be so hard to unlearn. And it sounds truthy: "Europe banned titanium dioxide, so it must cause harm!" However, the science is clear here. TiO_2 can't dissolve in water, and it most certainly would have to dissolve to get off the tampon string and into the vaginal mucosa. In addition, fabrics with TiO_2 have been tested by washing them repeatedly, and very little of the substance is released. Your tampon string isn't being agitated and exposed to detergent, as it would be in a washing machine; your mouth, on the other hand, goes through similar agitation when you're brushing your teeth, and yet TiO_2 is considered safe in toothpaste. Rest assured, the minute amount of TiO_2 on a tampon string isn't leaching into the vagina.

Also, cervical precancer and cancer are not caused by TiO_2; they are due to infection with specific strains of human papillomavirus (HPV). Tampons have never been implicated. The best way to protect against cervical cancer is to get vaccinated against HPV.

Are Organic Products Safer?

No study has ever demonstrated this. In fact, in some studies looking at residues, organic products fared worse. If you want to buy organic, buy organic, but there is no medical reason to do so for vaginal, uterine, ovarian, or hormonal health.

What About Period Product Hacks?

These involve using nonconventional menstrual products. None of these hacks are ever held to task by the media or so-called health influencers, yet these products have very real risks. (It's almost as if it was never about safety to begin with, you know?)

One that has been on the socials lately is inserting a makeup sponge, like the inexpensive disposable ones from the drugstore, into the vagina as a DIY tampon that can be used to absorb period blood during sex. Sometimes it's advertised as a hack used in adult films, which I think is supposed to make it look well vetted. These sponges are made of similar material to the Rely tampon—the one that was pulled from the market for causing menstrual toxic shock syndrome (mTSS)—so right out of the gate this seems like an idea fraught with issues. How this material interacts with vaginal bacteria is unknown, and when a sponge is compressed, it will release air into the vagina, which is a known contributor to mTSS. Although there are menstrual sponges sold in some countries using this material, I've been unable to find safety data on them. Also, sponges like this can get tucked up behind the cervix and become difficult to remove, and can potentially be left behind, leading to health concerns.

For those who want to try to reduce menstrual blood incursions into sex (not everyone has a navy-blue towel handy), the best option is a reusable or disposable menstrual disc. They're not likely to be 100 percent effective, but neither are sponges, and discs are infinitely safer.

Another period hack is sea sponges. Yes, the aquatic organisms that breathe and feed by filtering seawater. They are filled with air pockets (which is what makes them absorbent) and they expand in all directions, neither of which is ideal for an intravaginal menstrual product. In addition, they contain bacteria, dirt, sand, and other debris. Women who use sea sponges have significantly more bacteria, including *Staphylococcus aureus*, in their vagina during their periods than women who wear tampons or pads. And sea sponges are impossible to clean. If someone wanted to design exactly the wrong product to use in the vagina, they'd be hard-pressed to come up with something worse. I mean, air, widthwise expansion, bacteria, encouraging growth of *S. aureus*, and being impossible to clean—that's the royal flush of harmful vaginal poker. In the United States, it's illegal to sell sea sponges for menstrual use, and appropriately so.

The final period hack I want to address is crocheted or knit tampons (Gyno Etsy can be an . . . interesting place). Typically made of cotton, these are advertised as eco-friendly. There is no data on how this cotton might irritate the vagina or affect the growth of bacteria. Also, I'm not sure how crocheting cotton yarn into a tampon shape makes it better than just shoving a ball of yarn into the vagina and leaving the end hanging out. I mean, don't do that, but you get my point. I checked the absorbency of three knit tampons that I purchased from Etsy, and they all absorbed less than 5 ml (0.2 ounce).

If you need any more reason to not use a knit or crocheted tampon, I tried boiling one to see if it could be cleaned, and it fell apart.

Putting It All Together

When the latest myth, about titanium dioxide, made the rounds, I was infuriated. A week or so before that, the period hack about makeup sponges had gone viral, yet no health influencer raised any alarm, and no reporter wrote a story about it. Here was a period product that could pose a *real* health threat, and yet crickets. I guess they think that because an evil tampon company isn't behind it, it must be safe. Or perhaps they just know they won't get page clicks if they can't stoke the conspiracy theory outrage machine.

So how do you figure out what's true and what isn't the next time you hear a menstrual product myth? Because there will be many more to come over the years. Whenever you see a claim about a menstrual product, ask the following questions:

- *What is the source of the claim?* Trust reliable sources like the FDA, the CDC, and Health Canada—organizations that review data about safety—and reject propaganda from health influencers, naturopaths, and functional medicine physicians. The idea that the latter three have "secret knowledge" and know more than the former is laughable.
- *Were the tests conducted on single or multiple samples?* Be wary of sites that post data gathered by sending products away to be tested. They usually send only one sample, and the process isn't vetted in a peer-reviewed publication, so we don't know if the methodology is sound. When products are tested in studies to be published in peer-reviewed journals, multiple samples are usually tested, because there can easily be outliers.
- *Is the Environmental Working Group involved?* The EWG, an activist group that reports on toxic chemicals and pollutants, often overstates risks associated with everyday products (in one survey, 79% of toxicologist felt the EWG overstated risks from chemicals). You may be familiar with their "dirty dozen list" for fruits and vegetables, but a peer-reviewed study that evaluated this list states, "the methodology used to create the 'Dirty Dozen' list does not appear to follow any established scientific procedures."

- *Does the site mention dioxins?* If a site features fearmongering about dioxins in menstrual products, something we have good data on, then it is not invested in the science.
- *Does the claim use conspiracy theory language?* The suggestion that some mysterious and unnamed "they" are hiding something from you is a sure sign that you're looking at a myth. It is possible to pass on concerns about products in ways that don't tie into conspiracy theories.
- *Does it say you shouldn't put a menstrual product in your vagina?* Beware of purity culture as the driver, not science.
- *Does it say chemicals are bad?* From a rhetorical perspective, the word *chemical* is a devil term, meaning you are likely to assign it a negative connotation without any real scientific backing. As a corollary, does the source of the information regularly rail against "dangerous chemicals" and push for "natural" or "organic" products? Remember, so-called natural advocacy is a lucrative business model, so you should not trust it any more than Big Pharma or Big Chemical.
- *Does the site sell or recommend supplements?* Supplements are just untested pharmaceuticals. It is hypocritical to profit from untested products, which are often unsafe, all the while throwing shade at menstrual products with no proof of concern.

Bottom Line

- A tampon, menstrual cup, or menstrual disc cannot affect virginity. Virginity is a social construct, and there are no medical signs of virginity. Fears about vaginal menstrual products are often a product of purity culture.
- Don't get information about menstrual product safety from social media influencers. They're trying to provoke controversy, and stoking the fear machine gives them clicks.
- Tampons don't contain asbestos, the titanium dioxide in tampons is safe, and the dioxins found in tampons and pads are from the soil in which the raw materials are grown.
- Sea sponges, makeup sponges, and crocheted or knit tampons are unsafe and should never be used.
- It's illogical to get worked up over chemicals in tampons while ignoring greater sources of exposure to these and other, more dangerous chemicals.

Part 3

BLEEDING AND PAIN

15

A Primer on Abnormal Bleeding

Bleeding concerns are one of the most common reasons that people with periods seek medical care. During the reproductive years (ages eighteen to forty-five), up to 27 percent of women report abnormal bleeding patterns at some point, and that number rises to more than 75 percent over age forty-five. Whether it's heavy bleeding or irregular bleeding or bleeding between periods, the causes can be serious or not medically concerning. The impact on quality of life can be devastating or barely bothersome. Many people receive excellent health care, but for every person who receives great care, I hear from another one who has been dismissed. So, to make sure you know what is happening to your body, how to tell when you are receiving evidence-based medical care, and how to advocate for yourself when you are not, let's start with a primer on wonky periods, for lack of a better term. In the following chapters, we'll get more granular about the causes.

Menstrual bleeding can be abnormal in many ways and for many reasons. It can be too heavy, too light, too frequent, or too sporadic. Menstruation can even be so infrequent that it seems like it has stopped altogether, and there can be bleeding between periods. Sometimes people might experience many abnormal bleeding patterns at once. It can feel like you are a menstrual Goldilocks, perpetually looking for a mythical "just right."

There are many ways to classify abnormal bleeding. I just described menstruation based on what you might experience—your symptoms. The classification system we use in medicine (and I think it's good to learn this, as then you will know how your medical provider should be approaching your bleeding concerns) divides the causes of abnormal bleeding into two main categories: structural, meaning it's related to something physical that is happening to the uterus, and nonstructural, meaning something is acting upon the uterus to change bleeding. These main types of bleeding are further subdivided into groups using the mnemonic PALM-COEIN. Many articles about this system use photos or illustrations of a palm and a coin (the image usually looks very 1950s), so any magician who happened to stumble across one could be forgiven for thinking they were about to learn a bold new technique for palming a coin. Even though COEIN is spelled differently and neither a palm nor a coin has anything to do with abnormal uterine bleeding, and even though the mnemonic isn't particularly catchy, it seems to work.

The PALM part refers to structural issues that cause bleeding abnormalities:

- *Polyps:* Overgrowths of the endometrium—think of a chunk of uterine lining hanging by a stalk.
- *Adenomyosis:* A condition where the endometrium grows into the muscle of the uterus.
- *Leiomyomas:* Benign tumors of the uterus, also known as fibroids.
- *Malignancy:* Most often cancer of the endometrium, but cancer of the ovary, the muscle of the uterus, the cervix, or even the vagina can also cause abnormal bleeding.

The COEIN part refers to nonstructural causes:

- *Coagulopathy:* A disruption of the blood's ability to clot. This can be caused by a bleeding disorder or by medications.
- *Ovulatory:* Abnormal ovulation, typically infrequent (called oligo-ovulation).
- *Endometrial:* A disturbance in the lining of the uterus, possibly due to local changes in signaling chemicals, injury, infection, or even cancer.
- *Iatrogenic:* Related to medication, most often hormonal contraception. Steroid medications, either pills or injections, are another common

cause. Bleeding related to hormonal contraception is addressed in Chapters 23, 24, and 27.

- *Not otherwise classified:* There are times when we do a full, complete workup to the best of our ability and rule out other causes, but bleeding is still abnormal.

Structural   Nonstructural

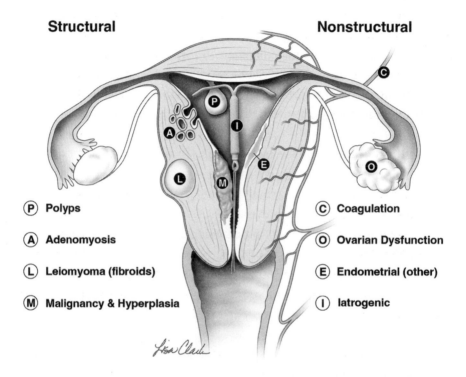

(P) **Polyps**   (C) **Coagulation**

(A) **Adenomyosis**   (O) **Ovarian Dysfunction**

(L) **Leiomyoma (fibroids)**   (E) **Endometrial (other)**

(M) **Malignancy & Hyperplasia**   (I) **Iatrogenic**

Figure 13 • *Causes of Abnormal Menstrual Bleeding (Illustration by Lisa A. Clark, MA, CMI)*

The Basic Biology

Structural issues with the uterus can lead to heavy periods and/or bleeding between periods (intermenstrual bleeding), but they won't change the regularity of the menstrual cycle. Because the frequency of menstruation depends on ovulation, an ovulatory change is the only thing that can alter it. Those are good starting points when you are considering what may be happening with your body. However, there are some caveats (always with the caveats). It's possible to have two medical conditions at the same time, one affecting the uterus and one affecting ovulation. One condition, polycystic ovarian syndrome (PCOS), can cause both heavy and irregular periods. And, to complicate matters further, it can sometimes be challenging to know if your menstruation is regular or not. For example, if you have a regular period but also breakthrough bleeding, it may seem like your period is irregular because it feels like you are bleeding all the time. It's also important to remember that irregular bleeding in the first and the last few years of menstruation is typical. It may still be heavy, and may need to be investigated and treated, but the irregular nature of menstruation during these times is not abnormal but expected.

Whenever someone has a bleeding concern, it's important to start with an open mind about all the potential causes, and then systematically rule out those that are unlikely or impossible and focus on those that are more likely.

What Kind of Bleeding Is Concerning?

Medically typical menstruation is considered to be bleeding that lasts for two to seven days, that occurs every twenty-four to thirty-eight, and where total blood loss is less than 80 ml (2.7 ounces). The medical definition of heavy bleeding is more than 80 ml during a menstrual cycle or bleeding for eight days or longer. It can be hard to quantify blood loss—it's not as if it's convenient to measure—so more practical ways to quantify blood loss as excessive include:

- Blood clots greater than 2 cm (0.7 inch).
- A sensation of gushing during a period.
- Needing to change menstrual products more than every one to two hours.
- Needing to double up on menstrual products.
- Soaking through menstrual products onto clothes or bedsheets.

While more than 80 ml over eight days or more is the strict medical definition, and this is important for studies, newer recommendations are to use a looser definition for heavy bleeding as blood loss that affects quality of life. This is important, as many cultural, social, and practical factors may impact what someone considers too heavy. For example, a fourteen-year-old girl who doesn't feel comfortable with tampons but wants to be on the swim team might want to not have a period at all. A twenty-year-old trans man who isn't taking testosterone might also prefer not to menstruate. A surgeon who operates for long hours might want to be able to make it through a six-hour surgery without leaking onto her clothes. Frankly, given modern medicine, there is no reason anyone needs to have a period if they don't want to, as long as they have an understanding of the risks of the therapy and can place those risks in context. That is the essence of informed care. Basically, if you think your period is too heavy, it is worth evaluating and seeking therapy, should you desire to do so.

I use both definitions in my practice. I ask about signs that blood loss is objectively excessive (such as soaking clothes) *and* ask if blood loss with menstruation is bothersome. I do both because it isn't uncommon for a patient with signs of excessive menstrual blood loss to tell me they are "normal" when asked about menstruation. When I reframe and ask how many days of bleeding, they often respond that it's more than seven days. And when I ask if they ever need to change their pad, tampon, or cup every one to two hours, I often hear, "Oh yes, but just for two days." What my patient means is, compared to their personal standard for their own body, their bleeding is normal. It's even possible they previously mentioned these heavy periods to a medical provider and were dismissed. If you have been told that soaking the bed the first night of your period is normal, and have never spoken with someone else about menstruation in a constructive way, how would you know otherwise?

Light periods that last less than two days are worth discussing with your health care provider. This can be completely normal and not a concern, but it can sometimes signify the start of several medical conditions, so it should be put in context with your health.

What about timing of and irregularity in menstruation? One or two late or early periods or one skipped period is almost never medically concerning (assuming no pregnancy) if you return to a cyclic pattern afterward. If you go ninety days between periods (two skipped periods), that should most certainly prompt a discussion with your medical provider if you are between the ages of eighteen and forty-five. If you are younger than eighteen or older than forty-five, this type of irregularity is expected. Between forty and forty-five is a bit of a gray zone, where the irregularity could be due to either early menopause or a medical condition. Investigation of irregular periods in this age range will depend on other symptoms.

Investigating the Issue

To understand what might be happening to your body and why, the first step is to consider your age, because irregular bleeding is typical in the first few years after the first period and in the last few years before the final period. Age also matters because the risk of endometrial cancer increases with age.

Regarding the bleeding issue, it's important for your health care provider to know if it is a new change or a long-standing problem, and specifically its pattern—whether it's heavy but regular, the same amount of flow but irregular, and so on. A menstrual calendar can be very helpful here. Share any changes in cramping or pelvic pressure or pain too, as some conditions, such as adenomyosis and fibroids, can be associated with a worsening of menstrual cramps. We also need to know if you have had bleeding issues before or are having bleeding issues unrelated to menstruation. For example, if you have had heavy bleeding after surgery, delivery, or dental work, or if you are bruising more easily or bleeding from your gums, share that information, as it raises concerns for a bleeding disorder.

General information about how you are feeling also matters, as well as how much you exercise and any change in stress levels. Some specific symptoms to mention if they apply to you are fatigue, hair loss, acne, increased hair growth on your face, arms, or abdomen, headaches, hot flashes, night sweats, vaginal dryness, and weight loss or gain. If you have a family history of fibroids or endometriosis, share that with your medical provider. And of course it is important to tell them what medications you are taking, including supplements, as some can lead to bleeding issues. If you have been vaccinated against HPV, let them know, as this dramatically lowers the chances of cervical precancer or cancer.

When the amount of blood lost isn't considered urgent, care for abnormal bleeding can often be started by video or phone call, or even via email, but an in-person exam will almost always eventually be needed. It's important to check your blood pressure and heart rate, and a general physical might offer clues for conditions such as polycystic ovarian syndrome or thyroid disorders. A pelvic exam can help identify some structural causes of bleeding, specifically fibroids, adenomyosis, and advanced cancer, and occasionally a large polyp might be seen protruding through the cervix. The exam can also tell us if bleeding is from the cervix rather than the uterus (due to infection, inflammation, or, rarely, cancer), or even from the vaginal walls (due to skin conditions or low estrogen).

Because the risk of all of these conditions, except for infection and inflammation, increases with age, a pelvic exam is less important, and may not even initially be needed, if you are in your teens or early twenties, depending on your bleeding pattern.

When the only concern is an irregular period, it is almost certainly due to an issue with ovulation. There are exceptions to the rule, and whether a pelvic exam is needed will depend on the individual situation. If a pelvic exam is too traumatic, an abdominal ultrasound (see page 201) can often provide a lot of information to get started with.

Think of the medical evaluation as a jigsaw puzzle: the cause of the bleeding is the picture, but when we start assembling the puzzle, we don't know what that final image will look like. Everything we do—the questions we ask, the individual components of a physical exam, and the tests we may order—are puzzle pieces. Sometimes the first few pieces give us a clear picture, but sometimes we need more pieces to see what's going on. Some pieces are more helpful than others, but even a negative test result is a piece of the puzzle, because knowing what you *don't* have is equally important.

Sometimes in medicine we immediately find causes, but other times it's all about learning what people don't have and then working from the short list of what is left and what makes the most sense.

Tests for Abnormal Bleeding

What blood tests you might need will depend on your bleeding issue and are addressed in the next few chapters. A cervical cancer screening should be completed (if it's not already up to date). Screening for gonorrhea and chlamydia is recommended for people under twenty-five and those who are spotting between periods. It's important to rule out pregnancy if sperm has been in, on, or around your body, as bleeding during early pregnancy is common.

An ultrasound is the most common test to evaluate abnormal bleeding; using sound waves, it can provide images of the uterus and ovaries without surgery. It is perhaps the best tool for looking at the ovaries, it is an excellent way to identify fibroids and ascertain the thickness of the endometrium, and it can sometimes detect adenomyosis and polyps. An ultrasound can also locate cysts on the ovaries, which are part of polycystic ovarian syndrome. There are three types of ultrasound tests:

- *Abdominal scan:* The ultrasound transducer, or probe, is placed on the lower abdomen to see the uterus. When the bladder is full, the urine inside it improves the quality of the images, which is why you are asked to have a full bladder if possible. The advantage of an abdominal scan is that a vaginal probe isn't needed, which is more comfortable for most people; the disadvantage is that the quality of the images is often not as good.
- *Vaginal scan:* When an ultrasound probe is inserted in the vagina, the images are typically superior, as the probe can get closer to structures. If an ultrasound is ordered for a gynecological reason, you should assume that a vaginal scan is part of the exam. For some, this procedure isn't uncomfortable or is a minor discomfort, but for others, it can be intrusive, triggering, and painful. If you have had pain with pelvic exams, with inserting a tampon or menstrual cup, or with vaginal penetration during sex, make sure your medical provider knows and tell the ultrasound tech. There are ways to help minimize pain, such as you inserting the ultrasound probe yourself. If it's too painful, then this part of the exam should be skipped and an alternative approach taken to get the necessary information.
- *Saline infusion sonogram (SIS):* A vaginal ultrasound is performed as a small amount of saline (salt water) is inserted into the uterus. Normally, the inside walls of the uterus are collapsed and touching each other; the saline fills the uterus just a little, so the walls separate. This can make it easier to see polyps and fibroids that are close to the uterine lining. A speculum is inserted into the vagina, a thin, soft, flexible catheter is inserted into the uterus through the cervix, and then the speculum is removed and the ultrasound probe is inserted.

A CT scan tends to be less useful for evaluating the uterus, but an MRI can be very helpful in evaluating fibroids and diagnosing adenomyosis. An MRI is painless and involves no radiation, but for some people with claustrophobia, it can be difficult. In that case, options might be antianxiety medication before the procedure or an open-sided MRI.

There are two common procedures that might be performed in the doctor's office: an endometrial biopsy and a hysteroscopy. These tests are used to get a sample of the lining of the uterus for a pathologist to evaluate for precancer, cancer, and signs of infection. With an endometrial biopsy, a thin, straw-like device is inserted into the uterus to collect tissue. The tissue retrieved this way can sometimes suggest a polyp, but an endometrial biopsy can't make that diagnosis very accurately, nor treat it. A hysteroscopy is like a souped-up endometrial biopsy with a camera. Instead of a flexible catheter, a thin operating telescope is used, as well as fluid to distend the uterus (like with the saline infusion sonagram), to allow the doctor to see inside the uterus and, depending on the equipment, remove polyps or direct a biopsy to a specific area of the uterus, and then also do an endometrial biopsy if needed.

Both procedures have advantages and disadvantages. An endometrial biopsy is typically faster, less painful, and less expensive. It can usually be done right away, so is more convenient, but there is no visual component, though it can be combined with a saline infusion sonagram to get more information. The advantage of the hysteroscopy is the visual component, and the ability (again, depending on the setup) to remove a polyp if one is seen—it's a "one and done" procedure. The downsides are more pain, higher cost, and less convenience, as sometimes a hysteroscopy needs to be scheduled at a specific time in the menstrual cycle.

Dilation and curettage is another option for getting a tissue sample from the lining of the uterus—think of it as a more aggressive endometrial biopsy. A D&C is too painful to be performed in the doctor's office; it requires an anesthesia provider and is typically done in a special procedure room or an operating room.

There are many permutations and combinations of testing, and ultimately, the best course of action for an individual patient will depend on many factors.

Pain with Endometrial Biopsy and Hysteroscopy

Pain experiences with endometrial biopsies and hysteroscopies vary from minimal cramping to excruciating pain. I know it may be hard to believe that these procedures can be relatively pain-free or mild for some people, but I'm one of them. I've had two endometrial biopsies and a hysteroscopy, and I thought the endometrial biopsies felt like minimal period cramping for a few minutes. The hysteroscopy was a little more uncomfortable but tolerable, and I went back to seeing patients afterward. On the other hand, I've worked with an OB/GYN who has had these procedures and found the endometrial biopsy so painful that, when she needed a hysteroscopy, she had it done in the operating room with an anesthetic. This is the uniqueness of pain.

In one study, pain with hysteroscopy was divided into two groups: those who found it to be more than a 5 on a scale of 0 to 10 (about 25 percent of people) and those who felt it was a 5 or less (the other 75 percent). Among the 25 percent with more pain, the average score was 7.7. Among the 75 percent with less pain, the average score was 2.2. Pain experiences vary a lot, and we need to give people the pain relief they require.

Pain with both endometrial biopsies and hysteroscopies can arise from many sources, including the speculum in the vagina, the instrument to steady the cervix, the passage of the instrument through the cervix, the uterus cramping in response to the stimulation, and even the uterine lining itself. We used to believe the endometrium didn't have nerve endings, so the actual sampling from the lining shouldn't be painful, but some people find this part excruciating, while others, like me, experience a brief cramp. It turns out that some people have more nerve endings in their endometrium than others, and hence are more likely to find the biopsy painful. People with conditions that cause pain, such as endometriosis and adenomyosis, are more likely to have more nerve fibers and experience pain with biopsy. People who have pain with sex or pelvic pain might also feel more pain during these procedures.

What's the best way to address the pain? It's a good idea to discuss a plan with your health care provider in advance. Knowing the range of experiences might inform the decisions you make about pain control. Options to consider during an endometrial biopsy include a TENS unit (see page 260 for more on these devices), lidocaine (a numbing medication) sprayed on the cervix, liquid lidocaine infused through the cervix into the uterus, NSAIDs (such as ibuprofen or naproxen sodium) or acetaminophen, the pain medication tramadol, and antianxiety medications (a class of drugs called benzodiazepines).

For a hysteroscopy, any of the above options except for liquid lidocaine (as it will be washed out with the fluid needed to fill the uterus) can be tried. A flexible hysteroscopy can be less painful, and sometimes the scope can be inserted without a speculum, which also reduces pain. A medication called misoprostol, given twelve hours before to soften the cervix, can sometimes help. If you are worried about pain or have previously had painful procedures, a hysteroscopy can be performed with an anesthesia provider to safely provide pain relief.

Some people ask about nitrous oxide (aka laughing gas) for pain control—you might be familiar with it from the dentist's office. One study shows that nitrous oxide performs about as well as a lidocaine injection into the cervix, but not all offices are set up to offer this option safely. For some people, it may not be safe to use nitrous oxide without a trained anesthesia provider; for others, it may be a good option where available.

Many people wonder why there aren't better options for pain control. When I trained, we had terrible data and many people suffered, but we have a lot of studies now—though we need more, as not all of them are of the highest quality. But we do now have many things to offer. Part of the issue is that there can be several sources of pain, and for many of them, there aren't really any great therapies. The nerves that supply the uterus (including the cervix) can't be blocked in the office in the same way that you can have a nerve block in the dentist's office to numb a portion of the mouth, so that is a big part of the issue. Also, inserting something through the vagina is far more invasive and triggering for many people than procedures elsewhere in the body .

Bleeding Pattern Bingo

Trying to figure out the cause of your bleeding issues can feel like a game of bleeding pattern bingo. Setting aside some rare causes that are beyond the scope of this book, here is a simplified framework you can use:

Table 4 • COMMON CAUSES OF ABNORMAL BLEEDING

SYMPTOM	COMMON POTENTIAL CAUSES
Heavy periods	Fibroids (leiomyomas), adenomyosis, polyps, PCOS, irregular ovulation, coagulopathy, teenage periods, menopause transition periods, cancer (malignancy)
Irregular periods	Teen periods, menopause transition periods, PCOS, irregular ovulation
Breakthrough bleeding/ mid-cycle bleeding	Polyps, cancer, conditions that affect the endometrium

SYMPTOM	COMMON POTENTIAL CAUSES
Bleeding after sex	Usually from the cervix, so it isn't menstrual bleeding per se; can be caused by chlamydia, inflammation from other causes, or cancer.

The body doesn't know these rules, though. Sometimes we see bleeding patterns that are atypical, for example, breakthrough bleeding with fibroids. At times it's easy to determine the cause of the problem, but sometimes we need to rule out causes one by one and then design therapy around the potential remaining causes.

Bottom Line

- Menstrual bleeding should be considered atypical if:
  - It is shorter than two days or longer than seven.
  - It is irregular for more than two cycles.
  - Ninety days elapse between bleedings.
  - There is bleeding between periods,
    or periods are heavy.
- A short list of likely causes for bleeding issues can often be determined with relatively little information.
- More than one condition can sometimes contribute to bleeding problems.
- An ultrasound can help diagnose many causes of abnormal bleeding but may not always be necessary.
- Sometimes it is necessary to get a sample of tissue from the lining of the uterus, and there are several options for pain control with these procedures.

16

Heavy Periods

Heavy bleeding can be a flow that's too heavy (think super-soaker), one that lasts longer than seven days, or both. It affects 20 to 30 percent of people who menstruate and is one of the most common reasons to see a gynecologist. Unfortunately, some people are dismissed by their health care provider with cringe-worthy platitudes along the lines of "That's the price of being a woman" (I threw up a little in my mouth writing that), with no acknowledgement that they have a real medical issue, which is completely invalidating and infuriating and leads to needless suffering. I touched on heavy bleeding in the previous chapter, and here we're going to take a deeper dive.

Heavy menstrual bleeding can happen anytime during one's menstrual life but is most common within the first few years after the first period and in the last few years before menopause (the menstrual bookends). Not only are heavy periods bothersome (leaking onto your clothes or mattress is a major hassle), but they can also be expensive—consider the cost of menstrual products, extra cleaning, medical appointments, medications, procedures, and missed work. Heavy menstrual bleeding can also lead to social isolation when people miss school or work or miss out on sports or other activities that bring joy. And, of course, the amount of blood loss can also be medically concerning, leading to a low blood count (anemia). I had anemia as a teen, and it led to years of suffering until I got the right therapy. It shouldn't be that way for anyone.

Heavy bleeding can sometimes be catastrophic, even life-threatening. The emergency management of heavy bleeding that might take you to the hospital is beyond the scope of this book.

Getting Started

As discussed in the previous chapter, in medicine we group bleeding concerns into conditions that affect the structure or shape of the uterus versus factors that act on the uterus, such as hormones or medications. Knowing this offers a window into how your medical provider might think, but you're probably not going to call up your doctor and say "Oh, hey, I think I've got a structural problem with team uterus." No, you are going to describe your bleeding pattern, and then your doctor should ask about other symptoms and your health in general. That information, combined with an exam and possibly some tests, will enable them to come up with a short list of causes for the bleeding and then offer therapy. Here we will use the same strategy, with the understanding that some conditions associated with irregular periods and breakthrough bleeding (covered in the next two chapters) can also cause heavy bleeding.

Polyps

A polyp is an overgrowth of the lining of the uterus—basically a chunk of endometrium hanging by a stalk. Polyps can be small, but at times they are so large they protrude through the cervix. The endometrium in a polyp doesn't have supporting tissue or appropriate blood vessels, and there is no surrounding muscle to help squeeze to stop bleeding, so polyps can lead to a variety of disordered bleeding patterns. Heavy bleeding is common, and some people experience bleeding between periods, ranging from spotting to a heavy flow.

We don't really know why polyps develop. It is likely because of a combination of genetics, hormones, and inflammation. If you consider all the cyclic trauma and repair in the endometrium, it doesn't seem far-fetched that some cells might get the wrong repair message and basically wing it, albeit incorrectly. One known cause is the medication tamoxifen, which is prescribed to treat breast cancer. Polyps are usually benign, but as we age there is a higher rate of cancer, and polyps associated with tamoxifen are more likely to be cancerous.

A polyp can sometimes be identified by ultrasound, but because the uterus is essentially collapsed, the polyp can blend in with the endometrium and easily be missed. An endometrial biopsy (a sample from the lining of the uterus) may find fragments of a polyp, which tells us to look for the whole thing and make sure there isn't more than one. If an ultrasound is ordered for heavy bleeding and no polyp is seen but suspicion is high, the next step is a saline infusion sonogram or a hysteroscopy (discussed in the previous chapter).

Treatment is removing the polyp, which is done through the cervix with a hysteroscopy. It's typically an easy procedure and, depending on the size of the polyp and other factors, can often be done in the office, though in some cases it may need to happen in the operating room. The decision about how to remove a polyp requires an individual approach.

Fibroids

Fibroids, known medically as leiomyomas, are benign (noncancerous) tumors of the myometrium. They can cause heavy bleeding and sometimes bleeding between periods, but 50 to 75 percent of fibroids just quietly hang out in the uterus, minding their own business, causing no symptoms. Having one or more fibroids doesn't necessarily mean they're the cause of your abnormal bleeding.

Fibroids are common—by the age of fifty, 70 percent of White women and over 80 percent of Black women will have at least one. They can range from the size of a tiny pebble to a watermelon. Fibroids can cause other health issues besides bleeding concerns. For example, they can aggravate menstrual cramps, and when they are large, they can create a sensation of pressure and even contribute to incontinence. If a fibroid outgrows its blood supply, it can be very painful. Some fibroids can affect fertility and lead to complications during pregnancy. Fibroids are more common as we age, so they are lower down on the list of possible causes of heavy bleeding for someone who is twenty and higher for someone who is forty. However, Black women are more likely to develop fibroids earlier in life, have multiple fibroids, and endure more severe symptoms.

Why do fibroids exist? That's a good question. We believe a fibroid develops when a stem cell in the myometrium gets triggered to divide . . . and then it keeps on dividing in an uncontrolled fashion. (Stem cells are special cells with the ability to turn into many other kinds of cells and are an important part of the body's repair mechanisms.) Think about what happens during pregnancy. Not only must the uterus make new muscle cells in order to grow, it must also be able to repair itself after being invaded by the placenta. Fibroids appear to be a corruption of the normal stem cell growth-and-repair mechanism.

The trigger for this dysregulated stem cell activity is likely a combination of factors. Genetics can play a role, which explains why some people with fibroids have a family history of them. However, new genetic mutations can also lead to fibroids, and these mutations aren't passed along to the next generation. Just because someone has fibroids doesn't mean their children will as well. There is growing evidence that people with fibroids are more likely to have high blood pressure, and the hypothesis is that both fibroids and high blood pressure involve abnormal signaling in smooth muscle, as blood vessels also have smooth muscle. For this reason, someone with fibroids should have their blood pressure checked regularly and, of course, treated if indicated.

Interestingly, fibroids are less common among people who have given birth, and the more pregnancies one has, the lower the risk of fibroids. After pregnancy, the body needs to remove most of the new muscle cells that were created; otherwise, each pregnancy would lead to a significantly larger uterus. It is hypothesized that during this process, potential fibroid seedlings may be jettisoned along with the muscle tissue.

Fibroids don't exist before puberty, and they typically shrink during menopause, so estrogen and progesterone clearly play a role, which may be why fibroids are more common in people who go through puberty earlier—an effect of a longer lifetime exposure to estrogen. Starting the birth control pill before the age of sixteen appears to slightly increase the risk of fibroids (but there's no increased risk for those who are older when they start), while the injectable contraceptive Depo-Provera, which doesn't contain estrogen, lowers the risk. Fibroids themselves can contain the enzyme aromatase, which allows them to convert other hormones into estrogen and essentially produce their own growth serum. Levels of aromatase in fibroids from Black women appear to be higher, which may partially explain their increased risk.

Other factors that may increase the risk of fibroids include:

- *Exposure to endocrine-disrupting chemicals.* For example, there is some evidence linking chemical hair straighteners (which contain these chemicals) with fibroids.

- *Obesity,* possibly because fatty tissue produces estrogen without a compensating increase in progesterone, or possibly because of the increased inflammation associated with obesity, or both.
- *Low levels of vitamin D.* The reason for this correlation isn't known, and there is no definitive evidence that supplementation will help. However, the risk of taking 1,000 IU of vitamin D a day is low, so that may be an acceptable option for people who are concerned about or at higher risk for fibroids, with the understanding that more data is needed.

Smoking cigarettes is associated with a lower incidence of fibroids, possibly because of its anti-estrogenic effect.

Fibroids don't transform into cancer. There is a rare cancer, called leiomyosarcoma, that looks like a fibroid, but the odds of this diagnosis are about one in one thousand or less. In general, if a tumor that appears to be a fibroid is growing more rapidly than expected, that increases the suspicion of this aggressive cancer.

We don't fully understand how fibroids cause abnormal uterine bleeding. There are likely multiple associations. Fibroids affect the uterine "chemical soup," meaning various growth factors, hormones, and inflammatory chemicals that are involved in triggering menstruation, repairing endometrium, and governing the behavior of blood vessels. A local chemical trigger would explain why smaller fibroids can cause devastating bleeding. Fibroids also affect blood flow to the uterus, and the physical presence of a fibroid may distort the endometrium and/or affect how the uterus contracts during menstruation. Although it's difficult to determine whether an individual fibroid is the cause of bleeding issues, fibroids that distort the endometrium and grow into it (submucosal fibroids) and those that are located primarily in the myometrium (myometrial—or intramural—fibroids) are far more likely to be the culprit than those close to the surface of the uterus that grow outwards (subserosal fibroids).

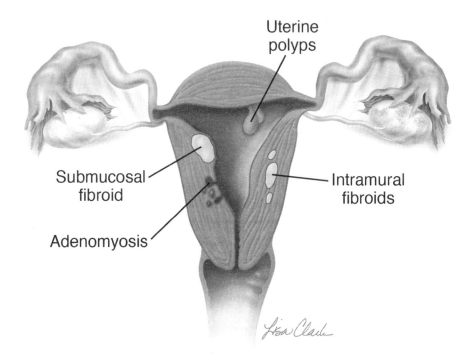

Figure 14 • *The Sources of Abnormal Bleeding: Fibroids, Polyps, and Adenomyosis (Illustration by Lisa A. Clark, MA, CMI)*

How are fibroids diagnosed? If the uterus is enlarged on exam, your health care provider should be suspicious, but sometimes it's not possible to tell with a pelvic exam, or a pelvic exam may not be possible or practical. An ultrasound is the most common way to make the diagnosis. A saline infusion sonogram and/or an MRI may be needed to get a more precise look at the location and size of fibroids, but these tests are usually needed only for planning surgeries and investigating infertility.

Adenomyosis

Adenomyosis is a condition where endometrium grows into the myometrium, causing the uterus to become a little larger. If you have a uterus, you probably intuitively understand why it might be painful to have endometrial cells trapped in the wall of the uterus. There isn't actual bleeding into the uterus (phew, right?), because the trapped cells don't function exactly like endometrium, but there is abnormal inflammation, and that's mayhem enough. Along with inflammation, the trapped endometrium is associated with abnormal blood vessels, which can impact tightly regulated chemical changes and affect how the uterus contracts during menstruation, leading to heavy bleeding. In addition, adenomyosis is associated with pelvic pain, infertility, and an increased risk of miscarriage, as well as pregnancy complications such as premature labor.

There are several theories about how adenomyosis develops. Endometrial tissue may work its way deeper into the muscle because of microtears created by trauma, for example, after delivery or surgery. Essentially, cracks develop that become a channel for the endometrium. Because adenomyosis is rarely seen in teens and increases with age, it's possible that cumulative trauma and inflammation (and yes, that includes "regular" menstruation) play a role. However, we have limited knowledge about adenomyosis in people under the age of thirty-five, and especially among teens and those in their early twenties, because a definitive diagnosis of adenomyosis requires a hysterectomy, and a much smaller percentage of people undergo a hysterectomy at such an early age. It is possible there is more adenomyosis among young people who have never been pregnant than we know.

Another theory is that the normal repair mechanisms of menstruation go awry, and a new, corrupted message instructs the endometrium to burrow too deeply. A third hypothesis is that cells left over from fetal development might remain dormant but trapped like little seeds in the myometrium, waiting to be triggered by trauma, inflammation, hormones, genetics, or something we don't yet understand. Endometrial tissue is quite industrious and can produce its own estrogen (I think of it as an overachiever, determined to prepare itself for pregnancy wherever it finds itself), so regardless of how these cells find themselves in the muscle of the uterus, they are determined to make it work.

It's interesting that repetitive injury, from menstruation and/or pregnancy, and the ability of the uterus to repair itself are involved in both fibroids and adenomyosis. The fact that these conditions become more common over the menstrual life span and appear to peak in the forties, suggests that the end of ovarian function (meaning menopause) ties in neatly with the uterus reaching the limit of its ability to incessantly repair itself. Many people wonder about extending ovarian function, but even if we could find a way to extend the life span of follicles and hence delay menopause, what would that mean for the uterus? What would fibroids or adenomyosis be like with ten or fifteen more years of ovulation? Menopause ends fertility, but it also ends fibroids and adenomyosis—painful and even disabling medical conditions that are essentially a side effect of the reproductive machinery over time. To have a uterus and ovaries is to walk the line between the potential for reproduction and trauma, and that can only go on for so long.

Ultrasound can sometimes, but not always, pick up changes that look like adenomyosis. The biggest role of ultrasound is to rule out other causes of heavy periods, especially fibroids. Adenomyosis can often be seen on an MRI scan, but an MRI is not essential to start treatment, as the first-line thera-pies are essentially the same as for fibroids. An MRI might be helpful if surgery is considered. Ultimately, a firm diagnosis can be made only with a biopsy of the uterus, but this is not recommended for a variety of technical reasons: it's difficult to do and the biopsy may miss the areas affected, giving a false impression the tissue is normal. Often a hysterectomy is performed for heavy bleeding with suspected adenomyosis, and then the diagnosis is confirmed after the fact, when the pathologist looks at the tissue under the microscope.

Blood-Clotting Concerns

When you injure a blood vessel, whether by skinning your knee or as part of menstruation, you trigger the coagulation cascade, a sequence of chemical reactions that combine to stop the bleeding. There are many steps in this process—so many that coagulation, or clotting, is one of the most complex things to learn in medicine, right up there with metabolism. In a nutshell, chemical signals trigger the injured blood vessel to squeeze, platelets become sticky and plug the opening, and fibrin (which can be thought of as glue) is produced. Fibrin plugs holes between the platelets and stabilizes them, allowing them to hold fast while the blood vessel repairs itself. (Understand this is a *very* simplified version of the process.) When any one of the steps is disrupted, the ability to stop bleeding is impaired. For example, bleeding disorders can arise if there are abnormalities in one of the many proteins required to form fibrin, if there aren't enough platelets, or if abnormal inflammation affects the blood vessel repair process.

There are several blood clotting conditions associated with heavy periods. The most common is von Willebrand disease (VWD), which is a deficiency of a protein needed for blood to clot. VWD is genetic, meaning it's inherited, and it's the most common bleeding disorder, affecting 1 percent of the population. VWD should be suspected if you have had heavy bleeding since your first period; in this situation, VWD is found in up to 24 percent of people.

A variety of medical conditions, including liver disease, kidney disease, and lupus, can interfere with the blood's ability to clot, as can certain medications, such as prescription blood thinners. Aspirin, a common over-the-counter medication, stops platelets from working and increases the risk of bleeding for about three weeks after you stop taking it. My dad used to feed me aspirin like candy for my painful and already heavy periods, and while it did help the pain a little in the short term, looking back I wonder how much it worsened my bleeding. Supplements such as garlic, gingko biloba, and vitamin E can also impair blood clotting.

A blood clotting issue should be considered if your periods have always been heavy, but also if you have other signs of abnormal bleeding—such as easy bruising, nosebleeds, or a history of excessive bleeding after dental work, after childbirth, or during surgery—or if you have a medical condition or are taking any medications that can affect blood clotting. Blood tests are the only way to identify a bleeding disorder.

Heavy Bleeding at the Menstrual Bookends

Although heavy bleeding is common in the first few years after the first period, that doesn't mean the blood loss is normal. The two most common causes are irregular ovulation and bleeding disorders (with VWD being the most common). Irregular ovulation can lead to heavy periods because the repair mechanisms and inflammation that are essential to stop bleeding each cycle are dependent on the normal sequence of hormones. Ovulation may be irregular for teens even when periods seem regular. About 30 percent of teens with heavy bleeding have a bleeding disorder, so blood testing is recommended. Regardless of the cause, the heavy bleeding should be treated.

Heavy bleeding is also common during the menopause transition, likely initially due to subtle changes in hormone levels affecting the endometrium, and then eventually caused by skipped ovulation. In many ways, it's a similar physiological process to the first few years of menstruation. ("Puberty is so nice, let's do it twice," said no one.) In addition, as we age, we are more likely to accumulate fibroids and adenomyosis.

Other Causes of Heavy Bleeding

Endometriosis is associated with heavier periods, likely due to inflammation, but subtle changes in hormones may also play a role. With endometriosis, periods are typically painful, so if adenomyosis is being considered as a potential cause, then endometriosis should be too. Thyroid abnormalities—both hypothyroidism and hyperthyroidism (an under- or overactive thyroid)—can both lead to heavy bleeding, so testing for these is usually recommended.

Obesity is also linked with heavy bleeding. Fatty tissue produces estrogen, which stimulates the uterine lining, as well as a variety of bioactive chemicals and inflammation, which can affect hormones and how the lining of the endometrium repairs. In addition, obesity is a risk factor for cancer of the uterus, which can sometimes cause heavy bleeding. Unfortunately, because of fatphobia, many people have their heavy periods dismissed as being weight-related without an evaluation for all the other potential causes. That is unacceptable. Although weight may play a role for some, everyone with heavy bleeding should be evaluated for all possible contributing factors.

Sometimes, even after a thorough evaluation, we fail to identify a cause for heavy menstrual bleeding, which is frustrating. In these cases, the abnormal bleeding may be due to minor fluctuations in hormones and/or inflammation that we don't yet have the technology to detect.

Tests for Heavy Bleeding

The testing to evaluate the cause of your heavy bleeding will depend on many factors, including your age; whether your periods have always been heavy or if this is new; whether there is reason to be concerned about a clotting disorder; your risk factors for endometrial cancer; whether your periods are irregular; and your other medical conditions, to name a few. In some cases, it may be appropriate to start treatment without much testing; in others, several tests may be needed first. Testing and treatment can also occur simultaneously. At a minimum, most people with heavy bleeding should have these two blood tests:

- *Complete blood count (CBC):* Also called a full blood count, this test for anemia essentially evaluates the amount of blood you have. It also tells us the number of platelets, which is important information for diagnosing bleeding disorders. The CBC helps you and your health care provider understand how urgent treatment is—how fast you need to stop the bleeding, from a medical perspective.

- *Ferritin:* Your ferritin level is a marker of how much iron is in your body. Because blood contains iron, menstrual blood loss is a cause of iron deficiency, and iron levels often drop before anemia develops. Not only is a low ferritin level an early warning sign of excessive blood loss, even without anemia low iron can cause fatigue, hair loss, and other symptoms. Iron deficiency is common; a recent study tells us that it affects almost 40 percent of American girls and women ages 12 to 21 years.

Other blood tests that your doctor may consider are:

- *Tests for a suspected bleeding disorder:* These include prothrombin time (PT) or international normalized ratio (INR)—different ways of looking at the same aspect of blood—partial thromboplastin time (PTT), and fibrinogen. If VWD or another bleeding disorder is suspected, there are specific tests for those. A consultation with a hematologist (a specialist in blood) may be a good idea, to ensure the correct tests are ordered. Ideally, these tests will be performed before you start hormonal contraception, which can affect their accuracy. In some cases, tests to evaluate the health of the liver and kidneys may be recommended, as liver and kidney disease can affect blood clotting.
- *Thyroid-stimulating hormone (TSH):* A test of this marker for thyroid function may be indicated to rule out thyroid conditions as a cause for the abnormal bleeding.

Many people wonder about checking their levels of estrogen and progesterone, but that doesn't typically help when it comes to heavy bleeding. A high estradiol level doesn't tell us if bleeding will be heavy or light. While the progesterone level in the second half of the cycle can inform us whether someone has ovulated, it reflects only what happened in that cycle; it is rarely, if ever, helpful in diagnosing the cause of heavy bleeding when periods are regular.

Other tests that may be indicated include an ultrasound, a saline infusion sonagram, and an endometrial biopsy to rule out cancer (more on that in the next chapter).

Therapy for Heavy Bleeding

Determining the best treatment for an individual isn't possible without knowing more about the person, their medical condition, and their test and ultrasound results, if those are needed. Also, different people have different treatment goals. Some might be happy with a 25 percent reduction in blood loss, while others want all bleeding to stop. Some want to preserve the option of pregnancy and others don't. For some conditions, there are multiple therapies; for others, we have only a few treatments, or even just one. For example, polyps require removal, but there are several options for fibroids.

One simple, inexpensive, yet underused therapy for heavy bleeding is non-steroidal anti-inflammatory drugs (NSAIDs)—think ibuprofen and naproxen. I feel this option is so underused it is almost fair to say it's a period hack "they" don't want you to know. These drugs work on prostaglandins and can reduce menstrual flow by 25 to 35 percent, and they are also helpful in reducing pain with periods. They work best if they can be started a day before menstruation begins and are then taken regularly for two to three days. The dose to reduce bleeding is higher than the typical over-the-counter (OTC) dose. For example, with ibuprofen, the OTC tablets are 200 mg, but the dose for heavy bleeding is 600 to 800 mg every eight hours. While NSAIDs do have a minor impact on platelet function, this is counterbalanced by their anti-inflammatory effect, and the net result is a reduction in blood flow. Not everyone can take NSAIDs; if you have a bleeding disorder such as VWD, have a stomach ulcer, and/or have had bariatric surgery, you should avoid them.

Another "on demand" medication, meaning one that you take just when you are bleeding, is tranexamic acid, which reduces bleeding by slowing the body's breakdown of blood clots. It is taken three times a day for five days, and most people have what is considered a "clinically meaningful reduction in bleeding," which is medical-speak for "people think this really helps." Another bonus is that it can be used by most people who can't take NSAIDs, even those who have VWD. While tranexamic acid requires a prescription in the United States and Canada (as of 2023), it's sold over the counter in many countries, including the United Kingdom, Sweden, and India. I hear awful stories in the United States of people scrambling to get a prescription and insurance approval every month, and it shouldn't be that way. My impression is that it's underused in the United States, but it's taken by 1 percent of women of reproductive age in Sweden, and I bet lack of OTC access plays a role in this disparity. I also wonder if some health care providers in the United States don't offer it because it's used in the hospital for severe bleeding (for example, during surgery), and I suspect some erroneously think of heavy periods as "not serious." (Heavy emphasis on *erroneously*.)

There is a theoretical concern that tranexamic acid could increase the risk of dangerous blood clots in the legs or lungs, but most studies haven't shown this to be true. In one study where tranexamic acid was used to prevent post-partum bleeding, over ten thousand women received the drug and there was no corresponding increase in blood clots. Considering that people are at the greatest risk for blood clots during the postpartum period, this research is very reassuring. Data from Sweden, where tranexamic acid has been sold over the counter for more than twenty years, also offers no suggestion of increased risk. However, in a recent review from Denmark, researchers tracked the records of women prescribed tranexamic acid and found a small increased risk of blood clots: for every 78,549 women who take the medication for five days, one might have a blood clot. To be clear, given the nature of this study, we don't know if this result was a true effect or an artifact of the study; given how rare the risk is, proving it either way is almost impossible with a clinical trial (the gold standard for detecting this kind of issue).

What does this mean for you? Most studies show no increased risk, but if there is one, it is likely very low. People should be reassured that tranexamic acid is a safe medication. Someone who has had a blood clot shouldn't take it, and people otherwise at higher risk for clots should discuss it with their doctor first. It's unclear whether tranexamic acid further increases the risk of blood clots for people who are also taking birth control pills, and while in general it's believed to be low-risk in this situation, it is something to talk over with your medical provider.

There are a variety of hormonal contraception options that can stop or reduce bleeding, such as the IUD and the pill. They work primarily because they include a class of hormones called progestins, which are synthetic versions of progesterone. Continuous exposure to a progestin results in a thin endometrium, so not only is there less lining to come out, fewer chemical mediators are released to trigger menstruation, meaning there is less bleeding from blood vessels. When the hormones are used daily with no break, there is no progesterone withdrawal, so no trigger for menstruation. A progestin can also be used by itself, rather than as part of hormonal contraception. It can be taken daily or just during the luteal phase, but it tends to be less effective at controlling bleeding when taken this way. Progestins can also be taken by people who want to delay a period in order to avoid bleeding at a specific time, for example, on vacation.

The IUD is probably the most effective of the hormonal options. The advantage is a high dose of the hormone in the uterus, where you need it, and a lower dose in the blood. The biggest potential issue is that an IUD may not fit in the uterus of someone with fibroids, so it's obviously a case-by-case solution. The pill works well for many people and can be taken daily to eliminate a period altogether. A bonus of Depo-Provera is that it can also prevent fibroids. The birth control implant is less effective at controlling bleeding and isn't typically recommended for this purpose.

With hormonal methods, the reduction in blood loss tends to increase over time, so bleeding after one year may be much better than after two to three months. These medications can also be used by people with VWD. Their individual benefits and risks are addressed in later chapters.

Another hormonal option is gonadotropin-releasing medications—GnRH antagonists and agonists—which stop the release of follicle-stimulating hormone from the pituitary. The follicles that show up to start each menstrual cycle after their almost year-long journey in the ovary get no stimulation from FSH, no estrogen is produced, and estrogen levels drop like they do in menopause, stopping bleeding. GnRH antagonists are preferred for this use, as they are taken orally and work faster than agonists. Both are typically combined with a small amount of estrogen and a progestin to prevent the symptoms and health considerations of early menopause without triggering bleeding. GnRH medications are primarily used for fibroids, either to shrink them before surgery or as a longer-term therapy to keep them from growing when surgery isn't desired or isn't an option. They can also be invaluable for preventing heavy menstrual bleeding during cancer therapy, as some cancers and chemotherapy can seriously impact blood clotting, leading to catastrophic bleeding. In addition, some data suggests that GnRH agonists can protect the ovaries from the toxic effects of chemotherapy, meaning they are more likely to recover function down the road, once the chemotherapy is stopped.

GnRH medications get a bad rap on social media, and I've even seen some doctors promote conspiracy theories about them, just as we see with vaccines. (Often these doctors profit from people not taking GnRH medications.) While it is true that GnRH medications can create all the side effects of a rapid meno-pause, which can be awful, those effects can be lessened significantly with the right medication. For many people, these medications are an excellent way to stop bleeding quickly, allowing for some breathing room to make decisions about a longer-term strategy. They can also be an important part of care for those who can't or don't want to have surgery. No one should feel forced to use GnRH medications, but lies about how they work or how they were approved are not any kind of answer.

In addition to medications, there are a number of procedures that may help reduce heavy bleeding. Here is a rundown of the procedures you might consider in consultation with your doctor:

- *Endometrial ablation:* This procedure, which involves burning the lining of the uterus, is ideally suited for people with heavy periods of undetermined cause or heavy bleeding in the menopause transition, but it may also be helpful for small fibroids and possibly for adenomyosis. An endometrial biopsy is essential beforehand, to rule out cancer. Endometrial ablation does not provide contraception, and when pregnancies do happen afterward, there is a high rate of serious complications, meaning future pregnancies are contraindicated. It's often discussed online as a "miracle procedure" we OB/GYNs are "keeping from you." The reality is that an endometrial ablation can reduce bleeding for many people, but it tends to be more effective for people forty-five years and older. It performs about as well as a hormonal IUD, from a bleeding perspective. It may not always be an option for someone with fibroids, depending on their size and location.
- *Myomectomy:* The surgical removal of a fibroid or fibroids, this procedure can sometimes be done with a hysteroscope (an operating telescope through the cervix), but it often requires what most people think of as traditional surgery, meaning the fibroids are removed through the belly. However, it can almost always be performed with laparoscopy (keyhole surgery), so the incisions are small and the surgery is minimally invasive. The best approach depends on the location and size of the fibroids. The chances someone will need more therapy for fibroids down the road after a myomectomy is between 10 and 25 percent, likely because of

fibroid seedlings that can't be seen at the time of surgery and subsequently grow. Depending on the location of the fibroid(s), a myomectomy may have implications for a future pregnancy.

- *Uterine artery embolization:* In this procedure, tiny particles of a special material are injected into the blood vessels that supply a fibroid, blocking its blood supply, which causes the fibroid to slowly die and hence shrink. The drop in blood supply causes a lot of inflammation, which can be extremely painful, so pain control is required. This procedure is typically done for fibroids but is being investigated for bleeding due to adenomyosis.

- *Fibroid ablation:* There are two different techniques for selectively targeting and destroying fibroid tissue. One uses ultrasound waves guided by an MRI scanner; the other uses radio frequency waves guided by ultrasound.

- *Hysterectomy:* A total hysterectomy—meaning removal of the entire uterus, including the cervix—is the only way to stop menstrual bleeding 100 percent. With a supracervical hysterectomy (often called a subtotal hysterectomy), the cervix is left behind, and a small amount of endometrium can sometimes remain attached to the cervix and can continue to menstruate. This is a subpar result if the goal is to eliminate bleeding altogether. There are different ways to perform a hysterectomy, but when possible, a vaginal hysterectomy is the preferred route. It isn't always possible if the uterus is enlarged with fibroids or for other reasons, such as scar tissue. There is no medical advantage to leaving the cervix, and studies show sexual function is the same whether or not the cervix is removed. The disadvantages of leaving the cervix behind are the risk of bleeding and the need for ongoing cervical cancer screening and treatment if testing is abnormal.

Bottom Line

- Heavy menstrual bleeding affects 20 to 30 percent of people who menstruate.
- Fibroids are the most common cause of heavy menstrual bleeding. Each fibroid develops from a single stem cell in the uterus.
- Adenomyosis is a condition where the lining of the uterus grows into the muscle. It is often associated with both heavy periods and painful periods.
- Anyone who has had heavy periods since they first started menstruating should be evaluated for conditions that affect the ability of the blood to clot.
- There are many treatment options for heavy bleeding. No one should suffer and go without therapy.

17

Bleeding Bingo: When Periods Stop, When They Become Irregular, and Breakthrough Bleeding

Sometimes it seems menstruation runs like the trains: "Schedule? What schedule?" Track changes, delays, cancellations—you name it! The causes of this menstrual chaos range from medically not concerning (although possibly personally problematic) to very serious. Unfortunately, many people who approach health care providers with menstrual concerns are dismissed or are given no real explanation about what is happening to their body. Often they are offered only one therapy, but people like, and deserve, choices where possible. It's not uncommon for me to hear about months or even years of menstrual disturbances and to have my patient or friend shrug their shoulders when I ask what they have been told by medical providers. That has got to change.

Finding Order in Chaos

There are many permutations and combinations when it comes to being off track schedule-wise, so how do you even begin to approach the issue?

It's a bit like an Impressionist painting. The individual cycle is just a dot of paint, but when you step back, you get a better view. Here, if we step back, we can see there are three main types of scheduling dysfunction: periods that stop, periods that are irregular, and breakthrough bleeding (meaning bleeding between periods). Understanding that there can be overlap (I know, always with the exceptions), once you know the basic pattern or patterns, you can start with what is most likely to be the top cause and then work from there.

As discussed in previous chapters, a normal menstrual cycle can ebb and flow from cycle to cycle by seven days in either direction, meaning one cycle may be twenty-five days and the next thirty, and this is of no medical concern. In general, we recommend a medical evaluation in the following situations:

- No period for ninety days.
- Periods that are outside of the twenty-four to thirty-eight day range for three cycles.
- Breakthrough bleeding.
- Bleeding after sex.

A few caveats:

- This chapter is primarily about periods that started and then problems developed. Periods that never started are a different matter and are beyond our scope.
- Hormonal contraception can cause periods to stop or to be irregular, and can cause breakthrough bleeding, and that is addressed in the chapters on contraception.
- Pregnancy obviously stops periods, but abnormal bleeding in pregnancy can be mistaken for menstruation. I didn't think I was pregnant because I was bleeding when I expected, but that was implantation bleeding . . . and I was pregnant with triplets! And yes, I'd been an OB/GYN for eight years at that point. It's always important to rule out pregnancy, especially when skipped or abnormal periods are relatively new. If you don't partner with someone who makes sperm, then this isn't part of the equation.
- Polyps, fibroids, and bleeding disorders were discussed in the previous chapter, and while irregular bleeding and breakthrough

bleeding are not "classic" for these conditions, lots of people have a uterus that hasn't read the gynecological literature. Symptoms are sometimes atypical, so these causes should always be considered.

- Polycystic ovarian syndrome (PCOS) is the most common cause of irregular bleeding. Because it affects so much more than bleeding, it has its own chapter, coming up next.

- Irregular bleeding for the first few years after your period starts and the last few years before it ends is typical, but it is still worth mentioning to your health care provider, because your personal medical history might change what we think about your irregular bleeding.

- This chapter will cover the most common causes of bleeding chaos. There are, of course, other conditions that are less common, and depending on your medical situation, those may also need to be considered.

Functional Hypothalamic Amenorrhea

Functional hypothalamic amenorrhea (FHA) is a condition where periods stop because of changes in the hypothalamus, the first "brain" in the brain-brain-ovary connection. Gonadotropin-releasing hormone (GnRH) release is diminished, resulting in a domino effect on the pituitary, reducing follicle-stimulating hormone (FSH) and luteinizing hormone (LH). Consequently, the follicles in the ovary receive no signal to develop, and as a result, no estrogen is produced and there is no menstruation. When periods stop, about 20 to 35 percent of the time the cause is FHA.

The triggers for FHA are disordered eating (including fasting, purging, a very low calorie intake, and eating disorders), weight loss, low body fat, excessive exercise, and psychological stress, which can all impact the chemical signaling required for the menstrual cycle. However, it's important to know that many people who have FHA are in what is considered a medically normal weight range. Genetic factors are also likely involved, meaning some people are more susceptible to these chemical changes than others.

Although one or two missed cycles isn't problematic, it's a different story when menstruation stops for years, or even a few months, because in this situation when menstruation stops, so does production of estrogen. A major concern is that the low estrogen of FHA might affect peak bone mass. We build bone until age twenty-seven or twenty-eight, then gradually draw on that bone bank for the rest of our lives. If FHA interferes with building the bone bank, it could increase the risk of osteoporosis. It's not yet known if FHA might have an impact on heart health like primary ovarian insufficiency. Additional consequences of FHA are infertility and vaginal dryness.

FHA should be considered whenever periods stop and when they are infrequent, especially when they are light. When someone has a lower weight and/or body mass index (BMI) and/or does intense physical training or has been exposed to a lot of stress, that adds to the suspicion. Blood tests will show low levels of both FSH and estradiol (and, of course, there should be no other cause for the stopped periods—so tests to rule out thyroid disorders, elevated prolactin, and diabetes are typically recommended). If someone with FHA has gone more than six months without a period, they need a bone density test to better understand their risk for osteoporosis.

The treatment for FHA involves targeting the cause, and that may not be easy. Working with a psychologist and cognitive behavioral training may help with stress. A registered dietician can help you understand what you need to eat to have enough fuel for menstruation. If you have an eating disorder, experts in this area can be invaluable.

Estrogen is also needed, to protect bone health. The preferred method used to be estrogen-containing birth control pills—they were easy, offered a significant amount of estrogen, and provided contraception to those who needed it, because even though ovulation is infrequent or temporarily absent, it can still happen with FHA, and pregnancy is possible. However, newer research suggests that, for people with FHA, oral ethinyl estradiol (the most common estrogen in the pill), and quite likely oral estrogens overall, increases the level of insulin-like growth factor 1 (IGF-1), which can interfere with bone development. (People who don't have FHA who are taking the pill do not experience this adverse effect.) Currently, the preferred way to replace estrogen is transdermal estradiol, typically a 100 μg patch, which provides the average level of estradiol released throughout the cycle. It's enough to protect bones, it doesn't increase IGF-1, and it doesn't increase the risk of blood clots. For people with a uterus, estrogen needs to be given with progesterone or a progestin (usually for twelve days a month) to prevent endometrial cancer. Transdermal estradiol in this dose isn't high enough to inhibit ovulation in most cases, and so if menstruation restarts that indicates the underlying issue is improving. The disadvantage of transdermal estradiol is that it provides no contraception for those who need it. When reversible contraception is needed, the copper IUD is the ideal choice, as its lack of hormones means you'll know when menstruation starts up.

The next best option is transdermal estradiol and a levonorgestrel IUD, as the hormones in the IUD will protect the uterus and provide contraception; the disadvantage is that the hormones in the IUD typically stop periods, so you can't rely on the return of periods to gauge improvement.

If an IUD is not an acceptable option for you, estrogen-containing contraception is another possibility, though it's less ideal from a medical perspective. You could try either the newer pill with estradiol valerate, which is closely related to estradiol (the main circulating natural estrogen), or the vaginal contraceptive ring, which avoids the oral route. I want to be clear: these methods are unstudied for FHA, but theoretically they may have less of an impact on IGF-1 than traditional estrogen-containing birth control pills.

Condoms are always an option for contraception, and for someone who is seeking out irreversible contraception, surgical sterilization is a possibility.

Relative Energy Deficiency in Sport

Relative energy deficiency in sport (RED-S), is a condition caused by low energy availability, meaning there are insufficient calories for the body to maintain health and function appropriately. From a menstrual standpoint, this can show up as infrequent periods or periods that stop, but there are widespread and serious implications beyond the uterus and ovaries. RED-S may be most known for harming bone health, but it's important to know that it can also affect many organ systems including the heart, the immune system, muscles, and the brain. RED-S can occur in men, but female athletes are at greater risk.

RED-S is a type of hypothalamic amenorrhea, but the cause here is energy deprivation—basically, you are burning more calories than you are taking in. The body needs a certain amount of energy to reproduce, and when that energy isn't forthcoming, it signals the hypothalamus to shut down reproduction: just like with HFA, GnRH is diminished, reducing FSH and LH and hence estrogen. The blood tests that confirm the diagnosis indicate low levels of FSH and estradiol. RED-S has the same consequences as FHA, although bone health appears to be at even greater risk.

The factors that go into assessing the severity of RED-S include energy intake (dietary restrictions or the presence of an eating disorder), BMI, age of first period, regularity of menstruation, bone density score, and history of stress fractures. Age of first period matters because when RED-S starts early, as it can for middle school and high school athletes, it can delay the onset of the first period. When this happens, there may be an even greater impact on bone health. Assessing the severity of RED-S is important in deciding on therapy, but also in determining if it is safe to continue training. One unique issue with RED-S is the fact that athletics may be a part of scholarships or be a career, and there are typically coaches and other professionals involved in training who need to be on board with the diagnosis and treatment.

Although any athlete can be affected, the risk seems highest for runners and dancers, possibly because low levels of body fat are desirable in those sports.

It's especially important to identify RED-S among teens, because fewer than six periods in a year at a young age can have an impact on maximum bone density. Screening for RED-S is why it's legitimate for schools to insist on medical clearance from a health care provider for sports. While it is appropriate for medical providers to ask about menstruation so they can determine whether it's physically safe to keep training at the same level, this information should not go to anyone else. People should be cleared or not cleared for sports—the school or government doesn't need to know the reason. Frighteningly, in Florida, the High School Athletic Association proposed mandatory reporting of menstrual cycles. In a country where abortion is legal and the government has no interest in regulating the comings and goings of the uterus, that might be a good way to monitor the impact of RED-S on a population level and provide an impetus for government-level initiatives to raise awareness and for legislation to protect female athletes from coaches and programs that seek to abuse them through inappropriate training. In a place like the United States, where abortion and sometimes even miscarriage can be criminalized, menstrual history could become a weapon for prosecution. Fortunately, after a justifiable uproar, the requirement for mandatory reporting of menstrual history was scrapped by Florida in early 2023. When reproductive health can be criminalized, it's simply not acceptable or safe for the government to have access to your menstrual history.

The management of RED-S is the same as for FHA, meaning transdermal estradiol and oral progesterone, with the addition of correcting the energy imbalance. Involving a physician and a registered dietician who specialize in the needs of athletes and/or an exercise physiologist can be helpful.

Can RED-S be diagnosed if you are on the pill? It's a good question.

Bleeding on the pill is triggered by the hormones in the medication, not hormones from ovulation. If you take the pill every day and don't get a period, that's to be expected and is not medically concerning, but now menstruation can't be used to identify someone at risk of RED-S. Similarly, if you take the pill 21 days on and 7 days off, the resulting menstruation isn't something that is reassuring about energy balance. This is important information for athletes, their health care providers, and coaches to know, so they don't misread the bleeding pattern in either direction. Levels of FSH are low with hormonal birth control, so they can't be used to make a diagnosis of RED-S (or FHA, for that matter), although a hormonal IUD typically doesn't impact FSH when it has been in place for longer than a year. Without periods to follow or an accurate FSH level to check, what to do? Risk of RED-S and need for contraception both require consideration, although the concern with an estrogen-containing contraceptive and RED-S is greater than with HFA, as the risk to bone health is greater with RED-S. Depo-Provera is definitely not recommended when RED-S is suspected, as it is associated with a lower bone mass.

If RED-S is suspected based on weight, training, or caloric intake or for any other reason, bone density should be checked, and that may help make a diagnosis for someone taking hormonal contraception. If the diagnosis is uncertain, then stopping hormonal contraception to monitor menstruation will likely be recommended. If periods don't restart after two months, then blood tests for RED-S can be done. However, if menstruation returns in two months or the test results are normal, that isn't necessarily an "all clear," as people with RED-S can have four or six periods a year. A longer time off hormones may be needed to make the diagnosis. In the meantime, if contraception is needed, non-hormonal methods are recommended. The finer details of diagnosing and managing RED-S in this situation are beyond our scope here.

Primary Ovarian Insufficiency

Primary ovarian insufficiency (POI) is a condition where ovulation, and hence menstruation, stops before the age of forty. It affects 1 percent of women. When I was in medical school, this condition was called premature ovarian failure or premature menopause, both of which are unacceptable terms. First, the word *failure* is awful here. It implies judgment, and women are judged enough already, thank you very much. Also, it's not as if the ovaries took a test and failed, you know? Finally, POI is not the same as menopause—for example, menopause is permanent, but up to 50 percent of people with POI will ovulate sporadically.

Diagnosing POI is important for several reasons. First, there are health concerns. The early drop in estrogen increases the risk of cardiovascular disease (heart attack and stroke), dementia, and osteoporosis. There is also a greater risk of anxiety and depression, as well as bothersome symptoms such as hot flashes, night sweats, insomnia, and vaginal dryness. Finally, POI can cause infertility.

For most people, the cause of POI is unknown and is probably related to many factors, but causes can include:

- Genetic reasons, which may have other health implications, so it's important to speak with a genetic counselor if you are diagnosed with POI.
- Autoimmune conditions, such as type 1 diabetes, lupus, and rheumatoid arthritis. POI can be an early sign of a rare and serious autoimmune disorder of the adrenal gland called autoimmune adrenal insufficiency. If the diagnosis of POI is confirmed, testing for autoimmune adrenal insufficiency is essential.
- Some forms of chemotherapy and radiation to the pelvis, as they can damage the primordial follicles in the ovary.
- Infections such as HIV, mumps, and tuberculosis.
- Smoking, because various toxins in cigarette smoke seem to damage the follicles. Some of these toxins can even be identified in the follicles.
- A hysterectomy, even though the ovaries are not removed, because of the postsurgical inflammation and changes to blood flow. Some surgeries on the ovary can also damage follicles.

Blood tests are needed to confirm POI. Estradiol levels will be low and FSH levels high. POI is the only menstrual condition that causes high FSH. The treatment for POI is the same as for FHA: estrogen replacement and a progestin (progestogen or progesterone) to protect the lining of the uterus, and transdermal estrogen is likely the best option for bone health.

For those who want to learn more about this condition, there is an entire chapter on POI in *The Menopause Manifesto*.

Endometrial Cancer

The prevalence of cancer of the endometrium is increasing rapidly. Each year in the United States almost as many women die of endometrial cancer as of ovarian cancer, yet it seems we rarely hear about it. There are several types. The most common, called endometrioid cancer, can be caused by exposure to estrogen when there is insufficient progesterone. Estrogen does not affect the risk of non-endometrioid cancer, which is more aggressive. Black women are at higher risk for non-endometrioid cancer.

Factors that increase the risk of endometrial cancer are conditions where the body doesn't make enough progesterone to counteract the estrogen, such as polycystic ovarian syndrome; taking estrogen without a progesterone or progestin; the drug tamoxifen; type 2 diabetes; and smoking. Risk increases with age, and genetic factors are involved in some endometrial cancers.

Obesity is a significant risk factor and is estimated to play a role in 40 percent of these cancers, and while BMI is a screening tool and not a good metric for health, it is important to know that a BMI greater than 40 is associated with a sevenfold increased risk of endometrial cancer. There are a variety of biochemical reasons, including the fact that fatty tissue produces estrogens; ovulation may be irregular, meaning enough progesterone is not being produced; and there is an association with insulin resistance and excess inflammation, both of which can encourage abnormal growth in cells. Understanding if you are at increased risk is important, as hormonal therapies can significantly lower the risk.

Bleeding patterns typically associated with endometrial cancer are periods less than twenty-one days apart; heavy bleeding or bleeding for eight days or longer; and breakthrough bleeding. The risk is higher if you're between the age of forty-five and menopause. However, bleeding patterns need to be put in context with all the risk factors. It's important not to dismiss a change in pattern or breakthrough bleeding as "just a thing," especially for Black women, who are at risk for a more aggressive cancer that doesn't have traditional risk factors. It's particularly important to test for cancer when abnormal bleeding is being treated but is persisting.

The only reliable way to rule out endometrial cancer before menopause is for your doctor to take a sample of tissue from the endometrium, most often with an endometrial biopsy, which is usually an in-office procedure, or with dilation and curettage (D&C), which is typically performed in an operating room. A hysteroscopy may also be recommended, depending on the bleeding pattern. See page 200 for more on these tests. An ultrasound is not helpful for identifying endometrial cancer for those who are still menstruating, because the lining of the uterus is typically thick from the menstrual cycle.

Endometrioid cancer can frequently be prevented by taking a progestin (a progesterone-like drug) or progesterone. Progestins are better than progesterone at targeting the effects of estrogen on the endometrium. The options include a levonorgestrel IUD, hormonal contraception, or a progestin taken in a cyclic fashion (every two weeks, to mimic the two weeks of progesterone exposure of a menstrual cycle). Weight loss for those who are obese can also lower the risk, as can exercise.

Treatment of endometrial cancer is beyond the scope of this book.

Endometrial Niche

While this sounds like a great name for a bookstore on gynecological health, it is actually a cause of intermenstrual bleeding that happens right after a period. It can seem like a longer period, where the second half is heavy spotting, or the bleeding can start again a few days after the period ends. This condition happens only after a cesarean section. Abnormal healing of the scar can produce an indent, or niche, in the endometrium and sometimes even the muscle beneath. Blood collects in the niche during menstruation and then continues to trickle out after the true period has ended.

If you have an endometrial niche, an abnormality may be seen on ultrasound or by hysteroscopy. There is no surgery to repair the divot, so therapy is geared toward controlling bleeding with hormonal medications or tranexamic acid. Those who have finished having children, or for whom childbearing isn't a choice, can consider endometrial ablation or a hysterectomy.

Other Medical Conditions

A variety of medical conditions can stop periods or make them irregular, either because they affect the hypothalamus or pituitary or cause inflammation. Some examples include:

- *Thyroid disorders:* Both an overactive and an underactive thyroid (hyperthyroidism and hypothyroidism) can be associated with irregular periods and periods that stop. Thyroid-stimulating hormone (TSH) levels should be checked in all cases of menstrual abnormality. The treatment involves addressing the underlying thyroid problem.

- *Hyperprolactinemia:* This condition, in which prolactin levels are high, can produce a variety of bleeding patterns, but the most common are infrequent periods or periods that seem to stop altogether. Many people are familiar with prolactin because of lactation, but it also plays an important role in the menstrual cycle; for example, during the luteal phase, it stimulates the production of progesterone. A high level of prolactin can inhibit GnRH and LH, stopping the oocyte from developing. High levels can be the result of a tumor of the pituitary gland or a side effect of some medications. Elevated prolactin levels are the cause of irregular bleeding patterns only about 1 percent of the time, but blood work is still recommended. When high prolactin is found, further investigation and treatment will depend on the level; commonly, the medication bromocriptine is prescribed, as it can return prolactin levels to normal.

- *Diabetes:* Both type 1 and type 2 diabetes are associated with disturbances in the menstrual cycle, most often irregular cycles, a longer cycle (thirty-one days or longer), and/or heavier bleeding. Inflammation and elevated insulin are two of the main contributors. Screening for diabetes is done with a blood test, either HbA1c, fasting glucose, or a two-hour glucose tolerance test.

- *Epilepsy:* This neurological condition is also associated with an increased risk of abnormal bleeding. One theory speculates that epilepsy has a direct effect on the hypothalamus. There is no specific testing to determine whether epilepsy is the cause of irregular bleeding, but ruling out other causes is important.

- *Obesity:* People with obesity are more likely to have irregular cycles. This may be because obesity is associated with insulin resistance, which can impact the follicles, and inflammation, which can affect how the endometrium repairs itself. However, your doctor should consider and test for all potential causes before assuming that weight is a contributing factor. If excess weight *is* possibly contributing to your abnormal bleeding pattern, hormonal contraception can help, as well as lower your cancer risk, and you can consider attempting weight loss, though I acknowledge that it is hard and may not be an option for some.

Medications

The connection between a medication and an irregular bleeding pattern can sometimes be very clear—the change in your bleeding pattern coincided with when you started taking the medication—but at other times, the side effects of medications appear gradually and you don't realize the association. The main medications to consider as potential culprits include:

- *Epilepsy drugs,* especially valproate. The exact reason is unknown.
- *Opioids,* which are believed to have an effect on GnRH. The result is irregular ovulation and overall lower levels of estrogen, which can also increase the risk of osteoporosis.
- *Psychiatric medications,* such as antipsychotics and antidepressants, which can increase levels of prolactin.
- *Steroids,* such as prednisone and cortisone, which when taken orally or as an injection (including nerve blocks), can disrupt signaling from the hypothalamus and the pituitary.
- *Supplements.* Some botanicals can boost the effect of certain blood thinners, increasing the risk of bleeding. Supplements can also be contaminated with other medications that may impact menstruation, such as estrogen, thyroid medication, steroids, and sometimes even designer steroids, meaning steroid drugs that have not been tested appropriately in humans.

If the medication that's triggering the abnormal bleeding can be stopped, then that is the number one treatment. If it can't, the next step is to consider a hormonal contraceptive, typically the pill, for cycle control. With opioids, treatment is the same as for FHA.

Infection

Infection in the endometrium can lead to irregular bleeding. Sexually transmitted infections (STIs) are among the most common causes, but in some parts of the world tuberculosis (TB) can be a cause. An infection can also develop after a procedure such as an abortion or hysteroscopy, and of course after childbirth. Testing for STIs and TB is indicated if you're at risk of exposure, and your uterus may or may not be tender when examined. Blood work may also be done, and sometimes an endometrial biopsy. The treatment is antibiotics, and in the case of tuberculosis, antituberculosis medications.

Bleeding after Sex

Postcoital bleeding—bleeding after sex—affects up to 12 percent of people, and it can be distressing. While many people with cancer of the cervix bleed after sex, most people who bleed after sex don't have cancer. The most frequent cause is something called a cervical ectropion, where the lining of the cervix protrudes into the vagina. These cells aren't meant to be exposed to the acidic environment of the vagina, so they can become inflamed and bleed easily when touched. About one-third of people who bleed after sex have an ectropion; it's more common in younger people, during pregnancy, and in those taking estrogen-containing contraception. It's benign, and it often goes away with age. Switching contraceptive methods to one without estrogen can sometimes help.

Other causes of postcoital bleeding include:

- *A polyp from the cervix.* This is usually quite easy to remove. Rarely, a polyp from the uterus could be the cause.
- *A sexually transmitted infection (STI),* specifically chlamydia, gonorrhea, or trichomoniasis. The infection creates inflammation, and then the friction of penetrative sex leads to bleeding.
- *Hormonal contraception.* In this case, light spotting related to contraception isn't noticed until it is essentially washed out by ejaculate (it doesn't take much blood to color something red).
- *Cancer of the cervix,* which is uncommon for someone who has been getting regular cervical cancer screening, especially if they have been vaccinated against HPV.

- *Lack of estrogen.* When estrogen levels are low, the cells in the vagina become thin, the tissue loses elasticity, and lubrication decreases, so friction can cause abrasions.
- *Skin conditions* that affect the vagina and the vaginal opening, such as lichen planus and lichen sclerosus.

Bottom Line

- Periods that stop, are consistently outside of the normal range, or are associated with breakthrough bleeding should be investigated.
- Functional hypothalamic amenorrhea is the most common cause of periods that stop; it is associated with low levels of estrogen. The risk of low bone density increases if the condition persists and goes untreated.
- Primary ovarian insufficiency is another possibility when periods space out or stop altogether. It affects 1 percent of women and is associated with elevated levels of FSH and low levels of estradiol.
- A variety of non-gynecological medical conditions can cause irregular bleeding, including thyroid disease, diabetes, and epilepsy. Medications can also be responsible.
- Endometrial cancer should always be considered with chaotic bleeding. While the risk is higher for those forty-five and older, rates are increasing for younger people. Risk factors include a long-standing bleeding issue, a history of not ovulating regularly, bleeding irregularities that have persisted despite therapy, and a BMI of thirty or more.

18

Polycystic Ovarian Syndrome

Polycystic ovarian syndrome (PCOS) affects 5 to 20 percent of reproductive-age women and is the most common hormone condition in this age group. The wide range is due to the varying definitions used for PCOS. Because it's a syndrome, meaning a collection of symptoms, features, and conditions that together make up the whole, there isn't one specific test that says "Yes, that is PCOS!" The sum of everything together, meaning how it affects the whole person, is what's most important. Even though PCOS is one of the most common medical conditions overall, it often goes undiagnosed and inadequately treated.

While experts are still wrestling over formal definitions of PCOS for studies, what you need to know is that it has two cardinal features. PCOS should be on the radar for anyone with either of these symptoms:

- *Evidence of elevated androgens* not caused by any other condition or medication. Androgens are hormones, like testosterone, that are often incorrectly thought of as "male" hormones. Higher-than-typical levels of androgens can cause excess hair growth over the lip and on the chin, chest, upper arms, upper neck, lower back, thighs, and abdomen. About 75 to 80 percent of women with this kind of excess hair growth have PCOS. High androgen levels can also cause acne and loss of hair on the head, and while PCOS should still be suspected here, there isn't as strong an association: about 20 to 40 percent of people with acne and 10 percent with hair loss will have PCOS.

- *Ovarian dysfunction,* meaning ovulation is irregular. This manifests as irregular and infrequent menstruation (which is why PCOS is in the section of the book dealing with abnormal bleeding). With PCOS, menstruation is typically at least thirty-five days apart, but people often have just two or three periods a year, and sometimes even fewer. The irregular bleeding is caused by infrequent ovulation; when there is estrogen but no progesterone, the lining can become unstable and can be triggered to bleed by inflammation or for other reasons. So bleeding shouldn't be considered proof of ovulation. The disordered ovulation of PCOS may be seen with an ultrasound as polycystic changes in the ovary. When ovulation is irregular, about 25 to 33 percent of the time it is because of PCOS.

The Complex Biochemical Changes of PCOS

Although the term *polycystic ovarian syndrome* makes it sound like this is a condition of the ovaries, it is about far more than the ovaries. In fact, some of the features of PCOS can persist even when the ovaries are removed. With PCOS, multiple complex biochemical changes occur throughout the body, including in the brain, pancreas, muscles, liver, adrenal glands, and adipose tissue (fat), as well as in the ovaries. Some of the key changes include the following:

- *Abnormal gonadotropin levels.* An abnormal release of gonadotropin-releasing hormone (GnRH) from the hypothalamus affects the release of follicle-stimulating hormone (FSH) and luteinizing hormone (LH) from the pituitary. One consequence is an increase in LH, which triggers the follicles to make excess androgens.
- *Disordered ovulation.* Remember, it takes three hundred days or so for a follicle to complete its developmental journey. With PCOS, there are abnormalities of development, and growing follicles stall out in the antral phase. They fill with fluid (hence their cyst-like appearance on ultrasound). The theca cells of the follicles grow abnormally, producing higher levels of androgens. The stuck

follicles also produce estradiol, but levels are typically in the normal range. Sometimes follicles do make it to ovulation, but it is typically irregular and often infrequent. The exact reason for the follicle traffic jam isn't known, but a myriad of genetic factors as well as abnormal levels of FSH, LH, testosterone, and insulin may all play a role. Interestingly, when a trans man takes testosterone, his ovaries may develop changes that look like PCOS on ultrasound.

- *Insulin resistance,* which affects 50 to 70 percent of women with PCOS. Insulin is a hormone essential for helping our cells use glucose. With insulin resistance, insulin has trouble doing its job, so the body makes more to compensate. While we don't know the exact causes, inflammation and genetic issues with how the body transports glucose may be contributing factors. Higher levels of insulin can have wide-ranging effects, such as triggering the follicles to produce more androgens, reducing the production of sex hormone binding globulin (see below), and increasing appetite. Insulin resistance also affects the muscles, liver, and adipose tissue. Some people with insulin resistance have darkening of the skin behind the neck, in the armpits, and on the inner thighs, called acanthosis nigricans.

- *Reduced sex hormone binding globulin.* SHBG, a carrier protein for hormones like testosterone and estrogen, is made in the liver. Reduction of SHBG appears to be caused by high levels of androgens and insulin. I think of SHBG as a bus. When hormones are on the bus, they aren't out on the streets, affecting the body. As far as the tissues are concerned, low levels of SHBG are like having higher levels of testosterone and estrogen. This effect is more pronounced for testosterone, which binds more tightly to SHBG, so when levels drop, more testosterone than estrogen is released into circulation.

- *Adipocytes (fat cells) behaving differently.* Altered production and/or function of communication molecules called adipocytokines contributes to insulin resistance and increased inflammation. Fatty tissue also converts testosterone to estrogen, which can impact the endometrium.

- *Increased production of androgens* by the adrenal glands, although the exact cause isn't understood. This affects about one-third of women with PCOS.

- *Chronic subacute inflammation* in the body, likely related to many aspects of PCOS.

How all these biological changes come together to produce PCOS isn't known. There has been a lot of research in the past decade, but right now what we know is kind of like having a list of ingredients for a recipe with limited information on quantities and cooking time and temperature. It isn't for want of trying. PCOS is highly complex, and animal models can take us only so far. It's not possible to sample the hormonal changes inside a follicle while it's inside a person, and it isn't ethical to remove healthy ovaries and ovaries with PCOS for a study, so researchers must rely on surgeries performed for other reasons and design experiments using this tissue. In addition, the past twenty-five years have opened the door to identifying and studying genes that control aspects of PCOS, something that was a dream when I was a medical student.

Here is an illustration of how some of the changes seen with PCOS work together:

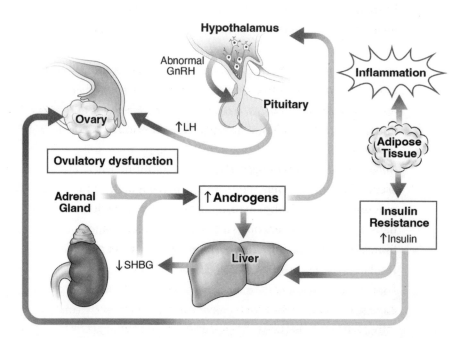

Figure 15 • *The Complex Interactions of PCOS (Illustration by Lisa A. Clark, MA, CMI)*

The role of obesity in PCOS is frequently misunderstood. Fatphobia has created a huge disservice, as people with obesity have been told erroneously that obesity caused their PCOS and the only answer is weight loss. Moreover, people who are not overweight have had their health concerns dismissed because they "can't possibly have PCOS." It's true that obesity can magnify many of the changes seen with PCOS; as a result, people with both obesity and PCOS are more likely to have severe symptoms than people with PCOS who don't have obesity. For that reason, people with both tend to be overrepresented in studies and among those who seek medical care for PCOS. However, when we use strict criteria to diagnose PCOS, it affects people equally, regardless of weight.

In addition to the classic symptoms of PCOS—irregular periods and signs of increased androgens—many other important health considerations can accompany it, including:

- *Type 2 diabetes,* which will affect 50 percent of women with PCOS by age forty.
- *High blood pressure,* which is associated with an increased risk of heart attack, stroke, dementia, and kidney disease.
- *Abnormal lipid profiles,* which increase the risk of heart disease.
- *Metabolic syndrome,* a condition where someone has three of the following: high blood pressure, high blood sugar, excess body fat around the waist, elevated LDL, and low HDL (LDL and HDL are lipids). Metabolic syndrome increases the risk of cardiovascular disease and diabetes. The risk of metabolic syndrome is doubled with PCOS.
- *Nonalcoholic fatty liver disease (NAFLD),* a condition where fat accumulates in the liver. About 20 to 30 percent of the time, NAFLD progresses to nonalcoholic steatohepatitis (NASH), which is essentially a more severe version associated with inflammation of the liver, cirrhosis (scarring), and, less commonly, cancer of the liver. NASH is a growing cause of liver transplants.
- *Precancer and cancer of the endometrium.* The follicles are producing estradiol and fatty tissue is creating estrone, but because ovulation is infrequent, there isn't enough progesterone to counteract this estrogen. Over time, the unopposed exposure to estrogen can lead to precancer and cancer of the endometrium, because estrogen causes cells to divide, and more divisions increase the risk of mutations. In

addition, there may be more potentially cancer-causing estrogen metabolites, and excess inflammation may also play a role.

- *Depression and anxiety*, especially for people with more androgens and elevated insulin. The burden of having a medical condition but being dismissed by medical providers and receiving inadequate care almost certainly plays a role.
- *Sleep apnea*, a condition with repeated obstruction of the airway during sleep. In addition to the impact of chronically disrupted sleep on mood and quality of life, sleep apnea is associated with many other medical concerns, such as an increased risk of heart problems and nocturia (getting up at night to go to the bathroom).
- *Pregnancy complications*, such as high blood pressure and diabetes.
- *Infertility*, primarily due to infrequent ovulation.

Testing for PCOS

Knowing you have PCOS is important because it's empowering to understand why your body is doing something, even when it's something unpleasant, such as having irregular periods or acne. But also, when you know your diagnosis, you can learn about all of the medical implications, advocate for the best therapies, and learn what is snake oil and what is science. Knowledge is power, given how many parts of your health can be touched by PCOS, not just now but over the years to come.

PCOS should *always* be considered with irregular periods and/or increased hair growth on the face and/or body, acne, or loss of hair. There are three different sets of formal criteria for diagnosis (it's research nitty-gritty stuff), but the most common criteria seem to be having two of the following three symptoms: infrequent ovulation, androgen excess (meaning excess hair growth) on exam or by lab testing, and polycystic ovaries on ultrasound.

Changes in the ovaries characteristic of PCOS can be seen on a pelvic ultrasound. However, if there is clear evidence of irregular ovulation and increased hair growth suggestive of PCOS, and periods aren't heavy, an ultrasound is unlikely to change the diagnosis and isn't typically needed. When the diagnosis of PCOS is in question, looking at the ovaries may help, and when periods are heavy, an ultrasound can help rule out other causes, such as fibroids. Like everything with PCOS, ultrasound results must be taken in context, because while 70 to 90 percent of women with PCOS have polycystic changes on ultrasound, about 25 percent of people without the condition will also have these changes. It's not whether you have polycystic changes; it's whether these changes could reasonably be part of PCOS, given your overall medical picture. One very important caveat: ultrasound is not useful for teens, because even up to eight years after the first period the normally developing ovary can look like an ovary with PCOS. Diagnosis of PCOS in teens, especially those younger than seventeen, is tricky and should be made only in consultation with an expert.

Blood tests are important to rule out other conditions that produce irregular ovulation and can mimic symptoms of PCOS. They may also be useful to confirm the diagnosis and can determine how PCOS might be affecting the body. Some of these tests include:

- *Follicle-stimulating hormone:* Irregular periods can also be seen with functional hypothalamic amenorrhea (FHA), primary ovarian insufficiency (POI), and other medical conditions discussed in the previous chapter. What we are looking for here is to make sure FSH levels aren't very high (possible POI) or low (possible FHA).
- *Luteinizing hormone:* LH is often elevated with PCOS but isn't always. This test isn't needed to make the diagnosis, but it may be helpful when things are uncertain. If LH levels are high compared to FSH, that favors PCOS.
- *Estradiol:* As with FSH, this test isn't to make the diagnosis of PCOS, where estradiol levels are typically normal or sometimes slightly elevated. But it's important to make sure they aren't very low, as that might signify another cause for the irregular bleeding.
- *Testosterone:* Levels of total and free testosterone are useful for confirming elevated androgens and ruling out a testosterone-producing tumor as the cause of increased hair growth on the face or body, or hair loss on the head. Increased hair growth is considered evidence enough of elevated androgens, so in that case testosterone levels are needed only to rule out another cause. However, acne and balding are not considered good evidence of elevated androgens; an elevated free testosterone level can help determine whether these changes are related to PCOS.

- *Other androgens:* Tests of androstenedione and DHEA-S are considered optional but can pick up high levels of androgens from the adrenal glands.
- *Anti-mullerian hormone:* AMH is typically elevated among women with PCOS. It's not a required test but may be useful when the diagnosis is in question. It is being investigated to see if it may be a better way to evaluate the ovaries for PCOS than an ultrasound.
- *Thyroid-stimulating hormone and prolactin:* It's important to exclude a thyroid condition and elevated prolactin.
- *17-hydroxyprogesterone (17-OHP):* A test of this hormone helps to rule out a condition of the adrenal glands called adult-onset congenital adrenal hyperplasia (CAH). While it's ideal to do the 17-OHP test in the follicular phase, before ovulation, predicting that timing can be challenging with irregular periods; a progesterone level clarifies whether 17-OHP is elevated due to ovulation or because of an adrenal condition.

PCOS is associated with insulin resistance, metabolic syndrome, and type 2 diabetes, so testing metabolic health is essential. Sadly, and inexcusably, these associations are often ignored. In addition to checking blood pressure, a lipid profile is recommended; typically, this includes tests of cholesterol, LDL, HDL, and triglyceride levels, done while fasting. Screening for diabetes is also essential. The recommended test is a two-hour glucose tolerance test: blood is taken, you drink a solution with 75 g of glucose, and then blood work is repeated two hours later. Other tests for diabetes—HbA1c, which measures average glucose in the blood over time, and fasting glucose level—can miss the glucose intolerance seen with PCOS. If these tests are normal, a two-hour glucose tolerance test should still be done. If two-hour glucose tolerance and lipids are normal, they should be rechecked every two years. People with metabolic syndrome or other signs of insulin resistance may need to have their liver evaluated for NAFLD or NASH. The risk for endometrial cancer should also be assessed when PCOS is diagnosed.

Why Does PCOS Exist?

PCOS is a genetic conundrum. Typically, conditions associated with both reduced fertility and worse health outcomes drift out of the population. Yet PCOS affects a significant percentage of the population, and the incidence has been stable for some time—not just hundreds of years, but likely thousands or maybe even tens of thousands.

Genes clearly play a role. Among identical twins, if one has PCOS, there is a 70 percent chance the other will also develop the condition; if your mother or sister has PCOS, there is a 30 to 50 percent chance you will develop it. Multiple genes associated with PCOS have been discovered, including those that control androgen production, insulin signaling, follicle development, and inflammation, to name a few. But PCOS isn't caused by just one of these genes; the most accurate explanation (though probably the most unsatisfying) is that PCOS is the result of a complex mix of genetics and epigenetics, which controls how genes are turned "on" or "off." It's possible some aspects of modern life, such as diet or exposure to endocrine-disrupting chemicals, may play a role in triggering these genes for some people. You might think about PCOS the way you think of height. Multiple variations in genes that affect our hormones, bone growth, cartilage, and overall health, as well as other factors, combine with our environment to determine our height, and the same principle is likely true for PCOS. It's important to know there isn't a single root cause, because there are many people making false claims about this on social media.

Once researchers knew some of the genes involved with PCOS, they could put on their detective caps and go digging through the genetic material left behind by our ancestors. It turns out some of these genes have been around for about sixty thousand years. Because PCOS has the same prevalence around the world today, the conclusion is that these genes are fairly stable. We also know that women with increased facial hair have been recorded throughout history, as far back as the time of Hippocrates. However, it isn't possible to know whether this excess hair was due to PCOS, tumors that were producing androgens, or other causes.

So how do we explain the persistence of a condition associated with reduced fertility and an increased risk of health issues such as heart disease? One theory is that PCOS offered an advantage to our ancestors. The higher testosterone levels may have led to more muscle mass or stronger bones, and the metabolic differences allowed increased fat storage, useful in times of famine and especially for having a successful pregnancy during a time of food shortage. The inflammation associated with PCOS might have been useful in priming the immune system to fight the onslaught of bacteria and viruses faced by our ancestors, who didn't have modern sanitation or medicine. In addition, PCOS is associated with a later menopause, which may have allowed additional time for childbearing into the forties, especially considering that disordered ovulation can improve over time for some people with PCOS. Lots of intriguing ideas, but an actual answer isn't yet possible with what we know.

Ancestral women may have had fewer physical consequences of PCOS. For example, most would have been more active than we are today, and physical activity reduces insulin resistance. Also, obesity was less common, and while obesity doesn't cause PCOS, it does increase the severity. We don't really know what PCOS might have looked like thousands of years ago.

Some experts have wondered about a biological advantage of PCOS for men. I know what you're thinking: How could a condition where a key component is disordered ovulation affect men? (Acknowledging that many trans men have ovaries.) Well, men have some of the same genes associated with PCOS. These genes don't give men PCOS; instead, they may be associated with increased reproductive success. This concept, where a trait improves fertility for one sex and decreases it for the other, is called sexual conflict. Basically, women with PCOS are sucking up the negative consequences, because if they pass on the genes that cause PCOS to a son, he may have more children. Sometimes I just want to punch evolution in the face.

Some General Treatment Strategies

The treatment for PCOS depends on several factors, including your most bothersome symptoms, metabolic concerns, risk of endometrial cancer, and desire to get pregnant. But there are some baseline measures that can be helpful regardless of symptoms, including exercise and diet. Exercise can reduce insulin resistance and improve high blood pressure. While everyone should focus on getting enough physical activity (at least 75 minutes of high-intensity activity or 150 minutes of moderate-intensity activity a week), regular exercise can be particularly beneficial if you have PCOS. Exercise can also help with depression and anxiety.

Diet may help the metabolic concerns associated with PCOS. Try to avoid foods that are high in saturated fat and/or added sugar; eat 25 g of fiber a day; try to get more protein from plant sources; increase your intake of foods that are believed be anti-inflammatory, such as fruits, vegetables, whole grains, and healthy, unsaturated fats (like olive oil and nuts); and eat at least two servings of fish a week. There is no robust data to recommend one diet over another, so the best strategy, as unsexy as it seems, is to eat a balanced diet, with less saturated fat, more fiber, and a good mix of vegetables (basically, the Mediterranean diet or any heart-healthy diet). Truthfully, it would be beneficial if we all ate like that.

If you have PCOS and are overweight, weight loss can be helpful, as obesity can amplify some of the biological changes associated with PCOS. I want to be clear here: weight loss is not required to treat PCOS, and other therapies can and should be started without it. However, you should know that disordered ovulation, excess hair growth, metabolic concerns, and the risk of endometrial cancer can improve with even a 5 to 10 percent weight loss. Because this can be a triggering conversation, your health care provider should ask if you feel comfortable discussing the potential impact of weight loss and should respect your wishes if you don't. For those interested in learning more, the best diet for weight loss is one you can follow. There is no hack to burn more fat; all diets work by restricting calories, whether you are formally counting calories, following a ketogenic diet, or trying intermittent fasting. In addition, there are newer weight-loss medications (glucagon-like peptide-1 receptor antagonists) that are truly game changers here, and there is also bariatric surgery.

For those with PCOS-related infertility, the best option is referral to a reproductive endocrinologist, who specializes in infertility therapy.

Medications for PCOS

There are a variety of medical options for treating PCOS. The estrogen-containing birth control pill is typically the first therapy recommended for people who aren't trying to get pregnant. This isn't because we are pushing the pill or can't be bothered to look for other therapies, as some people who recommend unstudied therapies claim. The truth is, there is a lot of evidence-based medicine supporting the pill, which seems to be more helpful than the patch or the ring (but both of those can be considered as well). Estrogen-containing contraceptives, especially the pill, treat some of the key disturbances seen with PCOS. The benefits include:

- Regulating menstruation (or eliminating it, if so desired).
- Protection against endometrial cancer, courtesy of the progestin.
- A decrease in LH, reducing androgen production by the ovaries.
- An increase in the carrier protein SHBG, so more testosterone is kept "on the bus" and inactive.
- Contraception, if needed.

No other therapy is as effective as the estrogen-containing birth control pill at lowering high levels of androgens, it's the best way to reduce excess hair growth or treat hair loss on the head, and it is an excellent treatment for acne. Offering the pill is sound science on the part of a health care provider; what is unacceptable is failing to explain how well this option has been studied, the many ways it can help, and the alternatives.

While some people have wondered if the pill can increase insulin resistance, recent studies have found no significant negative effects on blood glucose, insulin, or weight gain. For some people, the estrogen-containing pill can adversely affect lipid and triglyceride levels. Monitoring is necessary when the medication is first started; if there are concerning lipid changes, the pill can be stopped and those changes will reverse.

There is a common Internet lie that the pill can cause PCOS. This is biologically impossible, and in fact we have good data showing it treats many aspects of the condition. Yes, some people start the pill when they are fourteen or fifteen because of heavy periods, for contraception, or for acne, and after stopping it ten years later, they learn they have PCOS. What happened in these cases was that the pill was treating the PCOS, and once the treatment was stopped, the condition became apparent.

Can the pill interfere with the diagnosis of PCOS? While it's true that if someone has been on the pill for a long time, their ovaries might not show the polycystic changes and their excess facial hair growth, acne, and irregular periods may be well controlled, and that is a good thing. We also can't judge by levels of LH or testosterone. However, we can ask about their history. Many conditions can be diagnosed simply by listening to the patient's story. If they had irregular periods and excess facial hair before they started the pill, they almost certainly have PCOS and should have metabolic testing. (And if they have excessive facial hair or are balding despite being on the pill, that should prompt testing to rule out a testosterone-producing tumor.) Look, we don't tell people not to get their face waxed because one day we might need to look at their chin and upper lip to make a diagnosis of PCOS, and it's the same with the pill.

Other hormonal contraception options, including some pills, the Depo-Provera shot, and the implant, contain only progestins. While they do suppress ovulation and so will have some effect on reducing androgens, the impact is less, as without estrogen there is no change in SHBG. These medications are not well studied for PCOS, so their impact beyond controlling periods, protecting against endometrial cancer, and providing contraception is unknown. (These are all still worthy benefits!) The hormonal IUD will control bleeding, protect the uterus, and provide contraception, but it will not affect ovulation or how the ovary produces androgens. Progestins can also be given orally for twelve days a month to reduce the risk of cancer of the endometrium. This method will typically result in bleeding each time the medication is stopped. It won't provide contraception.

Another medication often used for PCOS is metformin, which increases insulin sensitivity, decreases insulin levels, decreases glucose production in the liver, and decreases absorption of glucose from the intestine. It can improve ovulation, reduce levels of androgens, and lead to some weight loss. For some, it can help control irregular bleeding and treat excess hair growth and acne, although the improvement is less than one would typically get from an estrogen-containing contraceptive. Metformin is a good option for people with PCOS who have metabolic concerns, as it can slow or stop progression to type 2 diabetes. Interestingly, many of the ways that metformin works on the body have led researchers to investigate it as an anti-aging drug. Side effects include gastrointestinal upset and diarrhea, although these are less common in lower doses and often go away over time. Metformin can also be associated with low levels of vitamin B_{12}, so monitoring may be needed. When insulin resistance is severe, other medications may be recommended.

Other common options for PCOS include:

- *Medications that block androgens:* The safest one is spironolactone. It can be used to reduce unwanted excess hair and to treat hair loss and acne. Flutamide and finasteride are other medications for excess hair growth, but they are associated with more safety concerns and can't be used by everyone.

- *Medications for acne:* These include benzoyl peroxide, topical retinoids, oral antibiotics, and oral retinoids. Oral retinoids can negatively affect the liver and may not be an option for everyone; they can also cause severe birth defects, so contraception is essential for those at risk of pregnancy.
- *Cosmetic therapies:* Excess hair growth can be treated with shaving, waxing, sugaring, and laser hair removal, as well as topical eflornithine hydrochloride.
- *Topical minoxidil:* This treatment can be used on the scalp for hair loss.

What About Natural Therapies?

Myo-inositol, a sugar the body makes from glucose, plays a role in how some steroid hormones bind to their receptors and in insulin metabolism. D-chiro-inositol (DCI) has the same atoms as myo-inositol, just arranged in a mirror image. Inositol products can be myo-inositol, DCI, or a combination of the two, but they can also contain other ingredients, such as vitamins and minerals.

There are many inositol-based products on the market that are touted as natural therapy for PCOS. However, these products are made in a lab—there is no inositol farm. There is some evidence that inositol products can improve ovulation, but overall, the studies are relatively low-quality (which is typical for supplements). Combining DCI with myo-inositol can decrease the ability to absorb myo-inositol, and some data suggests DCI can block the enzyme aromatase, which could lower estrogens and increase androgens. That's not ideal for PCOS. Given these potential issues and the fact that the data isn't great, inositol products are currently not recommended in medical society guidelines. For those who want to try them, myo-inositol seems to be the preferred option. Avoid products that contain added vitamins and minerals, as these additions may affect absorption and likely add nothing to the therapy. With supplements, it's always important to remember that the product may not contain what it claims to, owing to the lack of regulation. It is also possible for products to be contaminated with another drug, even metformin.

Magnesium supplements are promoted to decrease insulin resistance, as magnesium plays an important role in glucose metabolism. While it is true that, for people with type 2 diabetes and low levels of magnesium, supplementing the mineral can reduce insulin resistance, that doesn't mean people with PCOS will benefit from magnesium supplementation. Low magnesium is generally uncommon, but those who drink a lot of alcohol, who have kidney disease, or who have chronic diarrhea are at increased risk. Type 2 diabetes is a risk for low magnesium because of the complex ways glucose and magnesium metabolism interact. Someone with both type 2 diabetes and PCOS may benefit from a magnesium supplement if their levels are low, but the data to recommend it in other indications just isn't there.

Is PCOS Associated with Estrogen Dominance?

No. I'm not one for mincing words, and this is certainly no time to change that policy. *Estrogen dominance* isn't a medical term; it is gibberish. Typically, the term shows up in ploys to sell you unindicated tests, supplements, and diets, and sometimes to recommend topical progesterone, which is essentially a waste of money, because progesterone isn't absorbed well through the skin.

If PCOS were truly estrogen-dominant, levels of SHBG would be high and people with PCOS would not have high levels of androgens. In fact, PCOS isn't associated with very high levels of estrogen in the blood (they're typically normal, but sometimes slightly elevated during the follicular phase). The issue with estrogen in PCOS is that the lining of the uterus doesn't get enough progesterone to counteract the estrogen produced by the ovaries and other sources.

When you see the term *estrogen dominance* in reference to PCOS (or really anything related to human biology), translate it to *estrogen scam*. And if you see it on your social media feed, consider blocking the poster so you aren't exposed to any other disinformation. Bad information is like wolves: it travels in packs.

Final Thoughts

Many people with PCOS have been dismissed by their health care providers, which is unacceptable. Some are told the only treatment is weight loss; others are quickly offered the pill with no discussion about the goals of treatment, or even a full explanation of PCOS itself. Other people aren't offered the full range of therapies or a discussion of the benefits and risks of those therapies. And the metabolic aspects of PCOS often go unaddressed.

The answer to these very real problems is not found in lies and conspiracy theories or untested therapies. The answer is to insist that people are informed about all the health aspects of PCOS and are offered all the therapies, so they can decide what works for them. And those who sell unregulated products and tests must do better research so we can make recommendations about their products with confidence. We can guess why they are poorly studied: they are already profitable, so why risk proving that they add nothing to PCOS care? If someone truly believed what they were offering was helpful, wouldn't they use their profits to advance the science and help more people?

Bottom Line

- PCOS is the most common endocrine condition for women of reproductive age.
- PCOS is associated with irregular, infrequent ovulation, irregular menstrual cycles, high levels of androgens, and polycystic ovaries on ultrasound. Many people with PCOS also have insulin resistance.
- PCOS increases the risk of endometrial cancer, diabetes, and metabolic syndrome.
- Treatment of PCOS depends on many factors and needs to be individualized, but one universal therapy is exercise, as it improves insulin resistance.
- The first-line therapy for PCOS, when pregnancy isn't a consideration, is the estrogen-containing birth control pill, but there are other options as well.

19

Painful Periods

Painful menstrual cramps (dysmenorrhea) can affect health, quality of life, and ability to attend school and work. The impact goes far beyond an individual curled up on the couch with a heating pad. At least 10 to 20 percent of high school teens miss school because of menstrual discomfort, and an estimated $2 billion is lost annually in the United States *alone* because of missed work from painful periods, never mind the cumulative impact on education and earning potential. In short, period pain causes much suffering.

When it comes to painful periods, there is an epidemic of undertreatment. Women's pain is undertreated in general, as compared to men's, but painful periods have historically been seen as a "woman thing" and hence unimportant. Our patriarchal system has dismissed menstrual pain as both exaggerated and a sign of weakness, and at times, perversely, as something women deserve (punishment for "original sin," I suppose). I feel the need to pause here and point out the utter absurdity of the idea that women are too weak to tolerate menstruation, even though they stretch and tear to deliver a baby. The only way someone could reach this conclusion is if they had no interest in the experiences of being a woman and thought of women only as breeders. Which is likely a fairly accurate description of many supposedly learned medical men of yore.

The reverberations of this legacy are felt today in the inadequate research on the subject. Painful periods, which affect 50 to 60 percent of women for thirty-five or so years, are treated as a normal biological phenomenon (if the little ladies were just a little tougher, they could handle it). Meanwhile erectile dysfunction, which affects 50 to 60 percent of men for thirty-five or so years, is worthy of billions of dollars of funding, leading to multiple therapies and never-ending TV ads featuring people holding hands while in separate bathtubs on a hilltop. Like erectile dysfunction, painful periods can affect sex life, but erectile dysfunction doesn't affect one's school or job or leave them curled up in bed. Yes, it is enraging.

Unfortunately, we know very little about historical menstrual pain, but it is reasonable to wonder if it has always been this way or if pain with periods has increased over the past hundred years or so. A plausible hypothesis for this change is that now that we have increased exposure to endocrine-disrupting chemicals and an earlier age of the first period. There is mention of painful periods in the Hippocratic corpus from over two thousand years ago and in Chinese medicine from a thousand years ago, but it's mostly simple acknowledgement that menstrual pain existed, not of how common or impactful it was. Most historical writings about menstruation revolve around missed periods, because the egress of menstrual blood was considered essential to remove toxins and/or achieve balance for good health. Hence, much of historical medicine was about trying to bring on menstruation when it didn't happen and controlling heavy periods. Menstrual pain was also viewed in the context of how the body was understood at the time, being mostly a balance of the four humors (blood, phlegm, black bile, and yellow bile); within that paradigm, it was likely believed to be due to a backup of blocked blood.

The Ladies Dispensatory, first published in England in 1652, acknowledges that many women suffered from menstrual "difficulty and pain" and that heavy periods could be accompanied by "a most violent excruciating inward pain," which the author, Leonard Sowerby, concluded was due to "convulsive throws of the womb, violently pulling and stretching its ligaments from the parts in which they are inserted." While not physiologically correct, if you have ever had bad menstrual cramps, the visual of a blood-soaked Balrog-like monster fighting to break its chains might seem on point. Of regular menstruation Sowerby wrote, "Pains in the head, pains in the hips, the loins, the stomach, and the bowels, which latter resembles the Cholick, and Pains of the womb that have sometimes been compared to the pangs of Child Birth." (*Cholick* being colic, which is a pain that comes and goes in waves.) These descriptions tell me that Sowerby listened to women, because what he wrote is similar to what I hear in the office today (eighteenth-century vernacular aside). His therapies were a "thin diet," moderate exercise, bloodletting (if the blood was obstructed, it obviously needed to come out another way), cathartics (medicines that induce vomiting or diarrhea—again, fluid balance), and if the pain was especially bad, a variety of medicinal concoctions (some of which contained pennyroyal, which is toxic in any dose, so it's alarming to read with today's knowledge).

Given the mention of menstrual cramps in historical medical texts and the fact that Hadza women in Tanzania, who live a traditional hunter-gatherer lifestyle, report painful periods, it's reasonable to assume that painful menstrual cramps are a long-standing experience for humans.

Is there at least a point to menstrual pain, biologically speaking? Not that we know of. Other mammals that menstruate don't appear to have painful periods, but their menstrual flow is also lighter. Humans are unique in the volume of their menstrual blood, so we need a revved-up engine to stop the bleeding, and an unfortunate consequence is pain. As far as I can tell, this is just how the system works. Put another way, menstrual pain is a design flaw that almost half the population has been sucking up so humanity can continue. Evolution only needs to be "good enough," although that seems to apply disproportionately to bodies with a uterus. And not only has evolution required that those who reproduce bear greater physical burdens, whether they have children or not, but society also taxes them for it with lower pay, expensive childcare, and in many places, more medical expenses. It's no wonder the birth rates are declining in some countries: people are throwing their cards down on the reproductive table and saying "I'm out."

The Biology of Period Pain

Menstrual pain, also known as primary dysmenorrhea, typically doesn't start until ovulation, which often takes one to two years to occur regularly after the first menstrual period. This link with ovulation helps to clue us in to one of the major causes: prostaglandins, the class of chemicals released as the endometrium begins to detach from the lining of the uterus.

The reaction that leads to menstrual pain is a bit like a microscopic Rube Goldberg machine. The drop in progesterone when the corpus luteum reaches the end of its lifespan activates lysosomes, which are tiny structures inside endometrial cells. Think of lysosomes as a cell's cleanup crew: they're filled with acid and enzymes (proteins that can break structures down into smaller pieces) and they perform various functions, such as removing old parts of a cell, engulfing bacteria to kill them, and even helping a cell self-destruct when it has done its job for the body. Now activated, the lysosomes break down the membranes of the endometrial cells to help with removal, but this releases phospholipids, triggering the production of two groups of chemicals: prostaglandins and leukotrienes. Unrelated to what is happening inside the uterus, there is also an increase in levels of vasopressin, a hormone released by the pituitary.

The net effects of this prostaglandin-driven chemical soup are uterine contractions and a reduction in blood flow to the uterus (called ischemia). Both biological processes help stop the bleeding, but the downside is pain. Imagine squeezing your fist very tightly. The squeezing is painful (our proxy for the uterus squeezing), but if you squeeze tightly enough, blood flow to your fingers will drop, and that adds a secondary pain mechanism, as the decrease in oxygen leads to a buildup of chemicals that stimulate pain receptors.

So how much pressure is generated by a uterus that is squeezing during menstruation? I'm glad you asked! During menstruation, the baseline pressure in the uterus is about 10 mmHg, and there are typically three to four contractions per ten-minute interval. During the contractions, the pressure can easily get to 120 mmHg, which is the amount of pressure generated during the second stage of labor, when you are pushing. Yeah, let's pause to take that in.

If you've never experienced menstrual cramps or been in the second stage of labor, here's a reference point: when we inflate a blood pressure cuff and it's still sort of tight and you wish it would stop, that's about 120 mmHg.

The muscles around the vagina also contract to help move blood along, which may cause vaginal pain or pressure for some people. Moreover, the prostaglandins from the endometrium enter the bloodstream and can cause diarrhea for about 20 percent of people, only adding to the unpleasantness. Prostaglandins can also cause nausea and vomiting.

Why are some people's periods more painful than others? It seems some people produce more prostaglandins, and others may be more sensitive to their effects. People with primary dysmenorrhea can have one or more of the following:

- Increased baseline pressure in the uterus during menstruation.
- Increased frequency of contractions.

- More forceful contractions, with some as high as 200 mmHg (a blood pressure cuff at its tightest).
- Uncoordinated contractions in the uterus and the vagina. The muscles around the vagina also wrap around the rectum, which may cause menstrual-related anal pain for some.
- Tensed pelvic floor muscles. These muscles can tense up in reaction to pain, just as muscles do in other areas of the body, which may be an additional source of pain during menstruation. Some people may also feel this as pain in the rectum or heaviness, or even a sensation like something is falling out.

But wait, there's more. Think of the uterus as a toaster plugged into an outlet, which in our analogy is standing in for part of the spinal cord. Other "appliances"—the bladder, the muscles of the pelvic floor, some muscles of the bowel, and even some muscles of the belly wall—are plugged into the same outlet. Just as a short in a toaster can affect the outlet and everything else plugged into it, so can pain in an organ travel to another body part via shared connections in the nervous system. The medical term is *viscero-viscero sensitivity* when it's from the uterus to another organ, and *viscero-somatic sensitivity* when it's from the uterus to structures that are not organs, like the abdominal wall or pelvic floor muscles.

How do researchers know that pain can migrate? There are several studies. In one, investigators recruited women with painful periods and those without. A balloon was inserted into the rectum during menstruation and inflated to create stimulation. Women with painful periods had more pain from the balloon than those without. This sensitivity might manifest outside of a study in many ways. For example, people with dysmenorrhea may have painful bowel movements, pain with sex, or urinary urgency (meaning the need to empty the bladder more often) when they are on their period. We also see the consequence of this biology in the fact that painful periods are more common among people with interstitial cystitis, a pain condition that affects the bladder, and irritable bowel syndrome, a pain condition that affects the bowel.

Just like pain, inflammation can also travel along shared connections. This fact has been shown in elegantly designed studies where scientists took rats and introduced chemicals into their rectums to cause inflammation. The rats were then sacrificed and examined. Although the researchers had not touched the rats' bladders, the bladders were inflamed. To answer the question of how that happened, the researchers performed the same experiment on another set of rats, but this time, before introducing the chemical into the rectum, they severed the nerves in the spinal cord that allow the bowel and the bladder to communicate. The inflammation did not travel to the bladder, proving that the nerves provided the route for it. If the inflammation had been seeping through the tissues, cutting the nerves wouldn't have made a difference.

As pain travels along nerves to the spinal cord and the brain, it can change how the signal is interpreted along the way. The human nervous system has neuroplasticity, meaning it can adapt. Neuroplasticity is beneficial in many ways. For example, after a brain injury, other parts of the brain can adapt to regain lost function. But the process can also go awry when the signal is pain. With repeated exposure, cycle after cycle, to period pain, the nervous system changes. One of the effects is that pain is amplified, either locally at the source (called peripheral sensitization) or in the spinal cord and/or brain (called central sensitization). Basically, repeated exposure to pain can alter its volume in the parts of the nervous system that receive and interpret it.

What are some consequences? Local nerves become more sensitive to pain signals. For example, if you have painful periods, dilating the cervix may be more painful—something to consider when planning an IUD insertion. Data also shows that women with painful periods feel more pain with touch in areas of the body far from the uterus, like on the arm or back, and have a higher incidence of pain conditions affecting parts of the body not directly connected with the pelvis, including headaches and fibromyalgia. With peripheral and central sensitization, the discomfort is *not* made up or imaginary; very real changes are occurring that facilitate pain. This is another reason why treating period pain is important: pain begets more pain, and the legacy of undertreated painful menstrual periods can have widespread implications.

There is incredible biological complexity to menstrual pain, and it's only made more complicated because a healthy serving of misogyny and inadequate research are layered on top.

Investigations for Painful Periods

Painful periods can be "just because," meaning that it's simply how someone is wired, which I appreciate is an unsatisfying answer. But they can also be the result of other conditions, most commonly endometriosis and adenomyosis. When an investigation for other causes should start depends on how the pain responds to therapy and the likelihood of another cause. There is no hard and fast algorithm here, so many individual factors must be considered, such as age, when the painful periods started, response to previous therapies, findings on physical exam, and ultrasound results. For more on endometriosis, see Chapter 20, and head back to Chapter 16 for more on adenomyosis. Regardless of the cause, the first step for painful periods is to start therapy. Treatment won't interfere with the ability to investigate later, should that be needed.

How people approach pain varies so much from person to person. My experience, from treating painful periods for over thirty years, tells me it's almost impossible to predict who will want what therapy. Some people say, "Bring it on, all of it!" Others want to start with the least invasive treatment and move stepwise through them. Some people don't want to take any kind of medication; others live by the "better living through pharmacology" mantra. Goals for treating pain also vary. What one person might consider a success (say, a 20 percent reduction in pain), another might consider a failure. With these nuances in mind, the following sections cover the most evidence-based therapies to consider.

Heat

A hot water bottle, heating pad, or hot towel placed on the abdomen or lower back is a seemingly universal therapy for period pain. At one point or another, more than 50 percent of people with menstrual pain have tried it. There is some data here, although admittedly the quality of the studies is compromised because it's not possible to randomize people to a placebo: obviously you know if the device is hot or not. In the studies we do have, heat performs better than no therapy, which most people who have tried heat can probably confirm.

We don't know how heat works for menstrual pain. It penetrates about 1 cm (0.4 inch), so it reaches only superficial tissues, nerves, and muscles, not the uterus (and that's a good thing, as heating the pelvic organs could be dangerous). One possibility is that heat reduces spasm in the surface muscles where it is applied (abdomen or back), which have become involved in menstrual pain because of shared connections in the nervous system. Another hypothesis is that it has an impact on nerves via shared connections. Sensation, be it heat, light touch, or pain, travels along nerves from the source, and these nerves make a connection with other nerves in the spinal cord that will then take that sensation to the brain. If you think of the nerves as roads, where they connect is like a gate, and several roads converge on one gate in the spinal cord. Tactile stimulation, such as heat, can close the gate for pain, essentially overriding a painful message that shares the same connection. If the brain doesn't receive the signal, the pain hasn't happened. This is called the gate theory of pain. Because the muscles in the abdominal wall and low back have shared connections with the uterus, applying heat to them can close the pain gate. It's not a complete seal, so some pain gets through, but it seems to help many people.

There are issues with using heat, such as burns, which can be serious, and erythema ab igne, which is a mottled red or dark rash in a branching pattern. Erythema ab igne is caused by chronic exposure to heat that isn't hot enough to burn but is hot enough to damage the superficial blood vessels. To prevent burns, a heat source should never be above 40°C (104°F), but erythema ab igne can occur with lower temperatures—it can even happen from the heat of a laptop computer (it's related to both heat and duration of use, as well as repeated exposure). Erythema ad igne can reverse when it is mild, but over time the changes can become permanent. In addition to the cosmetic changes, there is even a risk of cancer associated with erythema ab igne.

To minimize injury from heat, always follow the manufacturer's directions, using the heat source for only fifteen to twenty minutes at a time (twenty minutes on and at least twenty minutes off is a good rule to remember). Do not sleep with a heat source, as exposure will be longer than twenty minutes, and if heat gets between you and the bed, it can't dissipate into the air, so more will be transferred to your skin. If you notice mottling on your skin, it's time to consider other therapies for pain.

The Forgotten Therapy: The TENS Unit

TENS stands for transcutaneous electrical nerve stimulation. A TENS unit is a small device that looks like a pager or smartphone (depending how antique the model). Worn close to your body, it is connected to the surface of the skin via wires and electrodes, sending an electrical current across the skin to the nerves. We don't know exactly how a TENS unit reduces pain, though there are several hypotheses. The main one is the gate theory discussed above, except here, the signal that closes the gate is vibration. That's why you rub your arm if you bang it—the vibration of rubbing closes the gate to the pain.

Data shows that a high-frequency setting (hfTENS) is helpful for period pain—up to 80 percent of people get some relief. There are two placement configurations to consider. The first is all four electrodes on the back: the upper ones on either side of the spine, about midway up the back (corresponding to what we call the T10–L1 level, to cover a group of nerves known as the inferior hypogastric plexus, which innervate the uterus), and the lower ones at or just below the level of the hip bones (to cover the nerves that supply the vagina, a region known as S2–S4). The other option is two electrodes on the back, in either the upper or lower position, and two on the lower abdomen. You can experiment to find the best configuration for you.

There are several settings for a TENS unit. The three you should know are:

- *Frequency:* The number of electrical pulses per second, measured in hertz. A typical setting for period pain is 80 hertz.
- *Pulse width:* The duration of each pulse. The typical setting for period pain is 200 to 250 µS (microseconds), but it could be increased to as much as 400 µS if that gives a better result.
- *Amplitude:* The intensity, or volume, of the pulse. It should be below 80 milliamperes.

These settings will get you started with a TENS unit, but there are other configurations to consider, and the advice of a physical therapist can be invaluable here. The stimulation should not be painful or result in muscle contractions.

Almost everyone can use a TENS unit, with a few exceptions. If you have a pacemaker, an implantable defibrillator, a heart condition, or epilepsy, check with your doctor before using TENS. Also, the electrodes shouldn't be placed over broken or infected skin.

I tell my patients that with a TENS unit they can take the edge off the pain. Most studies report a reduction of approximately 2 on an 11-point (meaning 0 to 10) pain scale. Many people find going from a 7 to a 5, for example, a meaningful improvement, especially given the lack of side effects. While there are expensive TENS units (over $100), the models in the $30 range work just fine.

Nonsteroidal Anti-inflammatory Drugs

First introduced in 1969, NSAIDs block the production of prostaglandins, one of the triggers for the domino effect that causes painful periods. NSAIDs with the common names ibuprofen and naproxen have been over-the-counter medications in the United States since 1983. They provide pain relief (analgesia) and also reduce inflammation, as their name implies, by inhibiting the enzyme cyclooxygenase, which is essential for forming prostaglandins (which are starting to sound like the villains of the story). There are two forms of cyclooxygenase, COX-1 and COX-2. Most over-the-counter NSAIDs work on both COX-1 and COX-2. COX-2 inhibitors were introduced in 1999 with the goal of reducing side effects (inhibiting COX-2 is more important for pain relief), but long-term use is associated with heart problems, so they are generally not recommended. Aspirin is an NSAID, but it should not be used for menstrual pain, as it blocks platelet function and can, paradoxically, increase bleeding.

This is one area in OB/GYN where we have excellent data (although there are still more trials for erectile dysfunction than for dysmenorrhea). When a review of NSAIDs for painful periods was published in 2015, there were eighty clinical trials to review, some comparing NSAIDs with a placebo and some comparing them with acetaminophen (Tylenol). The studies found that NSAIDs help about 80 percent of people, versus 18 percent for placebo. This doesn't mean they take pain away completely, but rather that they have a meaningful impact on pain. And remember, they can also reduce the volume of bleeding.

There is no data to suggest that one NSAID is better than another, so I typically suggest taking one you feel comfortable with or that has worked for you before when taken for other reasons. Overall, NSAIDs outperform acet-aminophen, so they should be the first choice of pain medication when they are an option. That doesn't mean it is unreasonable to take acetaminophen, and some people have side effects or medical conditions that preclude taking NSAIDs, including people with bleeding disorders or stomach ulcers and those who have had gastric bypass surgery. The biggest risks with NSAIDs are bleeding from the gastrointestinal tract and a potential for kidney injury. But when using these medications for menstrual pain, the risk is low because they are not being taken daily.

Some other points about NSAIDs:

- People are often told to take doses that are too low. Moreover, many NSAIDs work best with a loading dose—an initial higher dose that is dropped down for subsequent doses.
- Sometimes an NSAID works well for one person and not for another. If you try one and it doesn't help, try a different one.

- NSAIDs don't work for about 10 to 20 percent of people with period pain. This may be due to other causes of pain, such as endometriosis, but data tells us that some people may simply have NSAID-resistant pain.

Hormonal Contraception

Hormonal contraception is highly effective for painful periods. The primary method of action is thinning the endometrium (an effect of the progestin), resulting in less production of prostaglandins, but the progestin also inhibits COX-2. Many hormonal contraception methods can stop periods altogether, which is obviously a selling point: no period, no pain. All methods—pill, patch, ring, implant, injection, and IUD—appear equally effective. There isn't a lot of good head-to-head data, so choosing a method typically boils down to which one sounds right to you after hearing the pros and cons. There is more information on all of these methods in later chapters. In general, a three-month trial is recommended. If one method doesn't help, switching to another may well offer more improvement.

Other Medical Therapies

GnRH antagonists and agonists—medications that shut off ovulation temporarily—can be used for painful periods. With no developing follicles, there is no endometrium, no ovulation, and no prostaglandins. But given their side effects, these medications are typically considered only when endometriosis is suspected.

There are also three nonhormonal options that may work for people who can't tolerate other therapies or for whom those therapies have failed:

- *Nitroglycerin:* Also known as glyceryl trinitrate, nitroglycerine is a heart medication that can cause muscles to relax. In small studies, it had an impact on par with NSAIDs. Nitroglycerin is typically given as a patch. The big issue is that about a quarter of people develop headaches as a side effect.
- *Nifedipine:* Another heart medication, called a calcium channel blocker, nifedipine is believed to work for menstrual pain by

relaxing the uterus and dilating blood vessels. There aren't a lot of
studies. Side effects include a fast heart rate, palpitations, flushing,
and headache.

- *Sildenafil:* You may know this medication better as Viagra. Yup. It increases blood flow to the uterus, which can help because some menstrual pain is believed to be due to reduced blood flow. Small studies show that sildenafil might be useful, but the data isn't great, so it isn't something to think of as a first- or even second-line therapy. However, if you are really suffering, have tried several therapies, and are known not to have another cause for the pain, such as endometriosis, you could consider it.

Surgical Therapies

Endometrial ablation is a procedure that destroys the endometrium, and no endometrium means no source of prostaglandins. It is typically performed for heavy bleeding, but about 50 percent of people with both heavy bleeding and painful periods find it helpful for pain. Endometrial ablation is discussed further on page 220.

What about a hysterectomy as a therapy for dysmenorrhea? If you do not have endometriosis but simply painful periods, the answer is yes and no, and it depends. Over the years, gynecologists, especially in the United States, have been rightly accused of performing too many hysterectomies. The surgery was used to stop "undesirable" women from having children, to make money, or simply because no one listened and offered the right care. At one point, it was the most common elective surgical procedure in the United States. Even though hysterectomy rates are falling, thanks in part to hormonal IUDs, which are very effective at treating abnormal bleeding (the most common reason for the surgery) and period pain, a woman in the United States is far more likely to get a hysterectomy than in any other developed country. And no, it's not because American women are getting better care.

On the other hand, there are people who really suffer from period pain who have tried NSAIDs and continuous pills (or a patch or a ring) or a hormonal IUD and are still miserable. In this situation, a hysterectomy is a reasonable option if they are not interested in a future pregnancy. GnRH antagonists/agonists are also a possibility; I don't believe people should be required to try them before a hysterectomy, but they should be made aware of the option as part of informed consent.

A hysterectomy is a major surgical procedure, and complications are possible, so it's important to review all the risks. In addition, a hysterectomy (removing just the uterus, not the ovaries) can lower the age of menopause, which can have other health implications. There is nuance here that goes far beyond what I can offer in this book. Age, general health, and other risk factors for complications all play into the decision-making. What might be a relatively easy surgery for one person could be risky for another.

For people who decide a hysterectomy is right for them, the best procedure is usually a total hysterectomy, meaning the cervix is also removed, as well as removal of the oviducts, which are the source of many ovarian cancers. With a supracervical hysterectomy, where the cervix is left behind, 10 percent of people develop menstrual bleeding from the cervix, which is obviously undesirable and, because pain mechanisms are complex, could lead to persistent menstrual pain. There is no advantage to leaving the cervix, so it's best to make sure all the uterine sources of pain have been removed. A hysterectomy can often be accomplished vaginally (the preferred approach, leaving no scars on the abdomen) or laparoscopically (keyhole surgery with a telescope).

Final Thoughts

Because pain is complex, it is always possible that pelvic floor muscle spasm, irritable bowel syndrome, or painful bladder syndrome could be masquerading as painful periods or amplifying them. When initial therapies don't work, it is a good idea to revisit the diagnosis and not just assume it's refractory painful periods. A visit to a pelvic floor physical therapist may be in order, as well as a reevaluation of bladder and bowel symptoms. A urogynecologist or urologist (doctors who specialize in bladder health) and/or a gastroenterologist may need to be involved.

Bottom Line

- Painful periods are common and often undertreated.
- The primary cause of pain is related to prostaglandins and other chemicals released during menstruation.
- Some common features of painful periods are increased pressure in the uterus with menstrual cramps, more frequent contractions, and a higher resting level of spasm in the uterus.
- Painful periods can start a cascade of other events than can affect the nervous system.
- The first-line therapies for painful periods are NSAIDs and/or hormonal contraception, but some people also find a TENS unit helpful.

20

Endometriosis

Endometriosis is an inflammatory condition where tissue similar to the lining of the uterus grows outside the uterus, most often in the pelvic cavity but sometimes in areas not connected with the pelvis. It affects about 10 percent of women; worldwide, 190 million people are impacted. It is associated with painful periods, chronic pelvic pain (pain at times of the cycle other than menstruation), infertility, and a myriad of other painful and bothersome symptoms. About 24 to 35 percent of women with severe pelvic pain have endometriosis, and that number is even higher for teens, at 50 percent. Despite its prevalence, the average time it takes to get a diagnosis is seven years, and it's typical for a woman to see five doctors before she gets a diagnosis.

In addition to the suffering, endometriosis comes with a hefty price tag in the form of medical expenses, such as appointments, scans, medications, and surgery, as well as the ramifications of missed work and school. It's difficult to estimate the impact in a concrete sum; older data suggests an extra US$4,000 a year in health care costs alone. For perspective, this is on par with type 2 diabetes and rheumatoid arthritis. For many people, the amount is likely much higher. Endometriosis affects quality of life in many ways that are challenging to measure: fatigue, the impact on relationships of pain with sex, and the psychological impact of having one's pain repeatedly dismissed or downplayed, for example. For many women, endometriosis tragically and unacceptably means a life of pain.

Despite its toll, endometriosis is woefully underfunded. The National Institutes of Health in the United States had a $41.7 billion budget for research in 2022. Of that budget, just $16 million, or 0.038 percent, was allocated for endometriosis—an estimated $2.00 per patient per year. The equivalent funding for diabetes, which affects the same number of people, was $31.30. Crohn's disease, a painful inflammatory bowel disorder that, like endometriosis, can be devastating, affects about 0.3 percent of people and received $90 million in funding. During my medical lifetime, from when I entered medical school in 1986 to now, treatment options for both type 2 diabetes and Crohn's have increased significantly. We have not seen similar progress with endometriosis. This isn't about disease favorites, but it's a damning testimony to the importance of endometriosis, research-wise, and what society thinks of women with pain.

What Causes Endometriosis?

The short answer is, it is still an enigma. The long answer is that it is likely a complex mix of genetics and triggering environmental events that happen at key times, possibly even as a fetus. Because many women with endometriosis have it as teens, even with their first period, it's likely that the stage is often set before puberty.

One theory about endometriosis is a phenomenon called retrograde menstruation. With menstruation, some of the blood, which contains endometrial cells, heads backward out the oviducts into the pelvis and even the abdomen. A viral TikTok video about this left many people believing the uterus squirts a high volume of blood under pressure into the pelvic cavity; in reality, it's a small amount of blood, and it doesn't flow out under pressure, like a hose. The hypothesis is that some of the endometrial cells seed the pelvic and abdominal cavities and start to grow. However, endometriosis affects 10 percent of women and retrograde menstruation happens about 90 percent of the time, so if it is involved, there must be other factors as well, such as differences in the endometrial cells that make them more likely to take hold, or problems with the body's surveillance mechanisms for removing rogue cells. In other words, the issue isn't retrograde menstruation per se; if retrograde menstruation is involved, it's that plus something else.

Supporting points for retrograde menstruation being somehow involved are that endometriosis is most often found in places where blood would deposit, based on gravity and movement of fluid in the abdomen and pelvis, and that endometriosis is more common among people born with reproductive tract abnormalities that block the flow of blood out of the uterus, so more backs up into the pelvis and abdomen. Finally, we know that endometrial cells can be seeded elsewhere in the body through trauma—for example, during a C-section or even after a vaginal delivery—and endometriosis can then grow in the surgical scar or the site of the vaginal tear or episiotomy. Some researchers have postulated that the first uterine bleeding that can happen shortly after birth (triggered by the withdrawal of hormones when the baby is separated from the placenta) may play a role in seeding the pelvis. That would explain the presence of endometriosis from the first period. While only 5 percent of female babies have obvious bleeding, as many as 50 percent may have small amounts that go unrecognized. In addition, the neonatal uterus is structured in a way that favors retrograde menstruation.

Evidence against retrograde menstruation is phenomena such as endometriosis in the brain (which is very uncommon, but there is zero connection with the pelvis), in the lungs, in female fetuses, and in cisgender men. A theory that might explain these rare occurrences is that cells with the potential to become endometrium are present in a fetus either as stem cells or cells that were left behind as the uterus formed (remember, a male fetus initially has a Müllerian system—tissue with the potential to become endometrium), and these cells are later triggered. Perhaps the cells develop abnormalities that make them more likely to become endometriosis, or perhaps the body's surveillance mechanisms for this kind of mayhem are not working as they should. A final theory that might explain how endometriosis can end up in the lungs or the brain is that cells from the endometrium enter blood vessels or lymphatic channels.

Regardless of the origin of the cells destined to become endometriosis, they are different from regular endometrial cells, and their differences account for how the tissue grows and causes problems:

- *Abnormal inflammation:* Although the cycle of building and shedding endometrium in the uterus is inflammatory, it's controlled, so it doesn't spread beyond the lining and heals without scarring. With endometriosis, the inflammation is exaggerated—almost out of control at times—which can cause pain and scarring and even affect nerves.
- *Exposure to estrogen:* Estrogen likely plays a role in helping endometriosis cells stick and grow, and it may also impact inflammation.

Endometriosis cells can be more responsive to estrogen and can even manufacture their own; basically, they can keep the fires burning even when there is no fuel (estrogen) coming from elsewhere. Therefore, using medications to shut down estrogen production from the ovaries doesn't always work, and for some people, endometriosis persists even after the ovaries are removed or postmenopause.

- *Progesterone resistance:* As discussed in previous chapters, progesterone counteracts the effect of estrogen on the endometrium. With endometriosis, the tissue can be partially or even completely resistant to progesterone, which may contribute to its stickiness and abnormal growth, and also explains why progesterone or progestins (synthetic forms of progesterone) may not be effective therapy.

- *Abnormal blood vessels and nerves:* The inflammation (and likely other factors) causes blood vessels and nerves to grow in abnormal ways, which may not only fuel the growth of the endometriosis but also sensitize the nerves, increasing pain.

- *Genetic factors:* There is evidence that endometriosis cells have abnormalities in their DNA that favor their growth outside the uterus. In many ways, it is like a seed being genetically modified to grow in different soil. The genetic changes aren't necessarily the kind you inherit; many are epigenetic changes, meaning something changes how the genes are expressed. If you think of DNA as a book, a genetic change alters the words, while an epigenetic change alters how the words are read, even though what's on the page stays the same.

Let's put these elements together with some of the known risk factors for endometriosis:

- *Being born with a low birth weight:* This risk factor is especially associated with deep endometriosis. One explanation is that there appear to be similar signaling pathways for fetal growth and inflammation. Another possibility is abnormal development of tissues and blood vessels due to low birth weight, basically creating an environment that is more receptive to developing endometriosis.

- *Abnormalities of reproductive tract development:* These can cause a buildup of menstrual blood in the uterus and more backflow into the pelvis, increasing retrograde menstruation.

- *An earlier first period:* The theory here is an earlier exposure to high levels of estrogen.
- *A short menstrual cycle:* A cycle of less than twenty-six days may create more opportunities for retrograde menstruation.
- *A mother or sister with endometriosis:* While it's true that endometriosis runs in families—if someone has endometriosis, there is an increased chance their parent or sibling also does—it is rarely due to the inheritance of a single gene, as is the case for eye color. Rather, it's likely that several genes play a role in increasing vulnerability.
- *Endocrine-disrupting chemicals:* Diethylstilbestrol, a synthetic hormone that used to be given during pregnancy and is known to cause abnormalities of the reproductive tract, is associated with an increased risk of endometriosis. The data on other endocrine-disrupting chemicals is less clear (mostly because drawing cause and effect from the studies is difficult), but there is a fair bit of evidence implicating bisphenol-A (BPA) and phthalates.

What about food as a trigger? The data is conflicting, because not only is diet hard to study in general, but people with endometriosis may change their diet because of their pain. The best evidence suggests that people who eat more long-chain omega-3 fatty acids, which are anti-inflammatory, are less likely to develop endometriosis, and those who eat more trans fats, which are pro-inflammatory, are more likely to develop endometriosis. Overall, a diet high in omega-3s and low in trans fats is healthier for many reasons. Long-chain omega-3s are found only in some fish and algae, but other omega-3s, found in foods like chia seeds, walnuts, flax seeds, and canola oil, can be converted by the body into long-chain omega-3s.

Some people wonder if endometriosis is a relatively new condition or has been here all along but perhaps is getting worse. Another possibility is that it's been around for thousands of years and women have simply tolerated it. Getting a clear answer here is challenging. First, there is the long history of dismissing women's pain as a sign of mental illness or weakness. And as discussed in Chapter 12, women did not have space to write about their menstrual experiences. Finally, the ability to do surgery for diagnostic purposes (and have a patient survive) is relatively modern, as is the knowledge to call what was found endometriosis.

Some theorize that endometriosis may have been identified as early as the seventeenth century; others claim that Hippocrates and physicians of Ancient Egypt knew about it. But the source manuscripts don't describe what we consider to be endometriosis today, and translating ancient disease models to modern medicine is fraught with issues. The earliest feasible description in the medical literature is from 1860, and a definitive description was written in 1906 by Dr. Thomas Cullen. The disease was named in 1927 by Dr. John Sampson.

For many years, women with endometriosis were essentially blamed for having it. They were more likely to never get pregnant, so *obviously* (sarcasm font) the cause was delaying childbearing to pursue a career. (Delaying childbearing means more exposure to estrogen from menstrual cycles; if you are repeatedly pregnant and then breastfeeding, you have fewer cycles.) Of course, we now know that endometriosis is associated with infertility, so not getting pregnant is a consequence, not a cause. In addition, many people have endometriosis as teens, long before a supposedly "preventative" pregnancy would happen. Clearly this hypothesis is bunk, but it serves as a reminder that medicine can easily be perverted by patriarchal views on women and their place in society. If a theory positions women's contribution to society as breeders, and the solution to their issues as having sex with a penis, it props up a narrative that women are better off if they marry a man and don't work outside the home. Although many people make this choice, and for them it may be a worthy and desirable one, it's preposterous to suggest it is medically beneficial!

Many have speculated that endometriosis may indeed be a more modern disease, caused by an earlier onset of puberty, exposure to endocrine-disrupting chemicals, and/or changes in gut microbiome. While these theories each have some merit, we really don't know their validity.

The Carnage of Endometriosis

The abnormal tissue of endometriosis can grow on and into the uterus and ovaries, the bowel, the bladder, blood vessels, and nerves. In rare cases, as mentioned, it can even be found in the lungs and brain. Endometriosis can be located superficially or it can invade and grow deeply—to a depth of 5 mm (0.2 inch) or more. In many ways, the growth is like an out-of-control placenta or cancer, even growing through bowel and bladder. The resulting inflammation can produce scarring. Endometriosis can also produce cysts on the ovaries called endometriomas.

Endometriosis is categorized in stages from I to IV, based on the location and extent of the lesions, from lesser to greater. Although this scoring system can be useful in studies, it isn't of much use for people seeking care, because the severity of endometriosis in the body isn't related to the severity of symptoms. People can have minimal endometriosis, even just a few superficial lesions, and yet have terrible pain. Others can have stage IV endometriosis—a pelvis filled with endometriosis and scar tissue—and no pain. I remember a patient who had a hysterectomy for a reason unrelated to pain, yet widespread endometriosis was revealed during her surgery. I was shocked. Afterward, I made a point of asking about painful periods, as I worried she'd had her pain dismissed. But in fact she'd never even taken over-the-counter medications for period pain.

Moreover, where the endometriosis is located doesn't necessarily correlate to where the pain is felt, another counterintuitive concept. Someone can have all their endometriosis on the right side and feel it only on the left. And the disease doesn't progress in an orderly fashion from stage I through IV. When we look at people who have had repeat surgery, the endometriosis is fairly evenly split between regressing, staying the same, and progressing.

Pain is one of the most common symptoms of endometriosis. It can manifest as painful periods, pain outside of menstruation, pain with sex (especially with deep penetration), pain with bowel movements, and pain with urination. About 30 percent of women with endometriosis have pain that, unacceptably, the full complement of current therapies fails to treat adequately.

In a study I will always remember reading, a group of scientists opened the abdominal and pelvic cavities of rats. They implanted endometriosis in half the rats and just closed up the other half. Then painful things were done to the urinary systems of these rats, such as tying off the ureter (the tube from the kidney). The rats with endometriosis exhibited far more pain behaviors than those without. This tells us inflammation and pain from endometriosis can travel to the nerves, just as discussed on page 258 for painful periods, except here the inflammation and pain are likely greater. Hence, people with endometriosis experience a higher incidence of other pain conditions that share connections in the spinal cord, like irritable bowel syndrome, painful bladder syndrome, vulvodynia, and muscle spasm of the pelvic floor. They also have an increased risk of pain conditions not connected with the pelvis, such as migraines.

The important takeaway here is that endometriosis can cause pain in many complex ways. For some, the pain is related to the local lesions and the resulting inflammation and scar tissue. For others, it is more like a match that starts a fire; the pain persists even when all of the endometriosis is removed, just as a forest fire continues long after the match is extinguished.

Because endometriosis causes pain via different mechanisms that can be independent of ovulation, and because the tissue may not respond to hormones in the way the lining of the uterus does, endometriosis can cause pain right after the first period, unlike primary dysmenorrhea, which requires ovulation and withdrawal of progesterone to produce prostaglandins. This is something to consider if your periods were terribly painful from the get-go or within a few cycles, as it raises the chance that endometriosis could be involved.

Fatigue is a common symptom of endometriosis, and infertility is a common consequence, affecting up to 33 percent of sufferers. In addition, people with endometriosis are at higher risk for heart disease and early menopause, which has health consequences such as an increased risk of osteoporosis and dementia. Endometriosis is also linked with about a 50 percent higher risk of some less common ovarian cancers, although overall the risk is low (these cancers affect 1.3 percent of the general population and 1.8 percent of women with endometriosis). There is some suggestion that it may be associated with an increased risk of other cancers, including endometrial cancer, thyroid cancer, melanoma, and non-Hodgkin's lymphoma, as well as some autoimmune conditions such as lupus. However, the data isn't yet good enough to tell us whether these are true links. Endometriosis itself is not believed to be an autoimmune condition.

There are clearly many complexities we don't understand. Personally, I wonder if what we call endometriosis is perhaps different diseases, or at least different subtypes, that all look to us like endometriosis. At one time, headaches were headaches, but then with research (that's where money comes in), we learned there are several types, including migraine, tension, and cluster headaches, all caused by different phenomena and requiring different therapies.

How Do We Diagnose Endometriosis?

The older thinking was that surgery was required for diagnosis, not just looking at lesions in the pelvis and saying, "Yes, that looks like endometriosis." Studies told us that doctors could both over- and under-call endometriosis with the latter method, and biopsies were recommended so a pathologist could look at the tissue under the microscope and confirm endometriosis based on specific criteria. However, as we learned more about the widespread effects of endometriosis and the limits and consequences of surgery, we moved away from thinking of endometriosis as a surgical disease. We can now make a diagnosis based on symptoms, and possibly ultrasound and MRI, which are getting better at detecting endometriosis. This method is known as clinical diagnosis. Too often (in North America, anyway), surgery is equated with caring or listening, but doctors often make clinical diagnoses of serious conditions. For example, the diagnosis of migraines, at times a disabling pain condition, is based on talking with a patient and sometimes running scans to rule out other causes.

If you have severe period pain, pelvic pain that lasts longer than menstruation, pain with bowel movements, pain with deep vaginal penetration, bleeding from the rectum, or infertility, endometriosis is a possibility. Your medical provider should consider factors that might raise or lower the suspicion of endometriosis, and there is no excuse for anything longer than a six-month period for diagnosis (clinical or surgical). Factors that might raise the likelihood of endometriosis are period pain from the first period, heavy bleeding, fatigue, a family history of endometriosis, and/or a failure of NSAIDs or birth control pills to significantly help the pain. A pelvic exam can sometimes provide clues, such as tenderness deep inside the vagina or the presence of painful nodules, and if a uterus is retroflexed (see page 105), one possible reason is scarring from endometriosis.

Factors that raise the possibility of a different diagnosis are equally important. For example, although bleeding from the rectum can be seen with endometriosis, it isn't common, and other causes would need to be ruled out. Some bowel conditions, such as Crohn's disease, can cause abdominal and pelvic pain and bleeding from the rectum, so consultation with a gastroenterologist would be advisable. Similarly, someone with diarrhea (not just during their period) should be investigated for a bowel condition. A pelvic exam might reveal pelvic floor muscle spasm, which can cause severe pain, so referral to a pelvic floor physical therapist to treat the muscle pain would be recommended. Pelvic floor spasm can be painful enough that it can be mistaken for endometriosis pain. And, of course, people can have both: pain from endometriosis and pain from the pelvic floor. Adenomyosis can cause painful periods, but it is unlikely to cause other symptoms of endometriosis, such as fatigue and pain with bowel movements, and it is unlikely to be there from the first period.

To make sorting things out more challenging, some conditions that can cause pelvic pain—irritable bowel syndrome, painful bladder syndrome, and pelvic floor spasm—can worsen during menstruation because of the impact of hormone fluctuations on pain, in the same way that headaches can. Whether your pain is cyclic or not, keep these other causes in the back of your mind, because if therapies for endometriosis aren't helping, one possibility is that the symptoms aren't caused by endometriosis—though it's also possible that the therapies simply aren't working.

An ultrasound may be helpful, as it can identify endometriomas (cysts of endometriosis on the ovary) and often deeply infiltrating endometriosis, and it can rule out fibroids or a mass on the ovary as a cause for the pain. In some situations, an MRI may also be indicated, as it can pick up deep endometriosis. That doesn't mean an ultrasound and MRI are required to start therapy, or that if they are negative there is no endometriosis. Whether they should be ordered up front or only if treatment isn't helping is a decision you and your doctor should make together.

First-Line Medications

The initial therapies are the same as for painful periods and include an appropriate dose of NSAIDs (over-the-counter doses are too low), a TENS unit (see page 260), and if you have pelvic muscle spasm, a referral to a pelvic floor physical therapist. People who are trying to get pregnant can use these methods. If you've been trying to conceive for a year (or six months for those thirty-five years or older), then a referral to a reproductive endocrinologist is warranted. Management of infertility for those with endometriosis is beyond the scope of this book.

Hormonal contraception has an excellent track record for endometriosis and can be very effective for many of the symptoms, so it's considered the gold standard for initial treatment. The progestin (progesterone-like hormone) in these medications can reduce COX-2, decreasing prostaglandins, and inhibit the growth of endometriosis and reduce pain by limiting the ability of aromatase in the endometriosis to make estrogen, by decreasing inflammation, and by reducing the growth of abnormal blood vessels and nerves in endometriosis tissue. Many of the medications stop menstruation, which also reduces pain dramatically for many people. Options include:

- *Estrogen-containing oral contraceptives:* Even though they contain estrogen, their dominant effect is from progestin. They can be taken for twenty-one days, then stopped for seven days for a period, or can be taken continuously to stop menstruation. The latter option is typically preferred.
- *Oral contraceptives without estrogen:* These medications, which contain only progestins, are an option for people who can't take estrogen, although they are less well studied for endometriosis. Because spotting can trigger pain for some people, and spotting is more common with these medications, it's good to have a plan for this.
- *A levonorgestrel-containing IUD:* This can reduce or eliminate menstrual bleeding and shrink endometriosis lesions close to the uterus. Because the nervous system undergoes changes related to pain, a strategy for inserting the IUD that takes pain under consideration is advised.
- *An etonogestrel implant:* One study showed that this implant, another progestin-only method, can reduce pain from endometriosis by 68 percent. It has the highest risk of spotting of all the methods, which may be a consideration.
- *Depo-Provera:* This contraceptive injection is also very effective at treating pain, and by three cycles, 50 percent of people will have no periods.

There is no head-to-head data to compare these methods, so you might consider whether you want something that can easily be stopped (the pill, patch, or vaginal ring) or one that is long-acting (an IUD, an implant, or Depo-Provera), as well as your contraception needs (for example, if you're planning a pregnancy in a year, you might sway toward a more easily reversible method) and the medications' side-effect profiles, which are covered in detail in later chapters.

Progestins can also be given by themselves, meaning not as part of an approved method of hormonal contraception. The issue here is that there may be less suppression of ovulation and possibly more bothersome bleeding.

Hormonal contraception is evidence-based medicine for suspected and diagnosed endometriosis. There are some people who claim it "masks" the disease or doesn't treat the "root cause," but this tells me they don't understand the medicine. Not only do these medications reduce pain, a worthy goal, but they can also be considered disease-modifying drugs, given their impact on inflammation and abnormal growth of blood vessels and nerves. They can slow the progression of the disease and, after surgical removal, can delay its return.

In general, a six-month trial of hormonal contraception or progestins is recommended before moving on to other therapies. A good strategy is to check in with your doctor at three months to assess your improvement, how well the menstrual cycle is suppressed, and the incidence of spotting and other side effects. If there has been any change at three months, most experts recommend continuing to six, as the impact of the progestins can improve over time. Obviously, this general strategy needs to be individualized. For example, for a teen who is missing a lot of school because of pain, a three-month trial of medical therapy may be considered enough before moving on to surgery.

If hormonal contraception doesn't help, that doesn't mean you don't have endometriosis. As discussed earlier, some endometriosis lesions can make their own estrogen, and some are resistant to progesterone/progestins. In these cases, hormonal medications may not help, or may help only minimally.

Second-Line Medications

These drugs have more side effects and potential risks than NSAIDs, TENS units, and hormonal contraception, so in general they are recommended only when first-line medications are unsuccessful.

- *GnRH antagonists and agonists:* As discussed previously, these medications prevent the release of FSH from the pituitary and hence stop ovulation. Estrogen levels drop to the menopausal range, which cuts off one source of growth for endometriosis. In general, antagonists are recommended, as they are not associated with flares of pain, like agonists, and can be taken orally. GnRH medications can be combined with estrogen and a progestin in a dose high enough to prevent osteoporosis and counteract the menopause-like symptoms, but low enough that the estrogen doesn't stimulate endometriosis.
- *Aromatase inhibitors:* A class of medications that stop production of estrogen, aromatase inhibitors cause a dramatic reduction in estrogen and block aromatase, the enzyme that allows endometriosis to make its own estrogen. They can be given with oral contraceptives, progestins, or GnRH antagonists/agonists. They are often considered in situations where endometriosis persists after menopause. Side

effects can include all the symptoms of menopause, and long-term use is associated with osteoporosis, so monitoring is needed.

Surgery

Laparoscopic surgery is considered when first-line medical therapies don't help or don't help enough, or when they are not options. It's also not wrong to try second-line medical therapies before surgery. There is a lot of room for deciding the optimal surgical strategy.

The goal of surgery is to remove all visible endometriosis and correct scarring where possible. Surgery may be minimal for someone with small amounts of superficial endometriosis, or extensive when there is deep endometriosis, which can even enter the bowel or cause dangerous scarring around the ureter (the tube that connects the kidneys to the bladder). Surgery to remove deep endometriosis is quite specialized, and it isn't always possible to know the extent of the disease before operating; ideally, the gynecologist doing the procedure should have enough training to be comfortable with all levels of endometriosis. Removing endometriomas from the ovaries can have an impact on future fertility, so those who may wish to conceive should discuss this issue with their doctor as part of preoperative planning.

Overall, surgery tends to be more effective for pain related to deep endometriosis than for pain from superficial disease. That doesn't mean minimal endometriosis shouldn't be removed, but it is important to manage expectations. Some people get a great deal of long-lasting benefit from surgery, and others don't. When pain persists or returns soon after surgery, it is important to consider that there may be other causes, as discussed previously, such as pelvic floor muscle spasm or bladder pain syndrome.

Using hormonal medications after surgery can help reduce the risk of recurrence. One option, to avoid pain from the insertion, is to have a hormonal IUD inserted at the time of surgery.

Hysterectomy for Endometriosis

When medications and surgery have been suboptimal or ineffective for pain, a hysterectomy can be considered. Whether or not the ovaries should be removed at the same time is a complex decision based on many factors, including age, other medical conditions, the location and amount of residual endometriosis, and future fertility concerns (egg retrieval is still a possibility after a hysterectomy, for implantation in a gestational surrogate). Ovary removal before age forty-five is associated with an increased risk of heart disease, osteoporosis, and dementia, so hormone replacement therapy is indicated. Some people are concerned about how they might feel after their ovaries are removed or worry that they might feel poorly on hormone therapy. I've seen a few younger women who wish they hadn't had their ovaries removed, because of how they felt on hormone therapy. One option is a three-month trial of a GnRH medication before the surgery, as this mimics the hormonal experience of removing the ovaries. Hormone replacement therapy can (and should) be tried at the same time.

If you and your doctor make the decision to proceed with a hysterectomy, it's important to realize that active endometriosis may not, in fact, be the cause of your pain. In one study of women who had hysterectomies for endometriosis, only 43 percent actually had the disease. It's impossible to say whether the rest had been diagnosed incorrectly, meaning they never had endometriosis to begin with, or whether the endometriosis had been there previously and regressed. A hysterectomy is most effective for pelvic pain when endometriosis is present; for those with no endometriosis, the chance of improvement is much less.

Putting It All Together

In the past, endometriosis was considered a disease of lesions, and surgical therapy was emphasized. We now recognize it as a widespread inflammatory condition where surgery may be helpful for some people. When medical therapy isn't sufficient or isn't an option, surgery is recommended to completely remove endometriosis and associated scar tissue. However, surgery can also cause scar tissue, and the pain of surgery itself may provoke changes in the nervous system that amplify chronic pain, so repeated surgeries should be undertaken with careful consideration. If you are being pressured to have a repeat surgery when the previous surgery was done correctly (meaning all the endometriosis was removed), especially within one to two years of the previous surgery, I urge you to get a second opinion. It's important to have a comprehensive treatment plan for endometriosis, not just a surgical plan.

There are many permutations and combinations when it comes to treating endometriosis-related pain. Hormonal medications can be very helpful, but if the first one doesn't work, there are other options. Some people may want to try another first-line medication (for example, switching from the pill to the hormonal IUD); some, a second-line medical therapy; and others may want surgery. Some feel uncomfortable starting medications without surgery, and others are relieved they can have therapy without surgery. Some may want to proceed with surgery only if an MRI suggests deeply infiltrating endometriosis, the type more likely to respond to surgery. Because of these complexities and all the research gaps, doctors must rely on the basic principles of believing women about their pain, considering endometriosis as the cause, and starting therapy. Going forward, we desperately need tests that can better identify endometriosis without surgery and better tools to predict who will respond to which therapy, as well as better therapies.

Bottom Line

- Endometriosis affects about 10 percent of women. Common symptoms are painful periods, pelvic pain, pain with sex, pain with bowel movements, bladder pain, and infertility.
- The pain of endometriosis can be present from the first period or soon after.
- Hormonal contraception is the first-line therapy for endometriosis, but if it has not helped sufficiently after six months, other strategies should be considered.
- Surgery is no longer needed to diagnose endometriosis. As treatment, it tends to be most helpful for pain associated with deeply infiltrating endometriosis.
- It's important to consider other potential causes of pelvic pain, such as pelvic floor muscle spasm, irritable bowel syndrome, and nerve pain. These may coexist with endometriosis.

21

Alternative Therapies
for Menstrual Pain

Pain, as defined by the International Association for the Study of Pain, is an "unpleasant sensory and emotional experience" and "a personal experience that is influenced to varying degrees by biological, psychological, and social factors." It's the only sense that includes an emotional component. That doesn't mean it's in your head; rather, this definition encompasses the mind-body connection. As such, pain is not just the electrical signal the brain receives and interprets; many other factors, such as anxiety, depression, adverse childhood experiences, other pain conditions, sleep, stress, belief systems, and cultural factors, can all modify the pain experience in complex ways. Because of these complexities (and inadequate funding for studies), medicine doesn't always have answers, or the answers have side effects. Sometimes a well-studied therapy doesn't fit with an individual's belief systems. And many people have had their pain dismissed by medicine. So there are a number of reasons why people wish to try alternative approaches.

Treating a medical condition is in many ways like taking a trip. You are at point A, meaning in pain, and want to get to point B, less pain. Therapies are the routes between points A and B. Some routes have better maps than others, and some appear physically impossible—for example, going through a mountain where no tunnel exists. With medical care that has been studied, we can make statements like "Sixty-five percent of the time, if someone takes Highway 1, they can get from A to B, and we know this because several hundred people took that route and there was someone waiting at point B, counting how many made it through." Alternate routes are riskier. We can say, "Well, 50 percent of people said this route worked, but we don't have good evidence to show they made it to Point B." Or perhaps "That route looks like a shortcut that can't possibly work because that road doesn't exist." Alternative medical therapies are like these alternate routes. Some inhabit a medical gray zone, meaning the hypothesis is biologically plausible and hence intriguing, but the studies aren't good enough to make a recommendation for the therapy. Others have less plausible hypotheses and/or terrible data.

People sometimes think, "Well, if the hypothesis sounds good, why not?" The trouble is, lots of seemingly brilliant medical hypotheses turned out to be not just duds but harmful. One example is not eating peanuts until age one, to reduce peanut allergies. That sounds like it makes sense, right? We should wait until a baby's immune system can handle peanuts. So for years, that was the recommendation. As it turns out, that strategy *increases* the risk of peanut allergies. Another example is taking vitamin E to prevent heart disease. Researchers thought it was a good idea to test this hypothesis because people with diets higher in vitamin E seemed to be less likely to develop heart disease. And hey, vitamin E is an antioxidant, and vitamins must be safe: after all, they are natural and in food. That study came to an abrupt end because of worse outcomes for those who took vitamin E.

For doctors, alternative therapies are a difficult line to walk. Some are low-cost and low-risk, but some are expensive and time-consuming, and some, like vitamin E, have hidden risks. If the data were good, these therapies would be standard of care. Although many functional medicine providers and naturopaths do so with confidence, I couldn't look someone in the eye and recommend an untested and expensive "happy period" supplement. Alternative therapies are often promoted as "natural," which ties into the health halo of that word (*natural* being equated to *effective* and *safe*). However, there are no supplement trees or farms, so be wary of false advertising.

It's not wrong to try an alternative therapy. It's your body and your decision. What *is* wrong is for a medical provider to misrepresent the therapies. You can make an informed choice only if you are given accurate information. Consider two ways a health care provider might discuss turmeric for period pain:

1. "Turmeric is a good option for painful periods. It's an ancient therapy long used in traditional medicine, and it contains the powerful chemical curcumin."

2. "There are a few studies on turmeric for painful periods, but overall, they are low-quality, so it isn't possible to draw conclusions. The people who propose turmeric typically do so based on a substance it contains: curcumin. Some people recommend turmeric supplements, and others curcumin. It's debatable whether curcumin is biologically active (whether it does anything meaningful in the body), but even if it is, less than 1 percent of curcumin that is ingested enters the circulation. In addition, curcumin is removed from the bloodstream within minutes (it's meta-bolized very quickly), so even if it manages to be absorbed, it's not likely to hang around long enough to do anything. In higher-quality studies, curcumin has never been shown to be effective for any medical condition, and there are cases of liver failure associated with turmeric supplements."

If you were to decide to take turmeric for painful periods based on the first advice, you would be making an uninformed choice. But you wouldn't realize that, because you wouldn't know your medical provider didn't give you all the details. On the other hand, deciding to take turmeric after hearing the second description would be an informed choice. You'd have heard about the biological constraints, what research has shown and not shown, and potential downsides. It's easy to see why many people are attracted to the much shorter, more optimistic, but much less informative and ultimately unethical presentation.

With all of that in mind, here are some alternative options you might hear about and can consider for painful periods or endometriosis-related pain. For the record, I discuss some of them in the office, but I do so using the prin-ciples of informed consent that I just used for turmeric, which I suppose can be summed up as a "warts and all" approach.

Diet

Can diet affect painful periods? Maybe. And that's really a maaaaaaybe. Studies have linked a variety of diets and/or foods with less period pain: low-fat vege-tarian, higher in fruit, lower in legumes, lower in omega-6 fatty acids, lower in alcohol, lower in meat, higher in dairy. Some of these recommendations are contradictory, which is problematic. For example, vegetarians often eat legumes and omega-6s, so if a vegetarian diet is helpful, how is a diet higher in legumes and omega-6s harmful?

Diet data largely comes from observational studies, meaning people told researchers whether they had period pain and what they typically ate. Observational studies have a lot of issues. First, people's recall isn't always accurate. Second, we may not know who has endometriosis and who has painful periods. But even more importantly, what we eat is associated with a variety of factors that might affect pain and are unrelated to the actual food. For example, living in poverty can decrease the availability and afford-ability of fresh fruits and vegetables, and it can reduce access to health care, which can increase the risk of having untreated causes of pain. People with period pain may be more likely to choose ready-made meals because they are in too much pain to grocery shop and/or prepare food, but ready-made meals tend to be lower in fiber and contain seed oils, which have omega-6s. Or people with pain may feel comforted when they eat certain foods. Basically, diet can be linked with period pain in a myriad of ways, but not as a cause-and-effect kind of relationship. Finally, people have been eating very different diets around the world for millennia, and no culture seems immune from period pain.

To really answer the question about diet and menstrual-related pain, we need randomized studies, meaning one group is randomly assigned to one diet and another, almost identical group is assigned to a different diet, and then these two groups are followed to see if, over time, they report different levels of period pain. We just don't have this data.

Omega-6 fatty acids have been getting the villain treatment lately—being blamed for everything from type 2 diabetes to heart disease to brain fog and, yes, painful periods—and it's not uncommon to see period coaches and naturopaths vilifying seed oils because they are high in omega-6s. Omega-6 and omega-3 fatty acids are polyunsaturated fats that are essential for our bodies. Omega-6s are found in vegetable oils, nuts, and seeds; omega-3s are found in fish, vegetable oils, some nuts, flax seeds, flaxseed oil, and leafy vegetables. Some people believe omega-6s are inflammatory, and from a period standpoint, one theory is that the linoleic acid in omega-6s increases arachidonic acid, a necessary step in making prostaglandins, substances that cause painful periods. However, less than 1 percent of the linoleic acid in our food is converted into arachidonic acid, and arachidonic acid itself can be anti-inflammatory. Basically, it's complicated. But there are quality studies that don't link omega-6s with inflammation. In fact, they're associated with lower rates of heart disease, which suggests they aren't inflammatory.

It's important to remember that seed oils, the oils high in omega-6s, tend to be used in ultra-processed foods and fried foods in restaurants, which are linked with inflammatory health conditions. However, the omega-6s aren't the culprit; these foods also tend to have a lower nutritional value and are calorie-dense.

What about people who say they feel better, cramp-wise, after changing their diet? It's definitely possible to feel better within a few cycles after a dietary change. For example, if you increase your fiber intake, you are less likely to have constipation, and most people feel better when they aren't constipated (that's the understatement of the year). Improving diet quality may reduce bloating or heartburn, and again, that might make you feel better. Moreover, just the idea of self-care (and changing diet can be self-care) can make people feel better. It is also possible that changing diet affects pain in a way we have yet to understand.

The best we can say is that a traditional Western diet—one that is higher in calorie-dense, nutritionally poor foods, lower in fiber, and higher in saturated fat—is the least healthy diet overall. Trans fats are inflammatory and should be avoided for many health reasons. (They are banned in the United States and Canada but are still available in many countries.) Aiming for healthier diet choices is beneficial for many reasons, and if you are healthier overall, that may well be better for period pain. Given how many awful messages girls and women receive about their bodies, and the state of food policing, in the absence of high-quality data, my default is to simply consider these basics:

- Aim for at least 25 g of fiber a day. I really like this approach, as it adds something rather than taking something away. Foods high in fiber are associated with a low risk of breast cancer, colon cancer, and heart disease.
- Increase your intake of fruits and vegetables (this helps in the fiber department too).
- Try to eat two servings of fish a week (assuming you aren't vegetarian or vegan).
- Reduce animal fats. Swap in cooking oils for butter, introduce two to three vegan meals per week, choose leaner cuts of beef or eat

less beef, and switch out whole milk for 2% milk, skim milk, or even plant-based milks.

- Consult a registered dietician for good advice on dietary changes that are healthier overall. Personally, I'd take a hard pass on anyone who vilifies seed oils or sells supplements. Also avoid people who call themselves functional nutritionists, as that isn't a recognized branch of health care.
- Reduce alcohol intake. Not many people want to hear this, but overall, less is better.

Exercise

The data here is not the greatest, but overall, it seems that exercise may reduce the intensity of painful periods. Because of the low quality of the studies, we can't specify what type of exercise—whether aerobic, weightlifting, or some of both—or how many minutes is optimal. One theory is that exercise may reduce inflammatory mediators that are part of painful periods, but there is a lot of "maybe" and "possibly" here. However, we know exercise is beneficial for overall health, so it may be indirectly helpful for menstrual pain.

When I was a teen with painful cramps, if someone had said, "Well, you could treat your pain by exercising," I would have rolled my eyes. When my cramps were at their worst, any movement was painful. I've explained how pain can spread to other body parts, and for some that can be the abdominal wall. For me, it was often physically painful to stand up straight. In addition, given my menstrual diarrhea, there were times when I simply couldn't be far from a bathroom. I didn't exercise regularly, so telling me to start would have been as helpful as telling me to fly to the moon. However, when I began to get into running in my thirties, I did find that exercise was helpful when my cramps were uncomfortable but not excruciating. I don't know whether it was because exercise helped my mood and made me feel better that way, or because it provided a distraction (a valid therapy for pain), or because it lowered inflammatory mediators and directly reduced my pain. Over the years, the better I got at exercising, the more I could do it when I had cramps.

This is all anecdotal, and there are many other potential explanations, but if you suffer with bad cramps and don't exercise regularly, consider starting an exercise regimen on the days you don't have pain. Ideally, you'd get 150 minutes of moderate-intensity aerobic activity and two days of muscle strengthening activity a week. At the very least, this movement will make you healthier overall, and it will likely help your body deal with the stress of menstruation. If you find that exercise during your period helps, great, do it. If you find that it makes things worse, then don't do it.

Dietary Supplements

Despite what you might see on Instagram, Facebook, and TikTok, there is no quality evidence supporting supplements for painful periods. It's important to acknowledge that even the information I've included here is based on lower-quality studies.

There are two kinds of supplements: those that contain a single active ingredient (for example, magnesium or calcium) and those that contain multiple products (usually combinations of vitamins, minerals, and botanicals/herbs). Single-ingredient supplements that have been studied, may make some sense biologically, and seem low-risk include:

- *Magnesium:* 360 to 400 mg a day for three days, starting one day before the onset of bleeding. Magnesium can cause diarrhea, so keep that in mind.
- *Thiamine (vitamin B_1):* 100 mg daily.
- *Fish oil capsules:* 6 g (containing 1,080 mg EPA and 720 mg DHA), divided into two doses a day, or 2 g of krill oil a day.
- *Vitamin B_6:* 200 mg a day.
- *Ginger capsules:* 750 to 2,000 mg a day for the first three days of bleeding.

My advice to anyone who wants to try these products is to give it a go for three cycles, then decide if the benefit is worth it. If you do go this route, I suggest a brand like Nature Made (I get no money from them), which has affordable products that are USP verified, meaning the ingredients have been independently verified for quality and the bottle contains what is listed on the label.

A variety of companies and providers sell or recommend specific multi-ingredient supplements for menstrual pain, often with the bizarre names that imply your period is "broken." None of these products have been tested in a meaningful way, which is hypocritical, considering that the people who recommend them often accuse Big Pharma of dastardly deeds and hiding evidence and claim the birth control pill (a competitor to these supplements) is understudied. When it comes to these products, buyer beware. Supplements are a growing cause of liver failure, and you really have no idea what's in them. If the products are so effective, why don't the people who make them do high-quality studies so we can all learn? (I mean, we all know the answer. The results would undoubtedly negatively affect sales.)

Vaginal Steaming

This practice is offered as a cure for all manner of menstrual ills, from "unbalanced hormones" to "cleaning the womb" and period pain. The idea is that you squat over a pot of steaming herbs, and the steam (which contains volatile organic compounds, or VOCs) enters the vagina and does something. This "something" can apparently magically reduce cramps by who knows what mechanism, but I'm sure it has to do with "toxins." Interestingly, no one on TikTok who is concerned about VOCs in tampons seems to care about the VOCs here.

It's true, in ancient medicine vaginal steaming was used as a therapy . . . by practitioners who thought the uterus wandered around the body. If you accept vaginal steaming, you must also accept the belief system on which it is based, including some less-Instagram-friendly recipes. Think a disemboweled puppy stuffed with herbs and then burned for its smoke to fumigate the uterus.

It is biologically impossible for vaginal steaming to affect menstrual pain. Almost certainly, all of the steam will hit the vulva, putting the user at risk of burns (which have been reported). It's unlikely any steam will enter the vagina, but on the off chance it does, it would likely be harmful to the vaginal ecosystem. There is no biological mechanism for the volatiles in the steam to have any meaningful medical effect.

Acupuncture

Acupuncture is the practice of putting needles into the body at specific points based on meridians that are related to the flow of *qi*, a form of energy. Acupuncture is often held up as an ancient therapy, but ancient shouldn't be mistaken for effective. And the acupuncture performed today is almost certainly not the same as the ancient practice.

Despite its extensive use—worldwide, it's an almost $25-billion business annually—quality evidence supporting acupuncture is lacking. As far as painful periods are concerned, there are a few published studies, but most are of such low quality that no meaningful conclusions can be reached. While some people do report feeling better after acupuncture, spending time with a practitioner who listens and validates experiences is itself an intervention.

Although acupuncture is relatively benign, collapsed lungs have been reported in rare cases, and it can be time-consuming and expensive—this isn't a $10 bottle of magnesium that lasts three months. I don't recommend acupuncture, but when a patient asks for my opinion, I am truthful. I explain there are no quality studies for period pain, that the data for treating pain in general is low-quality, and that the bulk of it suggests a placebo response. If they want a referral, I am happy to make one. If someone simply asks for a referral for acupuncture and doesn't ask my opinion (as happens a fair bit), I am happy to make one. If someone were to tell me they wanted to pray for an end to their pain, an intervention based on divine energy, I would be supportive then too, but I wouldn't be recommending it to my patients.

Off Switches for Period Pain

An "on/off switch for period pain" doesn't exist. I know, it would be great. The manufacturer of Livia, the product that purports to be this magical switch, describes the product with language that is very similar to a TENS unit (for example, closing the "nerve gate" and "producing pain-fighting endorphins"). Based on its appearance and the information on the manufacturer's site, it seems like it's just a pretty TENS unit (see page 260). Currently, Livia sells for US$129. It looks like the settings are preset, so you cannot change frequency or pulse width to suit your own needs, as you can with a regular TENS unit. If you want to spend more because you like how the device looks, even though the settings can't be changed and hence it's likely to be less useful, that's a personal call. Are you getting anything better than a traditional TENS unit? Nope. Look, I spend a fair bit of money on shoes, but the people who make them don't tell me they are better at getting me from A to B than the $10 flats I picked up at Target.

Jovi

This is a skin patch, and the website claims, "When cramps kick in, an unbalanced electrical field is created at the source. (Looking at you, uterus . . .)." I've never read a medical description *quite* like that. Another claim, ". . . when placed on the source of your pain, the Jovi patch works to pick up the message your body is sending out, rerouting it and absorbing it like a sponge." This also doesn't make medical sense to me, and if the patch needs to go "on the source" "(Looking at you, uterus . . .)," why apply it to the skin?

Regarding the research, per the website, "Jovi is a general wellness product with hundreds of personal testimonials that back up our claims. We are in the process of seeking FDA approval and doing our best to meet their standards of claims. That is why you will not see clinical studies posted here until approved by the FDA. The Signal Relief technology that powers the Jovi Patch has undergone clinical testing with exciting results!" but the hyperlink goes to some data about muscle pain, not a peer-reviewed study on menstrual pain.

With a US$149 price tag, I believe you and your uterus deserve quality studies, not testimonials.

Cannabis

There is a popular myth that Queen Victoria used cannabis for her menstrual cramps, but it has been disproven by medical historians. Myths aside, cannabis has been used for pain for thousands of years, and our understanding of how it works and its effectiveness has been hampered by its illegality in many countries. The past few years have brought a significant change in opinions about cannabis, and in many places it is now legal. So we are now finally getting some data we can use to advise people about cannabis and pain. In fact, a review of the data by the National Academies of Sciences, Engineering, and Medicine concluded that cannabis has a moderate impact on pain.

Cannabis has over four hundred chemical compounds. The most abundant are THC (delta-9-tetrahydrocannabinol) and CBD (cannabidiol). Both act on the endocannabinoid system. Our understanding of this signaling system is far from complete, but we do know it has an important role in many bodily functions, including the menstrual cycle and pregnancy. The body produces natural endocannabinoids that interact with cannabinoid receptors, in the same way it makes estrogens that act on estrogen receptors. There are two endocannabinoid receptors that we know of: CB1, which is largely found in the nervous system, and CB2, which is mainly involved with the immune system. The endocannabinoid system plays an important role in the hypothalamic-pituitary-gonadal axis (the brain-brain-ovary connection), the development of follicles, ovulation, the function of the endometrium, and early development of the placenta.

We don't know how, or how well, cannabis might work for period cramps or endometriosis pain, but more and more people are using it for these purposes. It may be helpful via an effect on hormone levels or a direct impact on the endometrium, or it may work on pain processing in the brain. Given the lack of studies, it isn't possible to be specific about routes, doses, and percentages of THC and CBD for period or endometriosis pain. Some cannabis-based pharmaceuticals have been studied for other pain conditions that also involve muscle spasm, and they use a ratio of THC to CBD of either 2:1 or 1:1, so that is probably a reasonable place to start. Beyond that, it's difficult to make any recommendations.

Cannabis adversely affects the ability to safely drive or operate heavy equipment, which may limit its practical applications for many people.

Any discussion of cannabis would be incomplete without mentioning that it is an endocrine disruptor and its full effect on the reproductive system is unknown. Some studies have shown that it can impact the hypothalamus, the pituitary, and the ovaries; others have revealed changes in hormone levels and even negative effects on the developing follicle. I find it interesting that when cannabis comes up, these effects are rarely if ever mentioned. Does this mean people shouldn't use cannabis for pain? No. Pain itself has consequences in the body, and every medication has potential risks. But don't assume that, because cannabis is a plant, it has no negative impact on reproductive hormones. There is simply a lot we don't know.

For teens and those in their early twenties who use cannabis ten or more times a month, there is a risk of potential effects on the brain. And although the risk of dependence and addiction is lower with cannabis than with opioids and alcohol, the possibility does exist. There are concerns about use in pregnancy causing low birth weight and abnormal neurological development for newborns. And in many places, cannabis isn't legal, so that is a legitimate concern as well.

As for the best route, smoking or vaporizing produces faster results that tend to be more predictable, and the effects typically last two to three hours. With edibles, it takes longer for the cannabinoids to get into the bloodstream, but the effects tend to last longer.

What about vaginal administration? There are a wide variety of vaginal suppositories, tinctures, and even tampons containing either THC alone or THC and CBD for sale. Many people who promote these products do so with the claim that vaginal mucosa has the highest concentration of cannabinoid receptors in the human body, apart from the brain. I know of no scientifically credible data to support this assertion, and I double-checked with an expert in the area. I despise this kind of sciencey-sounding truthiness. Regardless, when you have painful periods, it's not the lining of the vagina you want to target for therapy. Suppose the goal is to treat period cramps or endometriosis-related pain. In that case, the research that exists, such as it is, supports getting cannabis into the bloodstream via inhalation or ingestion. While it's true that many medications can be absorbed from the vagina into the bloodstream, and this route has advantages in some cases, we don't know if THC or CBD is absorbed well from the vagina.

There is also the potential for a negative effect on the vaginal ecosystem. Cannabinoids have antimicrobial activities, but we don't know what that means for healthy bacteria in the vagina. We shouldn't assume that vaginal administration is beneficial or even neutral. One study tells us that people who use marijuana for any reason are more likely to have yeast in their vagina. While we can't extrapolate this study to what might happen with vaginal use, it's not exactly reassuring. The potential impact of vaginal cannabis products on the vaginal ecosystem must be evaluated, especially as the people who make these products are promoting them for regular use.

There is simply no data to back up the wild claims you might read or hear about vaginal cannabis products. The onus is on those selling the products to do the research and prove their safety and efficacy. We've already seen with the Rely tampon how something that seems like a great idea can turn out to be bad for the vagina.

The Three-Cycle Trial

With any product for period pain, three cycles is generally a long enough trial to determine if you are experiencing a benefit. I encourage people to ask themselves three questions about their cycle, and write down the answers, before they embark on any new therapy for pain, whether it's an alternative therapy or a well-studied treatment:

- How many days a week does pain interfere with my quality of life?
- When I have pain, what is its maximum score out of 10, with 0 being no pain and 10 the worst pain ever?
- When I have pain, how does it interfere with my quality of life?

Three cycles after starting therapy, revisit these questions and compare the answers. Also make note of any side effects. (Obviously, if the side effects are bad, don't wait three cycles to stop!) It isn't uncommon for me to see people who are unsure whether therapy has helped, but when they look at the objective information they have collected, they realize they have had more or less benefit than they suspected. It's human nature. People sometimes stop a therapy because they think it didn't help, and then, a month later, I hear, "You know, now that I've stopped, I feel much worse." Conversely, I see people who think the treatment is helping, and then, by cycle four or five, they realize it isn't. This supports the idea of revisiting the questions at six and nine months. It's important to remember that there is a very real placebo effect with medications—and interestingly, more expensive medications tend to have a stronger placebo effect.

Bottom Line

- When you're looking for less traditional options for treating menstrual pain and/or pain from endometriosis, it's important to look at the possible risks. Many people who advertise alternative products are not forthcoming about the potential downsides.
- No quality data supports a specific diet for menstrual pain, but overall, a healthy diet may help people feel better and is certainly better for overall health.
- Of the supplements for menstrual pain, magnesium and omega-3s have the best supporting evidence and are low-risk.
- Livia is an expensive TENS unit, and Jovi is a fairy tale.
- Cannabis may be an option for menstrual pain and endometriosis-related pain, although the data is limited.

Part 4

CONTRACEPTION AND ABORTION

The History of Hormonal Contraception

Historically, people have used a variety of products to prevent conception, from animal dung inserted vaginally to herbal teas to spells. The first condom appears to have been made of linen and was used to prevent transmission of syphilis; its effectiveness for pregnancy prevention is unknown. When the process to vulcanize rubber was patented in 1844, it paved the way for the first rubber condom (hence the slang *rubbers*) in 1855. In 1886, an English pharmacist, Walter Rendell, sold vaginal suppositories made of quinine and cacao butter—the first commercially available medical contraceptive. Again, effectiveness unknown. Diaphragms became available in the 1880s, but how well these early devices worked remains a mystery.

One of the issues with developing and studying new contraceptives in the United States and Canada was legality. In the United States, the Comstock Act of 1873 criminalized birth control, making it illegal to provide education about contraception or to disseminate contraception across state lines. In 1892, Canada criminalized the dissemination of information about contraception, as well as selling contraception or distributing it for free. Why develop a contraceptive if you can't legally sell it and it could land you in jail? Restrictive laws don't just hurt people at the time, they also hamper research, potentially impacting future generations.

Without contraception, women often resorted to douches, with the mistaken idea that the chemicals might kill sperm or induce an abortion. These products were marketed for "feminine hygiene," to bypass the laws about contraception, and they had awful slogans, such as this one for Lysol: "She was a jewel of a wife . . . with just one flaw. She was guilty of the 'ONE NEGLECT' that mars many marriages." The message was clear to women of the day: neglecting to keep the number of babies in check, whether they had a say in having sex or not, was *their* problem. Douches were also dangerous, but to what branch of the government do you complain when your clandestine contraceptive doesn't work?

The history of hormonal contraception is fascinating, and I highly recommend reading *The Birth of the Pill* by Jonathan Eig, which is impeccably researched, is a great read, and provided vital reference material for this chapter.

The Idea

During the time when contraception was illegal, Margaret Sanger, who would later go on to found Planned Parenthood, came up with the term *birth control*—the revolutionary idea that a woman could and should be able to control when she gave birth. Sanger was passionately pro-contraception. She wanted women to be liberated from the financial and physical burdens of multiple pregnancies and to be allowed the same sexual freedom as men, meaning to have sex for pleasure, without the fear of pregnancy. According to Sanger, "No woman can call herself free who does not own and control her own body. No woman can call herself free until she can choose consciously whether she will or will not be a mother." Although Sanger was vehemently in favor of birth control, she was anti-abortion, and Planned Parenthood did not start offering abortions until three years after her death.

Sanger educated women about birth control and distributed condoms and diaphragms. In 1914, threatened with arrest, she fled the United States for England without her husband, who served her thirty-day sentence for her. (I know, right?) When she returned, she opened a birth control clinic in Brooklyn, once again distributing condoms and a diaphragm-like device, but this time under the guise that the device had a medical purpose: to support the uterus. She was arrested. She eventually divorced her first husband and married a wealthy man, who provided the funds to allow her to pursue the dream of a birth control pill. It had to be a pill—something that was discreet, easy, and under a woman's own control. A pill of one's own.

Sanger was also instrumental in changing laws about birth control. In 1932, a box of diaphragms sent to her from a Japanese physician was seized by the postal service. Sanger challenged the seizure in court, arguing that it impeded medical progress. Surprisingly, the New York State Board of Appeals agreed; if a physician was involved, it became legal in New York to mail not just information about contraception, but contraceptives themselves. However, contraception was still illegal in over half the states.

Sanger would talk about birth control with anyone who would listen. She worked with leaders in the Black community and believed Black women would feel more comfortable in a clinic in their own community staffed by Black medical providers. But she also spoke with the women's auxiliary branch of the Ku Klux Klan to get support for her cause, and any association with that group is deplorable. Sanger had racist views about Black people and supported the eugenics movement. Although these ideas were tragically common (compulsory sterilization was even constitutional at the time), that doesn't excuse her racism. We must acknowledge the history so this harmful legacy isn't perpetuated today. Sanger's story reminds us that birth control offers an attractive Trojan horse for racism and eugenics. Therefore, studies on contraception and programs that offer contraception must follow rigorous codes of ethics and meet the needs of all communities. Everyone deserves access to contraception, but it's equally important that no one have contraception pushed on them.

The Scientist

Sanger approached scientist after scientist to find someone to help her with her quest, but she was repeatedly turned down, possibly because the science was believed to be too complex, but also likely because birth control was still illegal in thirty states. Many scientists didn't want to engage with the topic of contraception because it was a "private" matter, and I'm sure there were also many who didn't believe in sexual liberation for women.

In 1950, when she was seventy-one years old, Sanger met Dr. Gregory Goodwin Pincus, a scientist studying reproduction in rabbits. By 1936 he had successfully performed in vitro fertilization on a rabbit and had coaxed rabbit eggs into embryos without sperm, a process called parthenogenesis. It's not hyperbole to say he was brilliant; at the time, he was likely the foremost expert on ovulation. I mean, making an embryo without sperm in 1936 was an incredible act of science. Pincus courted the press, but among scientists a desire for fame was frowned upon, and it eventually backfired: his research left him labeled a modern Dr. Frankenstein (undoubtedly also because of antisemitism). Despite his stunning scientific achievements, he was forced to leave Harvard, where he had been working, and had difficulty securing another university appointment. Eventually, he found a place at Clark University in Massachusetts, setting up the Worcester Foundation for Experimental Biology, a private lab to study hormones, something that really wasn't being done at the time.

When Sanger met Pincus, she found not just the brain power but the scientific curiosity to complete the task. At this point, Pincus knew progesterone was nature's contraceptive: it didn't just prepare the uterus for implantation, it also shut down follicle development. Remember, the LH surge is exquisitely sensitive to progesterone, because once pregnancy has occurred, the body has no need for ovulation. So Pincus had a candidate hormone, progesterone, but still had several major hurdles to overcome. He had to prove it suppressed ovulation in an animal model, and that it could do so when given orally. Then he needed to test it in humans. The tests would require a lot of progesterone, which was cost-prohibitive at the time.

As luck would have it, a new method for making hormones had just become available. Until this point, hormones were extracted from animal ovaries and urine, or from human urine. It takes a lot of urine to get a little bit of hormone, which must then be purified in the lab. But all that changed when Dr. Russell Earl Marker discovered that diosgenin, a chemical found in a yam in Mexico, could be converted into progesterone via a process that bears his name today: the Marker degradation. Pincus went to work with this newfound supply of progesterone and found that it did indeed effectively prevent ovulation in rabbits and rats. And not just as an injection—it also worked as a pill.

A contraceptive pill was possible.

The Money

Drug development is extraordinarily expensive, more than Sanger could finance on her own. There can be many false starts, and rabbit holes can go on for years before you realize you've spent a lot of money getting hopelessly off track and need to start over. Scientists, lab spaces, and raw ingredients are also expensive, and human trials even more so. As luck would have it, around the time Pincus discovered that progesterone worked in rabbits, Sanger received a letter from Katharine Dexter McCormick, a widow and one of the richest women in the world. She wanted to support birth control research.

The Doctor

Rabbits only get you so far. Ultimately, a birth control pill had to be tried in women, but Pincus wasn't a medical doctor. They needed an open-minded physician with access to female patients. Enter Dr. John Rock, an OB/GYN who was in many ways ahead of his time. Unlike his peers, who thought infertility was always caused by the woman (I know you're simply shocked by this), he believed men could be responsible for infertility. He also believed a pregnant woman's life was more important than that of her fetus. Despite being Catholic, he supported abortion and taught women the "rhythm method," the earliest fertility awareness method. He was also a pioneer of in vitro fertilization, which is how he came to know Pincus. Sanger was distrustful because Rock was Catholic, but Pincus persuaded her to include Rock in their efforts.

Rock decided to give progesterone and estrogen to some of his infertility patients to see what happened. Why he added estrogen isn't clear. Rock was honest with the women, telling them the hormones wouldn't help their infertility, but it was work that might help in the eventual goal of treating infertility (that was possibly a stretch). It was the 1950s, and consent for research was essentially nonexistent. Doctors sometimes simply gave women medications with vague information that they were trying something new or attempting to advance care. It's hard to imagine this today, but many people—especially women—just did what their doctor recommended, with few if any questions. The more vulnerable the population, the more likely they were to be used as guinea pigs, with little consideration for safety.

Fortunately, no one died from the hormones and no one got pregnant, although thirteen of the women became pregnant shortly after stopping the drugs. This became known as the Rock rebound: the belief that fertility may be enhanced after the ovaries are suppressed for a while. Another takeaway was that the hormones stopped menstruation; consequently, many women thought they were pregnant and were upset when they found out they weren't. Pincus and Rock decided the answer was to stop the progesterone for a few days each month to allow for menstruation. And that is the origin story of the placebo pills in oral contraception.

The Studies

With a hormone regimen that hadn't killed or caused any major adverse side effects for any of the eighty women who took it, the next step was larger-scale studies. They were hampered by the fact that contraception was still illegal in Massachusetts, where Pincus and Rock were based. The work-around? They claimed to be working on a fertility treatment. They told the women that the medication would shut down their ovaries so they couldn't get pregnant, that they might feel pregnant (an effect of the hormones and the missed menstruation), and that when they stopped the medication their chance of pregnancy would be higher. Although the scientists might have believed in the Rock rebound, this study would not be considered even remotely ethical by today's standards.

Two trials with progesterone were carried out, eventually totaling sixty patients over three cycles. Rock and Pincus also managed to convince some nurses to try their progesterone protocol. The women took 200 mg or 300 mg of progesterone a day, with twenty-one days on treatment and seven days off. It was a cumbersome study; the women collected daily urine samples for hormone monitoring, and half of them also checked their temperature and collected daily vaginal swabs to be analyzed under the microscope for the effect of the hormones. The protocols and some of the side effects were so onerous that half of the participants dropped out. Among those stalwarts who stuck it out, 15 percent ovulated. Not a success.

Looking back, it's not surprising this regimen failed. Progesterone is absorbed poorly by mouth, and this dose wouldn't have been enough to completely suppress ovulation.

Getting enough women for their studies was proving to be a challenge. The only women who had been willing to do exactly what Rock asked of them were those with infertility who had been led to believe the procedure might help them. This only highlights that false hopes can be a way to take advantage of a vulnerable population, especially since the women enrolled didn't know the potential risks or if the Rock rebound was a true or spurious finding.

Women started asking questions about the medication: Is it safe? Will it affect my fertility down the road? And neither Pincus nor Rock had answers. So they looked for a population with no other option but to participate and gave progesterone to sixteen psychotic patients in an asylum. (Yes, really.) Pincus and Rock defended it as legitimate research, claiming there was evidence that progesterone might be useful for psychosis, which looks like wishful thinking on their part. Given the general lack of knowledge about hormones and about mental health at the time, trying progesterone for psychosis wasn't necessarily problematic in and of itself. You can understand how family members would be desperate enough to consent to a novel therapy when nothing else was available. But though Pincus said the patients themselves were willing, they couldn't have truly consented by today's standards. This research was what we would now call a phase-one study, meaning preliminary work, and today it can be performed only on healthy volunteers where there is no risk of coercion, and these volunteers are compensated for their time and the potential risk.

I don't buy Pincus's claim that this was a side study on psychosis. The women were required to have endometrial biopsies, a sampling of tissue from the lining of the uterus that can feel like a cramp for some but can be excruciating for others. Information from endometrial biopsies wouldn't have been needed for a study on psychosis, but it would have been important for evaluating the impact on ovulation and designing a birth control pill. In addition, in 1957, the medical journal *The Lancet* reported on a lecture given by Pincus about his work on the pill where he specifically mentioned the study on "patients in a mental hospital"; if that study were for other reasons, it would have been phrased differently. We also now know that McCormick gave money to the hospital for painting and furniture, which undoubtedly helped paved the way for the work, something that would be considered highly unethical today.

Even some physicians of the day considered this kind of research on vulnerable patients unacceptable. When Dr. James Milne read about it, he wrote to *The Lancet*, "this use as guinea pigs of chronic psychotic patients who are not able to give or withhold valid permission for experiments in psychological research of this type must be as repugnant to many of your readers as it is to me."

Around this time, some of the scientists working with Pincus started giving progesterone to their wives—sometimes for contraception and sometimes to stop periods. But a few patients from asylums and private practice amounted to no more than preliminary safety studies. Besides, the progesterone didn't reliably suppress ovulation. Pincus and Rock needed something that acted like progesterone on the brain and the uterus but could bypass the issue in the gut that was preventing absorption. As luck would have it, drugs with that potential were by then in investigative stages.

The ability to make progesterone in large amounts via the Marker degradation opened the door to more tinkering (a woefully inadequate word for such intricate research) with hormones by pharmaceutical companies, leading to a new class of drugs called progestins. Progestins act like progesterone in some ways; specifically, they suppress the LH surge and counteract the effect of estrogen on the uterus. But progestins, it turned out, also have some key differences from progesterone. Not only are they easily absorbed when taken by mouth, but they are more potent in countering estrogen's effect on the lining of the uterus and more effective at inhibiting ovulation. In addition, they thicken the cervical mucus, preventing sperm from making it to the uterus (often referred to as making the cervical mucus inhospitable to sperm, which sounds like the sperm were coming over for tea but were passive-aggressively disinvited at the door).

There were two candidate progestins, norgestimate and norethynodrel. Animal studies showed that norethynodrel, the product being developed by the pharmaceutical company Searle, had fewer side effects. So norethynodrel it was. The first studies were on a small scale, with a few women in Dr. Rock's private practice and a trial in Puerto Rico. In 1954, contraception was legal in Puerto Rico, and about 16 percent of Puerto Rican women had already had a surgical sterilization, so the idea of contraception was societally acceptable. In addition, the investigators felt that, given the poverty and typical large family size of people on the island, recruitment would be easy. The idea of traveling to another region and looking for a vulnerable population to bear the potential risks of a barely tested drug that can't be borne by women in your own region is medical colonialism and it is abhorrent.

Initially they started with twenty-three medical students who were "convinced" to take norethynodrel and complete the rigorous follow-up, including vaginal smears, daily temperature monitoring, and urine samples. Pincus and Rock felt the students could be trusted to take the pill and would be motivated to complete the study, but one wonders if there were barely veiled threats about grade retaliation if the study wasn't done correctly. Even so, over half of the women dropped out, and many of the samples from the remaining participants were incomplete or contaminated. Eventually, the doctors were able to recruit over two hundred women for a larger study of their candidate pill, now named Enovid. The pregnancy rate was 17 percent, which they explained away as inconsistent pill-taking. The truth seems impossible to determine. Was the pill taken inconsistently, or did it just not work as well as they had hoped? Another troubling issue was that about 10 percent of the women dropped out because of the side effects.

More patients were enrolled and, curiously, the pregnancy rates this time were lower, but there were significant side effects, including breakthrough bleeding, nausea, and headaches. And then a mistake was uncovered: the norethynodrel from Searle was contaminated with an estrogen called mestranol. Pincus assumed mestranol must have been the cause of the side effects, so new batches of norethynodrel were obtained and double-checked to ensure they were pure progestin. To Pincus's surprise, most of the side effects remained and the irregular bleeding worsened, as did the impact on ovulation. The serendipitous estrogen had not only improved the contraceptive's efficacy but had also reduced irregular bleeding. Pincus and Rock decided the pill should have an estrogen as well. The final formulation for Enovid they tested was 10 mg norethynodrel and 0.15 mg mestranol. To put this dose of estrogen in perspective, 0.15 mg is 150 µg, which is equivalent to the estrogen in three to five of today's pills. So it's understandable that people had side effects!

The Approval

With a year's worth of data, Pincus convinced Searle to submit Enovid to the FDA. But there was a catch. Because contraception was still illegal in seventeen states, they would seek approval for it as a treatment for painful periods, irregular bleeding, and infertility, based on the Rock rebound idea. In 1957, the FDA approved Enovid for bleeding concerns and infertility. Listed as a side effect? Preventing ovulation, which certainly didn't hurt sales! *Warning, this drug prevents pregnancy.* It was approved in Canada in 1960, but only for treating bleeding issues, and in the United Kingdom in 1961 as contraception, but only for married women.

In 1959, with tens of thousands of women taking Enovid, Searle went back to the FDA to get approval to market the drug for contraception. This time they encountered more opposition, in the form of Dr. Pasquale DeFelice, an OB/GYN resident who was working for the FDA. He questioned the data, as there had been only 130 patients in the contraception study, and only 66 had taken the pill for twenty-four months; most had used it for just several months. How could it be safe? He took the unusual step of questioning fellow OB/GYNs, who seemed to be narrowly in favor of approving Enovid as contraception. On May 9, 1960, it was official: the first birth control pill was approved. And by 1961, four hundred thousand women were taking Enovid in the United States alone.

I sometimes wonder how so many people tolerated that much estrogen, but when abortion was illegal and you probably knew one or more people, some young girls, who had had awful clandestine abortions or who had been sent away to have a baby, only to come back in shame, the side effects might have seemed mild compared to what society had in store for you. Thinking back to my own cramps, heavy bleeding, and menstrual diarrhea, I probably would have tried Enovid if it had been my only option. Perspective is helpful.

The Legacy

I often see memes about the pill being a "seventy-year experiment on women." It sounds truthy (maybe even more so considering the history I've just relayed), but it isn't accurate. It's true that there were significant ethical issues with some of the studies that we wouldn't accept today. And even though Puerto Rican women bore the potential risks of studies of the first pill, there was no investment in making the approved pill available for women in Puerto Rico. When the studies were closed, the supply of pills disappeared, and they couldn't enjoy the results of their efforts.

But this history doesn't mean the pill we have today is experimental or unsafe. We now have decades of quality research and require institutional review boards and ethics committees. We recognize that vulnerable populations—for example, people with intellectual disabilities, children, those affected by racism, poverty, and homelessness, and those who are desperate for treatment—are more vulnerable to exploitation, and safeguards must be in place to guarantee informed consent and safety. In addition, financial compensation for participating can't be high enough that it might be a form of coercion.

The pill is probably one of the most studied medications in the world. It is excellent contraception and can dramatically improve quality of life for many people whose medical conditions are due to or affected by their menstrual cycle, such as painful periods, endometriosis, heavy periods, polycystic ovarian syndrome, and PMDD, just to name a few.

Another important legacy of the hormonal contraceptive pill is financial. One study estimated that by the 1990s the pill was responsible for 30 percent of the narrowing of the gender wage gap. The pill literally changed societal norms and life trajectories as more women went to college and entered the workforce. Sometimes I think about the tens of thousands (hundreds of thousands?) of women in the 1960s and early 1970s who weren't forced into an awful marriage or onto a dirty table in a back alley because they had access to the pill. And it wasn't just women who could now see a different future for themselves; those who hired them did as well.

Research for the pill begat the hormonal IUD and the contraceptive implant and injection. Without the pill, we might not have so many hormonal contraceptive options today.

Are there things about the pill we don't know? Undoubtedly, just as there are things we don't yet know about antibiotics. For example, we are only beginning to unravel how antibiotics impact the microbiome. But no one would say we should stop using penicillin until we fully understand the complicated relationship between it and the microbiome! We should always be reevaluating older medications as new concerns arise or new technology is developed. In response to new data, researchers have been continually lowering the dose of the pill and finding new delivery systems (patch, vaginal ring, implants, injections, IUDs), as well as developing new hormones. That's a testament to the ongoing efforts to improve the safety of these medications, reduce their side effects, and improve their contraceptive efficacy.

In fact, hormonal contraception has never been safer.

Bottom Line

- A birth control pill was the idea of Margaret Sanger, who wanted women to have control of their sexuality and enjoy reproductive freedom. Sanger has a complicated legacy involving racism and eugenics that we must be mindful of going forward so we don't repeat past mistakes.
- Dr. Pincus and his research team realized that progesterone was a natural contraceptive, and this epiphany became the basis for his work on designing a birth control pill.
- Much of the original background research on the pill exploited vulnerable populations.
- Two key steps in designing the pill were the discovery of progestins and the inadvertent addition of estrogen.
- Some of the original research on the birth control pill was far below standards we would accept today, but we now have decades of quality research to inform medical advice about hormonal contraception.

23

Estrogen-Containing Contraceptives: The Modern Pill, Patch, and Ring

Hormonal contraception has come a long way since it was first introduced in 1957. Doses of estrogen are much lower, there are several different estrogens and progestins to choose from, and the hormones are now formulated so they can be delivered into the bloodstream across the skin via a patch or from the vagina via a ring. While the original Enovid was one-size-fits-everyone (which works about as well in medicine as it does in clothing: it's better than nothing if it's all you have), today's permutations and combinations of hormones and delivery systems mean you can personalize your search to find the estrogen-containing contraceptive (ECC) with the best fit.

Over the past thirty or so years, amazing work has been done to improve the safety of the pill, reduce side effects, and create more options. But misinformation thrives because historically medicine has done an awful job of explaining hormonal contraceptives. Conversations with health care providers are often limited to "Here, take this," as opposed to "Here are the options. This is why I think an ECC might be best for you; now let's review the science that supports that position." In truth, many other medications, from fluconazole (Diflucan) for yeast infections to medications for high blood pressure, are offered with the same brusque prescription. But for many people, contraception feels more intimate and the lack of information more dismissive. These are medications that people use daily, often for years, so it's understandable and wonderful that they want to know more. And they should. You can't be an informed patient and make an empowered choice without accurate information.

The truth is, the estrogen-containing pill, patch, and ring are excellent medications. Like any medication, they are not for everyone, but as a class of drugs they are not evil or harmful. As a comparative example, I can't take NSAIDs because I have kidney disease, people who have had bariatric surgery also shouldn't use them, and for some people they can even contribute to stomach ulcers. But these truths should not take away from the fact that, for most people, when used as directed, NSAIDs are fantastic medications.

The Basics

ECCs are delivered into the bloodstream in different ways—through the gastrointestinal tract, across the skin, or across the vaginal mucosa—but these medications are all similar in how they work, their benefits, and their risks. All ECCs consist of an estrogen and a progestin, and they provide contraception in several ways:

- *Suppressing FSH and LH:* Follicles start to develop and produce estradiol each cycle, but without a rise in follicle-stimulating hormone and luteinizing hormone, they get to cycle day 3 and then hang out. Eventually they time out (they can only be held "on ice" for so long) and are reabsorbed by the body. Both hormones contribute to FSH and LH suppression.
- *Preventing the LH surge:* If a follicle escapes past day 3 (life always tries to find a way), it's unlikely to ovulate because the hormones, primarily the progestin, suppress the LH surge.
- *Thickening the cervical mucus:* This progestin-driven effect means sperm can't get from the vagina into the uterus.
- *Affecting movement of sperm and egg in the oviduct:* Basically, both hormones help prevent the egg and the sperm from meeting, although how much this contributes isn't known.

These effects would make excellent names for punk rock bands if some-one were so inclined. I imagine a battle of the bands with music by Inhospitable to Sperm, the GnRH Suppressors, Crashing the LH Surge, and Sperm and the Highway to Nowhere.

Progestins also thin the endometrium. Some have wondered if that could be a mechanism of contraception. If so, it would be a post-fertilization effect, and to someone who considers a fertilized ovum to be a life, it could be con-strued as abortion. I want to emphasize that medicine does not consider a fertilized ovum a life. In any case, there is no proof that the thinned lining prevents conception. People can be assured that ECCs prevent the egg and sperm from meeting.

The typical failure rate of ECCs is four to seven per hundred users per year. While some failures may be due to forgetting a pill, a small percentage of people are what we call fast metabolizers, meaning they break down the hormones faster. For them, it's like taking a lower dose, so the ECC may have a higher failure rate. There are no commercially available tests to predict this risk.

The Estrogen

The original estrogen used in the pill, mestranol, was abandoned because of fears, later disproven, that it caused tumors. Mestranol is converted by the body into ethinyl estradiol, which was selected as the replacement estrogen in the pill, and later as the estrogen in the patch and the ring. Ethinyl estradiol is absorbed easily, resists being metabolized by the liver, and is a potent estrogen. In addition, it has an especially strong effect on the endometrium, so it's very effective at preventing progestin-induced irregular bleeding. Like Liam Neeson in the movie *Taken*, ethinyl estradiol has a very particular set of skills. Because it is so effective and inexpensive, it took decades for researchers to come up with candidates that might be acceptable alternatives.

The dose of ethinyl estradiol in ECC pills ranges from 10 μg to 35 μg, or micrograms (35 μg is a low-dose pill and 10 to 25 μg ultra-low-dose pills). Pills with 50 μg are still made, but they are considered high-dose pills and should be used only in some situations where heavy bleeding needs to be stopped urgently; they should not be taken daily for contraception. Lowering the dose to 10 or 20 μg may reduce estrogen-related side effects and complications, but the data here isn't great. Lowering the dose also increases the risk of irregular bleeding. Because many of the side effects and all of the serious risks associated with ECCs are related to the dose of estrogen, if you don't have a compelling reason to use a 35 µg pill, a 20 µg pill is a good place to start.

Depending on the brand, the patches release 30 to 35 µg of ethinyl estradiol a day, and the two rings on the market release 13 to 15 µg ethinyl estradiol a day, but they are not directly equivalent to the pill dose-wise (µg to µg). With an oral medication, hormone levels rise rapidly and fall in a twenty-four-hour cycle; with the patch and ring, the hormones are absorbed and then stay at a constant level. Taking these factors into consideration, the ring results in overall lower levels of estrogen in the blood than a 30 µg pill, and the patch results in higher levels.

Although the risk of serious complications from ethinyl estradiol is rare, researchers have worked hard to find estrogens with even lower risks and reduced side effects. Refining any medication based on new knowledge or technology is a worthy goal. The studies have led to three new estrogens that are closely related to estrogens made by the body:

- *Estradiol valerate:* A chemically modified version of 17 beta-estradiol, the estrogen made by the ovary. The modification, through a process called esterification, improves absorption from the gut. When the estrogen reaches the liver, instead of being rendered largely ineffective, it's converted back to 17 beta-estradiol.
- *Micronized 17 beta-estradiol:* A form of 17 beta-estradiol modified by micronization, a process that makes the hormone's particles smaller (like converting tiny pebbles into sand). Micronization also improves absorption.
- *Esterol:* The estrogen made by the fetal liver, found in the body during pregnancy.

When ethinyl estradiol is metabolized by the liver, it encourages the liver to make proteins that increase the ability of the blood to clot, and it decreases proteins that break down clots. It also increases proteins that promote inflammation. Estradiol valerate, micronized 17 beta-estradiol, and esterol *may* be less likely to produce these effects—with a heavy emphasis on *may*, because we don't know for sure. They are not as potent as ethinyl estradiol and they are removed from the body a little faster, so they *may* have reduced estrogen-related side effects, such as nausea and headache, for people who are sensitive to estrogen. Esterol is purported to have no activity on breast tissue, so it might be an option for people who experience breast tenderness on the pill. We don't yet know whether the very low risk of breast cancer with ECCs will be even lower with esterol. There are a lot of ifs and maybes here, as a lot of what we know is based on animal studies, which do not always translate into the same effects in humans.

The Progestin

Progestins are synthetic hormones with many progesterone-like properties. Together with progesterone, they are known collectively as progestogens. Progestins are made in a lab, using testosterone, progesterone, or spironolactone (itself derived from progesterone) as the starting hormone. If we go back to the key-and-lock analogy, with sex steroids acting as the key and their receptors on cells the lock, the idea with novel synthetic compounds is to try to remove the part of the key that causes side effects and complications or leads to breakdown by the liver, while improving the part that is beneficial, for example, the effect on the endometrium.

Progestins derived from testosterone retain some testosterone-like activity when tested in the lab. Studies over the years have tried to rid these progestins of their testosterone heritage and make them a closer duplicate of progesterone. Examples of the resulting "low testosterone" progestins include desogestrel and gestodene. Progestins derived from progesterone and spironolactone (which is a diuretic, or water pill, that also blocks the effect of testosterone) have no testosterone-like activity.

Although there are differences between progestins in the lab, a lot of what we hear is pharmaceutical company jargon designed to show their progestin is "better," meaning it has less of a testosterone-like effect. I get it from a marketing standpoint. But how a progestin affects one specific aspect of rat endometrium in a culture dish (or whatever test is used) doesn't reflect what happens to a human uterus inside a person. Until recently, all ECCs contained ethinyl estradiol, so the only difference from brand to brand was the progestin. As a result, companies leaned into "my progestin is better than your progestin" testing, but no studies were done to show that any of it mattered in humans. There is no head-to-head data to say pill A with progestin A is superior to pill B with progestin B for a given specific reason.

Here's what you need to know: the estrogen typically counteracts any potential effect from the testosterone used to make the progestin, so the net effect is what we call estrogenic. However, if someone is struggling with a side effect—for example, if they feel their acne is worse—we might say, "Okay, let's try a pill that is supposed to have less of a testosterone-like effect." And if someone is struggling with irregular bleeding, we might say, "Let's try one of the older progestins, because they may be better for bleeding."

Progestins may be meaningfully different when it comes to blood clotting. Progestins by themselves appear to have no impact on the clotting system, but ECCs with the "low-testosterone" progestins desogestrel, gestodene, drospirenone, and cyproterone acetate (derived from spironolactone) may be associated with a higher rate of blood clots—up to a twofold increase— compared to pills with "older" progestins like levonorgestrel and norgestrel. One theory is that because the newer progestins are less testosterone-like, they don't counteract the effect of estrogen on the clotting system as well. The studies here conflict, with some showing an increased risk of blood clots and others not showing it. Because the risk of blood clots is very low, it's not an easy phenomenon to study.

The Benefits of ECCs

Besides the contraceptive effectiveness of ECCs and the rapid return to fertility within four weeks after discontinuing use, they have numerous health benefits. Although they contain estrogen, the progestin dominates, so the endometrium thins out. By one year after starting an ECC, 20 percent of people will have no periods; by two years, that number increases to 37 percent. Among those who continue to menstruate, bleeding is lighter overall, meaning less blood loss per month. So ECCs are very effective for heavy bleeding. The reduction in blood loss also improves iron-deficiency anemia because you are no longer donating blood to the environment thirteen or so times a year.

The lack of ovulation and thinned endometrium mean fewer prostaglandins, so ECCs are also an effective therapy for painful periods and menstrual diarrhea, and the progestin can suppress endometriosis and adenomyosis, conditions that can cause painful periods and pelvic pain. ECCs can be taken continuously, which can also be very helpful: eliminating bleeding altogether is great for heavy periods and painful periods. When ECCs are taken this way, the endometrium simply doesn't develop; there's no need to worry that it's hanging around going bad or accumulating harmful substances.

Because ECCs stop ovulation and hence prevent the fluctuation in hormones, they can be very beneficial for people with medical conditions triggered by menstruation, such as menstrual migraines, premenstrual syndrome, and premenstrual mood dysphoric disorder.

ECCs can also treat conditions associated with testosterone overactivity, such as acne and PCOS. There are two mechanisms for this: one is the estrogen itself; the other is the fact that estrogen increases production of sex hormone binding globulin, which carries estrogen and testosterone. As discussed on page 239, I think of SHBG as a bus. When a hormone is on the bus (bound to SHBG), it's inactive; as soon as it leaves the bus (becomes unbound), it is free to interact with the body. When SHBG levels are high, more hormones are bound, and vice versa. But there's a catch. Testosterone binds more strongly to SHBG than estrogen, so when SHBG levels go up, more testosterone boards the bus relative to estrogen, meaning less testosterone is available to interact with tissues, reducing its impact. Increasing SHBG doesn't affect the levels of testosterone or estrogen, just the ratio of available to unavailable hormone. Estrogen's effect on SHBG is another reason why it probably doesn't matter for most people if the progestin in an ECC has more testosterone-like qualities in a lab.

Other benefits of ECCs include:

- A fourfold reduction in the risk of bacterial vaginosis, likely because the estrogen promotes the growth of lactobacilli.
- A reduced risk of fibrocystic breast changes, cysts, and fibroadenomas (benign tumors).
- A reduced rate of ovarian cysts.
- Longer and thicker hair on the head, because estrogen prolongs its growing phase, but a reduced rate of hair growth on the face.
- A 40 percent reduction in the risk of endometrial cancer.
- A 27 percent reduction in the risk of ovarian cancer.
- A reduced rate of colon cancer.

Like all forms of effective contraception, ECCs are also associated with reductions in maternal mortality because of the reduced number of pregnancies, and they can give people time to improve medical conditions for a safer pregnancy.

The Safety of ECCs

All medications have risks, and ECCs are no exception. In the United States they are given a black box warning, due to the risk of blood clots, but this risk must be put into perspective. A black box warning doesn't mean no one should take the medication; it's like a road sign about a potential danger ahead. And let's be real: pregnancy should have a black box warning. In the United States especially, a woman is far safer being on the pill than being pregnant. The risk of death and serious complications, such as blood clots, stroke, needing a blood transfusion, incontinence, and postpartum depression, JUST TO NAME A FEW (yes, I'm yelling), is significant. We should be trying to fix the atrocious rate of maternal mortality, but the point still holds. I have yet to see a naturopath, "functional medicine" provider, or "health influencer" who incorrectly hypes the risk of ECCs and also addresses the risks of a pregnancy that might happen because someone was frightened away from their contraception. That tells me that as long as your body is in servitude to the patriarchy, the greater risk of pregnancy is perfectly acceptable. If a less effective contraception method than ECCs is chosen, the risks of that other method must include the risks inherent with pregnancy.

ECCs are much safer than many activities that don't come with dire warnings of doom. The risk of dying from an ECC for a non-smoker between the ages of fifteen and thirty-four is 0.06 in 100,000. They are more likely to die from being struck by lightning, and they have about the same risk of dying from a miscarriage. In the United States, deaths from gun violence, car accidents, COVID-19, or pregnancies that go to term are all far more common than deaths from ECCs. Risks jump for smokers aged thirty-five and older, which is why ECCs are not recommended for this group.

The biggest medical risk associated with ECCs is cardiovascular disease, including dangerous blood clots in veins and arteries, heart attack, and stroke. Of all these outcomes, the most common is a blood clot in a vein, which can travel to the lungs and cause a pulmonary embolism, which is potentially fatal. Fortunately, fatalities from blood clots are rare (see Table 5). The risk appears to be highest for people in their first year on an ECC; the exact reason isn't known, but this fact is often reassuring to people who have happily been on the pill for years and then see an Instagram post from someone over-hyping the risks.

Table 5 • RISK OF BLOOD CLOTS CAUSING DEATH

FACTOR	RISK OF DEATH
Baseline risk as a woman	1–5/10,000 per year
ECC pill, ring*	3–7/10,000 per year
ECC pill with desogestrel**, norgestimate patch	7–12/10,000 per year
Pregnancy	5–20/10,000 pregnancies
First three weeks after delivery	40–65/10,000 pregnancies

* There is less data on the ring, but risk-wise it seems comparable to the older pills.
** The data showing this higher risk isn't robust, so this is a "possibly" rather than "definitively."

It's not possible here to address how every medical condition is affected by ECCs. I encourage anyone with a health condition, including those who smoke, to look up the Medical Eligibility Criteria for Contraceptives to see if there are any concerns related to their situation. Enter "medical eligibility criteria for contraceptives" and "CDC" or "WHO" into your browser, and it should come up. The CDC also has the U.S. criteria available as a free app (abbreviated as CDC MEC) for Apple and Android devices, and it's easy to search by medical conditions and contraception methods.

Many of the contraindications and relative contraindications revolve around factors that affect the risk of blood clots, heart attack, and stroke, as they can be cumulative with the pill. Age increases the risk of blood clots, but unless other risk factors are involved, such as smoking, age alone isn't a contraindication. Healthy people can continue to take the pill until age fifty-five. ECCs are not a safe option for smokers aged thirty-five and older, or for those with the following medical conditions:

- High blood pressure.
- Migraines with aura.
- A blood clotting disorder.
- Heart disease.
- Vascular disease due to diabetes or lupus.
- Breast cancer, current or a previous diagnosis

Other conditions that increase the risk of blood clots, stroke, and heart attacks include low HDL cholesterol, high LDL cholesterol, high triglycerides, diabetes (without vascular disease), migraines without aura, and obesity. Sometimes people have several of these conditions, and while each on its own may not be significant enough to recommend against contraception with estrogen, taken all together it might be a different story. Because age also affects risk, these factors may mean something different risk-wise at age twenty than what they mean at age forty-five.

What about breast cancer? There is a 25 percent increase in the risk of breast cancer with ECCs, and while that sounds dramatic and scary, the risk for women under age forty-five is so low that even with a 25 percent increase, it's still minimal. For example, if ten thousand women take an estrogen-containing pill for five years and stop by age thirty, in this time frame there will be forty-four cases of breast cancer unrelated to the pill and five cases related to the pill. The risk drops back down to the baseline by five years after stopping the pill. You know what else causes breast cancer, though it's almost never discussed? Pregnancy. And likely by the same mechanisms as the pill. Most experts believe breast cancer happens because the hormones encourage a small tumor that is already present to grow. Think of it as a seed already planted in soil; like water for a seed, the hormones in the contraception activate the cancer. This is very different from a tumor caused de novo, meaning no seed was there to begin with, which is what we see with cigarettes and lung cancer; even after someone stops smoking, the risk of cancer remains elevated because smoking planted the seeds.

One other consideration with the pill is that it's not a good option for people who have had bariatric surgery, as that can affect absorption. For more on the potential risks of ECCs, and the mythology about those risks, see Chapter 30.

Starting and Cycling

Initially, ECCs were given as a set of twenty-one active pills, each with the same amount of hormone, and seven placebo pills. The first package was to be started the Sunday after bleeding began (if it began on a Sunday, that was the day to start). The advantage of this method was a uniform approach, and "Sunday start" was catchy, but someone who was involved in pill research in the 1970s told me that many researchers and doctors thought anything else would be too confusing for women. As if. It sounds like something dreamed up by someone who has never menstruated and has a low opinion of women. A Sunday start also meant the withdrawal menstruation would likely start on a Monday or Tuesday and be over with by the following weekend. You know, so no one had to miss their weekly Saturday sex because of "Aunt Flo." Women once again needing to manage men's disgust with their normal bodily functions.

The downside of the Sunday start approach, besides the patriarchy, was that those who started bleeding on Monday would start their first pill on day 7 (the following Sunday), which meant they might ovulate in that first cycle, as it takes seven days for the contraceptive effect to kick in. Six days is plenty of time for a dominant follicle to be well on its way, and the pill might not be able to stop the LH surge. Also, the waiting led to many people not starting at all, leaving them with an unmet need for contraception.

We now have great research supporting a quick start, which is starting the pill, patch, or ring on the day of the prescription, regardless of the day of the cycle. This significantly increases the number of people who continue to use their contraception and reduces the need for backup contraception to just seven days. If a pregnancy test is negative and you don't think you are pregnant, the ECC can be started that day. If you've had unprotected sex in the previous five days, you can take emergency contraception and start the ECC at the same time.

As described in Chapter 22, the first pill had a hormone-free interval of seven days to induce menstrual bleeding, because many women thought they were pregnant when the pill stopped their period. However, since then we've learned that a follicle can sometimes start to develop in a seven-day hormone-free interval, possibly reducing the contraceptive's efficacy. This discovery has led to packages with twenty-four active pills and three placebo pills, which still allows for a withdrawal bleed but improves efficacy and also reduces the risk of abnormal bleeding. With the patch, a new one is applied each week, with one week off out of every four, and with the ring, it's three weeks of wearing the ring, then one week off.

With all ECC methods, it's also completely fine, and often preferred, to skip the placebo pills or the hormone-free week. The advantages of continuous use are no menstruation and no hormone fluctuations. There are pills that are specifically packaged for this use (for example, eighty-four active pills), but with any monophasic pills you can simply skip the placebos and start a new pack. There is nothing harmful about skipping periods this way.

The endometrium doesn't build up; it simply doesn't develop. When you stop the medication, menstruation will return. The biggest issue with continuous use is the risk of irregular bleeding. It really varies: some people can take the pill continuously for thirty-five years and never have spotting or get a period; others need to have a period every three to four packs as a preventative strategy against irregular bleeding; and some people get irregular bleeding if they try to skip even one period.

The Nuances of Patches and Rings

Patches are as effective as the pill. The estrogen used is ethinyl estradiol, and there are a variety of different progestins. Availability of the options depends on where you live.

- *Xulane and Zafemy:* Release 35 µg ethinyl estradiol and 150 µg norelgestromin per day. Currently sold in the United States.
- *Evra:* Releases 35 µg ethinyl estradiol and 200 µg norelgestromin per day. Available in Canada, the United Kingdom, and Europe.
- *Twirla:* Releases 30 µg ethinyl estradiol and 120 µg levonorgestrel per day. Currently sold in the United Kingdom.
- *Lisvy:* Releases 13 µg ethinyl estradiol and 60 µg gestodene per day. Available in Europe.

There are a few considerations with patches. Estrogen levels are a little higher, which may account for the slightly higher rate of breast pain, headaches, and nausea. The patches may also have a slightly higher rate of blood clots. One concerning issue is that they seem to be less effective and riskier with higher body weights, and depending on the patch (some use BMI and others weight), people with a BMI over 30 or weight over 90 kg (198 pounds) cannot use it. This restriction excludes a large percentage of the population who might want to use a patch. And it's a potential inconvenience, considering that people often gain weight as they age and might have to change contraceptive methods.

Contraceptive rings are impregnated with hormones that are released slowly into the vagina, where they are absorbed across the vaginal mucosa into the bloodstream. They include:

- *NuvaRing (brand name) or EluRyng (generic):* Releases 15 µg ethinyl estradiol and 120 µg etonogestrel per day. The ring is worn for three weeks, then either it's removed for a week or a new one is inserted for continuous use. There is enough hormone in a ring for a two-week grace period, so if you choose to use it continuously, you don't have to change it every three weeks; you could change it every four or even five weeks to save money.

- *Annovera:* Releases 13 µg ethinyl estradiol and 150 µg segesterone per day. One ring can be used for an entire year, or thirteen cycles. The ring is placed in the vagina for three weeks, then removed for a week to allow for a withdrawal bleed. When not in use, it is washed and stored in the provided compact. It can be kept at room temperature between uses, as long as that's 30°C (86°F) or less. Theoretically, this ring could be used continuously, meaning you don't take it out for a year, but there is no data on this yet, as it's so new. According to the package insert in the United States, "The safety and efficacy of ANNOVERA™ in females with a BMI >29 kg/m² has not been adequately evaluated"; the reason is that during the studies there were two blood clots among women with a BMI greater than 29, so they stopped enrolling women with a BMI >29. As a result, it's unknown how effective and safe this method is for those women, which is unfortunate.

Here are some other ring-unique issues:

- Rings can be left in or removed for vaginal sex. If removed, the NuvaRing or EluRyng can only be out for three hours; otherwise, backup contraception is needed for the next seven days. The Annovera ring can only be out of the vagina for two hours out of twenty-one days or backup contraception is needed for a week.
- Tampons don't affect absorption of the hormones, but the ring may come out while you're removing a tampon.
- Oil-based and silicone-based vaginal medications, lubricants, and moisturizers should be avoided. Some vaginal yeast medications and vaginal clindamycin are oil-based.
- Rings are associated with toxic shock syndrome, though it is rare and the risk is likely not higher than with tampons.

- Rings increase vaginal discharge, which can sometimes be mistaken for an infection.
- The risk of blood clots is believed to be the same as with estrogen-containing pills, but there is an asterisk with the etonogestrel rings. Desogestrel is metabolized by the body into etonogestrel, so there is a theoretical concern that there could be a slightly higher risk of blood clots, as is seen with desogestrel-containing pills.

Managing Bleeding and Side Effects

As I've noted, irregular bleeding can be a side effect of ECCs, typically due to the relative dominance of the progestin and its effect on the endometrium. Irregular bleeding is common in the first three cycles and often resolves on its own. If that bleeding is annoying or if it persists, it's important to know that you don't have to suffer and suck it up. Strategies to manage bleeding include:

- *A five-day course of ibuprofen or a similar NSAID:* There is really no reason not to try this one immediately. After all, we have modern medicine for a reason.
- *Switching pills:* If the bleeding irregularities are persistent, options include increasing the dose of estrogen to 35 μg of ethinyl estradiol, if the current pill has less estrogen, and then waiting another two to three months; trying an option with twenty-four days of active pills; or trying a pill with a different progestin. The risk of bleeding with the newer estrogens isn't well known, but since they are not as strong as ethinyl estradiol, logically this doesn't seem like the right switch—although that doesn't mean it's completely unreasonable. For whatever reason, some pills just work better for some people, and science can't quite explain it. My theory is that people have minor variations in how they metabolize specific hormones. For the patch or ring, switching doses or hormones isn't currently an option.

With persistent bleeding, it's a good idea to consider other potential causes, including all the causes of irregular bleeding addressed in previous chapters. Sometimes two things do happen at once.

Breast pain, nausea, and headaches are other side effects that are seen with ECCs, although they are uncommon, affecting only 1 to 2 percent of people.

They are typically due to the estrogen dose. Other EEC concerns are addressed in Chapter 30.

Which Pill, Patch, or Ring Should I Use?

Choosing can be like trying to decide on dinner at the Cheesecake Factory—too many options! Isn't there a prix fixe? In the United States, there are currently more than seventy pills on the market, and because these products are never studied against each other in a meaningful way, it's impossible to know which is the "best." Some people go to the doctor with a specific brand in mind and say, "I want pill X" or "I want the patch"; unless there is a pressing reason to select a different pill or method, what they want is the best one for them. Studies tell us that the choice people want is the one they are most likely to keep using. (File that under things that seem obvious now but might not have been to patriarchal men who "knew best.") It's obviously important for doctors to discuss the BMI/weight restrictions for people who want the patch, and the fact that the dose of estrogen is a little higher. With the patch and the newer ECCs with gestodene and desogestrel, the slightly increased risk of blood clots isn't definitive, so as part of informed consent I simply explain that there may be a slightly higher risk but that these are still incredibly safe medications.

So-called biphasic and triphasic pills were introduced in the 1980s. With these pills, the estrogen and progestin doses weren't the same in each pill; rather, they contained either two different doses (biphasic) or three (triphasic). This approach was theoretically designed to slightly reduce the cumulative exposure to hormones, reduce the risk of abnormal bleeding, and mimic natural fluctuations in estrogen and progesterone. But there was never any real proof that the varying doses were of value, outside of the ability to market the pills as something new and sciencey. It was all bogus. Biphasic and triphasic pills offer zero advantage, and they can be problematic for anyone who wants to take pills continuously, as that can't be accomplished unless the dose of hormones is the same in every pill. There is zero reason to prescribe these pills, and I do so only if it's the specific pill that someone loves.

The patch and the ring are good options when remembering a daily pill or swallowing a pill is challenging. Another advantage of the patch and the ring is that the hormone levels are stable. With a pill, estrogen and progestin levels shoot up after the medication is absorbed, then plummet back down before the next dose. A greater stability in hormone levels might be beneficial for someone with PMS when the pill isn't helping. The patch and ring may have less of an effect on sexual function, so the small percentage of people who feel that an ECC pill has affected libido or sexual function may want to explore those options.

In the United States, when someone wants a pill, the sad fact is that the first thing doctors do is consult the insurance formulary to see what is covered at a reasonable price. If there are several options available, here are some things to consider:

- *Estrogen dose:* I usually recommend a 20 µg ethinyl estradiol pill, but if you have previously experienced irregular bleeding on an ECC, I might suggest a 30 to 35 µg pill. For people who have previously had issues with nausea or breast tenderness on the pill, or who have cycle-related breast tenderness, I might suggest a 10 µg pill, with a warning about the increased risk of bleeding; if that is a concern, then I recommend a 20 µg pill. A ring might also be an option for symptoms that may be related to estrogen dose.
- *Type of estrogen:* A pill with one of the newer estrogens might be a good option if you have had nausea with estrogen or have concerns about breast tenderness.
- *Type of progestin:* If you have PMS/PMDD and a lot of bloating, a pill with drospirenone seems to be uniquely effective.
- *Twenty-one-day vs. twenty-four-day vs. continuous:* Options with twenty-four days of active pills protect more against escape ovulation and hence are slightly more effective than twenty-one-day pills, and they tend to have a more favorable bleeding profile. Continuous pills are also likely more effective, as there is no break in hormones. So the question is whether you want to have a period.
- *Brand-name vs. generic:* Brand-name pills are no better than the equivalent generic. Choose a generic where possible and save money.
- *Pills with added goodies:* There are pills with iron and with calcium, but there is no data to suggest they are more beneficial than pills that don't contain supplements. Iron can cause constipation, so keep that in mind from a side-effect standpoint. If you have anemia, you can take an iron supplement, which works best when taken

every other day, and then stop when you no longer need it. In general, adding minerals to pills is more marketing than medicine.

And finally, you are not married to your ECC. You can always switch.

What If I Miss a Pill or Forget My Ring or Patch?

It happens. What you should do when and if you need backup contraception is typically covered in the product monograph—that big packet of papers that comes with the prescription. You can keep one tucked away or find it online by searching for "Product monograph FDA" and then the name of your contraceptive. Take a screenshot and save it to your phone under Favorites so you always have it with you. Another option is to search "missed pills OCPs" (short for oral contraceptive pills) and either "CDC" or "NHS" (the National Health Service in the United Kingdom); excellent pages will come up. Bookmark or take a screenshot. The CDC page has a great chart that lends itself to saving on your phone. Don't get advice on this subject from period apps.

Set a reminder to take the pill or change the patch or ring, or download a contraceptive reminder app. Life gets busy. If I missed a pill, I often had breakthrough bleeding, so the negative reinforcement forced me to take mine daily, but that isn't necessarily the best strategy! One study of electronic pill packages that recorded when pills were removed revealed an average number of 4.7 missed pills per package over three packages, even though the study participants thought they'd only missed one. This study may not be applicable to all women—the average age was twenty-two and the demographic was mostly White and had a high school education—but it is likely that missed pills are more common than we think. Remembering to change a vaginal ring every three weeks is not intuitive, and neither is twenty-four days of active pills and a three-day break, so many people benefit from an external reminder. I started using an app for my menopausal hormone therapy because I take my progesterone at night, so sometimes I'd take it really late and there were many mornings when I was staring at the pill bottle thinking, "Did I or didn't I?"

Bottom Line

- Estrogen-containing contraceptives include pills, patches, and rings, and there are many permutations and combinations of hormones.
- Almost all of the risks, which are rare, are related to estrogen. The serious risks are blood clots, heart attack, and stroke.
- The patches and some pills may have slightly higher rates of blood clots, but this is not definitive.
- Bleeding irregularities are the most common side effect of ECCs, and they often improve with time.
- There are some nuances in estrogen dose, type of estrogen, and type of progestin that may be important for some people.

24

Progestin-Only Methods

Progestin-only contraceptives quickly followed after Enovid was approved. Some of the research was driven by the hunt for therapies for cancer of the uterus and treatment of heavy or irregular menstrual bleeding, which can both be helped by progestins, but there was also a desire to eliminate serious complications of the pill, which are largely estrogen-related, and to make hormonal contraception available to more people, as estrogen is related to almost every medical reason someone can't take the pill.

Today we have four widely available progestin-only methods: pills, implants, an injection, and an IUD. The progestin IUD is addressed in Chapter 27; here, we will focus on the pills, the implants, and the injection, which all work by inhibiting ovulation (primarily by inhibiting the LH surge, although some methods may have an impact on FSH as well) and by thickening the cervical mucus. Like estrogen-containing contraception, these medications also have use beyond their contraceptive action. Heavy bleeding, fibroids, and painful periods are just a few of the reasons people might use them other than contraception.

The only absolute contraindication to progestin-only contraceptives is currently having breast cancer or having had it within the past five years. However, there are a few conditions with which these medications are generally not recommended: systemic lupus erythematosus (SLE) with antiphospholipid antibody syndrome, advanced liver disease, some liver tumors, and a current or previous diagnosis of breast cancer. Also, as with the estrogen-containing pill, a progestin-only pill is generally not recommended for people who've had bariatric surgery, as it may not be absorbed well enough to work.

The limited restrictions mean progestin-only methods are open to many people who otherwise couldn't use ECCs, including smokers over thirty-five, people who have migraines with aura, and those with heart disease or high blood pressure, to name a few. Regardless, it's always important to review your unique medical situation with your health care provider and check the CDC's Medical Eligibility Criteria for Contraception (see page 318). The risks of blood clots, stroke, and changes in blood pressure, while generally low with the estrogen-containing pill, aren't concerns at all with the progestin-only pill. In addition, people who experience estrogen-related side effects from the pill, such as breast pain, nausea, headaches, and yeast infections, won't have these issues with progestin-only methods. There is less data on the non-contraception health benefits of progestin-only contraception, though we know they reduce the risk of endometrial cancer and likely also the risk of ovarian cancer.

What's the catch? Almost everything comes with a trade-off. In return for greater safety, progestin-only methods have a higher rate of irregular bleeding, and the early progestin-only pills may have had a higher pregnancy rate. With those caveats in mind, let's jump in.

Progestin-Only Pills

The first progestin-only pills, also called minipills, were introduced in the late 1960s. They had less progestin—or a mini dose compared to an estrogen-containing pill—hence the nickname "minipill." The lower dose seems counterintuitive, but it was the first attempt to lower the risks of blood clots and other side effects, like nausea and headache; at the time, it wasn't clear whether the estrogen or the progestin was the source of the issues. There were a couple of false starts until a norgestimate pill was introduced in the early 1970s. This formulation is still available today.

The issue with the original minipills is that the progestin used is quickly removed from the body, and the dose is believed to be just barely enough to suppress ovulation and thicken the cervical mucus. Just as with an estrogen pill, the follicles that are recruited each cycle stall out at day 3. If the progestin level drops a little—for example, if you take a pill several hours later than the day before—the contraceptive effects might be compromised. So the recommendations are to take this type of minipill within the same three-hour window each day to avoid reduced contraception efficacy (this idea that these pills are sensitive enough to need a three-hour window is controversial medically, but with contraception we typically err on the side of caution). The inconvenience of a three-hour window and a fear that the pills might be less effective kept many people from choosing them. The good news is that there are now two progestin-only pills with longer-acting progestins, desogestrel and drospirenone, and studies show that they don't have a strict three-hour window. With the desogestrel pill there is a twelve-hour window and the drospirenone pill has a twenty-four hour window, which creates a lot more breathing room.

The advantages of progestin-only pills are that they are not associated with an increased risk of blood clots and won't raise blood pressure or trigger migraines or cause any of the estrogen-related complications or effects seen with the estrogen-containing pill. So they're a great option for people with heart disease, migraines, or a history of blood clots. They may also help reduce sickle cell crises for people with sickle cell anemia. As for disadvantages, irregular bleeding is more common with progestin-only pills than with estrogen-containing pills, though we don't really know how much more.

The pregnancy rate with progestin-only pills is 4 to 7 percent. The options include:

- *Norethindrone 350 µg:* Brands of this minipill include Micronor, Nor-QD, and Noriday. These pills carry the theoretical three-hour-window concern (see above). Each pack has twenty-eight pills, and the all the pills are active, so one must be taken every day.
- *Levonorgestrel 30 µg:* A minipill with the same three-hour-window issue. Brand names include Microval and Microlut. Each pack has twenty-eight active pills.
- *Desogestrel 75 µg:* Also a minipill, but a newer one. The brand, Cerazette, is available in Canada, the United Kingdom, and France, but not in the United States as of July 2023. Desogestrel is very effective at suppressing ovulation, so there is no concern about the three-hour window. There are twenty-eight active pills in a pack, so one pill is taken daily.
- *Drospirenone 4 mg:* Not a minipill, as the dose of progestin is higher than in an estrogen-containing pill. The brand name is Slynd. It can

raise potassium levels for people whose medical conditions or other medications put them at risk for this; they should have their potassium level checked after their first cycle on the pill. There are twenty-four active pills and four placebo pills per package; the four hormone-free days are supposed to reduce bleeding concerns. There is also no concern about a three-hour window.

Implants

With implants, a long-acting reversible contraception method, silastic rods deliver progestin to the body in a constant, steady supply. In the United States, the only option currently available is Nexplanon, which is a single rod containing the progestin etonogestrel. In other countries, Implanon, also a single rod of etonogestrel, may still be available. The only difference is that Nexplanon contains small amounts of barium sulfate, so it can be seen with X-rays as well as ultrasound and MRI; Implanon can be seen only with ultrasound and MRI. Thus, in the rare case where an implant migrates, there are more imaging options for finding the Nexplanon. Nexplanon is also easier to insert correctly than Implanon. Systems with two rods, Jadelle and Levoplant, are available in some places but not in the United States. Both contain levonorgestrel.

Nexplanon is 4 cm (1.6 inches) long and 2 mm (0.1 inch) wide, about the size of a matchstick, and contains 68 mg of etonogestrel, which is a metabolite of desogestrel, a hormone that is also used in some oral contraceptives and in the NuvaRing. It's effective regardless of weight or BMI. The implant is placed in the upper arm and is inserted and removed with a short outpatient procedure that typically takes a few minutes. Nexplanon and Implanon are approved for three years of use, but studies show they are effective for five years. The Jadelle and Levoplant systems are effective for five years. Most of the focus below is on Nexplanon and Implanon, as they have the same medication, dose, and delivery system, but much of the information also applies to the other systems.

Nexplanon and Implanon work by very effectively suppressing the LH surge, preventing ovulation. They were designed to release an amount of etonogestrel that is 100 percent effective at suppressing ovulation for the first thirty months. Etonogestrel also makes cervical mucus hostile to sperm, so as the level of hormone drops slightly over time, there is a built-in backup method of contraception. You might be wondering if the implants are so effective at suppressing ovulation that they cause a temporary menopause. In the first few months, follicles in the ovary are completely suppressed and estradiol levels do drop, but the ovary recovers, and by six months, estradiol levels return to normal for the early part of the menstrual cycle. At that point, just as with the pill, follicles are recruited and produce estrogen but there is no LH surge, so they disappear. Progesterone levels remain low, as there is no ovulation.

Pregnancies with the contraceptive implants are exceedingly rare. With Nexplanon, the rate is 0.38 percent, and most of the pregnancies that do happen occur in close proximity to the time of insertion, meaning the individual was already a few days pregnant when the insertion took place (before a pregnancy test would be positive) or did not use backup protection for the first week (it takes seven days for the contraceptive effect to kick in). The implants can be placed anytime you know you aren't pregnant, including right after delivery. Once the implant is removed, fertility returns quickly; by two months after removal, baseline fertility is restored. It's possible to have an old rod removed and a new one inserted on the same day.

The right hormone levels are essential for the implants to provide adequate suppression of ovulation, so it's important to be mindful of medications that can increase how etonogestrel is metabolized, as these drugs can make the implant less effective. Some medications for epilepsy and for HIV can have this effect; if you take medications for these conditions, or if you start them once you have an implant already in place, be sure to let your medical provider know. St. John's wort can also have this effect, so it should be avoided with an implant.

The implants do not seem to have a negative impact on metabolism. In a study that compared people who used an implant with those who used the copper IUD, there was no difference in weight gain. And because the follicles develop and produce estrogen, there is no increased risk of osteoporosis with prolonged use.

Advantages of the implants (besides worry-free contraception for almost everyone, with no limitations based on weight or BMI) include a reduction in painful periods—about 80 percent of people report an improvement in menstrual cramps, and implants can also be effective for treating pain related to endometriosis. The effect on acne varies, with some reporting an improvement but others a worsening. The implants can also decrease painful sickle cell crises.

The downsides, aside from low risks of pain and bruising with insertion, include a very small risk of migration, meaning the implant travels under the skin, which can make it harder to remove. In very rare cases, it can end up in a place where removal is challenging, like the armpit. But I want to stress how rare this is. The biggest issue most people have is irregular bleeding. Just as with birth control pills, bleeding is common in the first three months; in fact, two-thirds of people will call their bleeding pattern unsatisfactory. But by six months, about 22 percent of people have no bleeding and 34 percent have infrequent spotting. On average, those who have more bleeding bleed about the same number of days as they did prior to the implant—it's just that, with the implant, it tends to be irregular, which can, of course, be distressing. By six months after insertion, only one-third of people say their bleeding pattern is still unsatisfactory, but obviously "unsatisfactory" means different things to different people. If your period meant ten days of flooding and now, two months after the implant, you spot unpredictably for six days a month, you might welcome the change, whereas someone whose period was two days long might find the same amount of blood loss via irregular spotting worse. Eventually, 11 to 14 percent of people get the implant removed because of bleeding.

It's impossible to predict who will have issues with abnormal bleeding, who will get intermittent light spotting, and whose periods will stop after the implant. The only factor that has been linked with more disordered bleeding is a lower BMI, although the reason isn't known. One hypothesis is that etonogestrel levels are higher in people with low BMI—the smaller you are, the smaller the volume in which the medication disperses—which may have a greater effect on the uterine lining.

There are strategies to reduce the bleeding, but sadly these are often underprescribed. Irregular bleeding should not be simply brushed off. People shouldn't have to put up with side effects that can be managed, and bleeding issues can lead them to switch to other methods of contraception or even to go without, increasing their risk of an unplanned pregnancy. For more information, see the section "How to Manage Troublesome Bleeding" on page 336. Everyone should have the right dose of ibuprofen on hand when the implant is inserted, so they can start taking it immediately if they get bleeding issues.

Depo-Provera

Also known as the birth control shot, this contraceptive method is an injection of a progestin called medroxyprogesterone acetate (MPA), brand name Depo-Provera and typically abbreviated DMPA (the *D* is for *depot*, meaning injection). MPA was first approved by the FDA in 1959 and was initially used to treat heavy bleeding. The injection can be given into the muscle (intramuscular) or underneath the skin (subcutaneous) every thirteen weeks. The failure rate when the injection is received every thirteen weeks or less is 0.2 percent, but the typical failure rate is 4 percent, as people don't always get subsequent injections within the required time frame. Depo-Provera can be given anytime during the cycle. After the first injection, it takes seven days to become effective, so those who are sexually active and don't use a backup contraceptive in that first week are at risk for pregnancy. There is a little wiggle room regarding dosing—you can go up to fifteen weeks between injections without needing a backup method.

Besides the benefits of reliable contraception, after one injection up to 30 percent of users will no longer have periods; by one year that number is close to 50 percent; and by five years it is 80 percent. Many people like this added bonus, and it is great for those with heavy periods, iron-deficiency anemia, and painful periods. Depo-Provera is also effective therapy for endometriosis, and there is good data that it can shrink fibroids. People with sickle cell disease tend to have fewer crises. For people with epilepsy, there are no anti-seizure medications that affect how the injection works, unlike with the birth control pill and the rod. Depo-Provera is also associated with a reduced risk of endometrial and ovarian cancer, and it is neutral for breast cancer.

Like all medications, Depo-Provera has side effects. The most common one is irregular bleeding. Some people bleed unpredictably until their periods eventually stop; for others, the bleeding is persistent. Overall, 70 percent of people will have irregular bleeding in the first year. The longer you are on Depo-Provera, the more likely it is that the bleeding will stop. As with the implants, there are interventions that can reduce the bleeding (see page 336).

Another issue with Depo-Provera is a delay in return to fertility. Some people will get pregnant as soon as fifteen weeks after their last injection, but for others it takes almost a year to return to baseline fertility—something to consider if you hope to get pregnant soon after stopping birth control.

Depo-Provera is associated with weight gain for some people, an average of 4 kg (9 pounds), versus 2.3 kg (5 pounds) for those who used a copper IUD with no hormones. However, averages don't tell us the whole picture. It turns out that only a small subset of people gain weight with Depo-Provera, and those who do tend to start adding weight within the first three to six months; for them, the average gain is 10.9 kg (24 pounds). Meaning if you don't gain weight initially, it's not likely to be a concern for you, but if you do, this may be something to discuss with your provider.

Other risks with Depo-Provera include a transient drop in bone density that recovers when the medication is stopped (this is the black box warning), a temporary adverse effect on cholesterol and lipids, and vaginal dryness, which can be treated with vaginal estrogen. Some concern has been raised about an increased risk of contracting HIV if exposed, but the data here isn't solid enough for a definitive statement. Many people talk about a link between depression and Depo-Provera—so much so that it's become a medical truthism, meaning something that sounds medically plausible but isn't backed up by data. There is no good evidence linking Depo-Provera with depression, and having depression isn't a contraindication to starting it.

Depo-Provera has received a lot of bad press. Whenever I post about it online, inevitably there is a chorus from people who hate it. However, I receive an equal number of private messages from people who love Depo-Provera but are ashamed to admit it in public. It's not a crime against feminism to like a contraceptive, hate a contraceptive, or have no strong feelings either way. But your experiences are not generalizable to your friend or your neighbor or anyone who reads your Twitter post or Instagram comment. The most you can say is that it worked or didn't work for you. Social media may reflect bias sampling, and people who have negative experiences are more likely to post publicly. What I have seen in my practice over the years is a mirror of the replies I get on social media: some people love Depo-Provera and some hate it.

At one year 43 percent of people have stopped Depo-Provera, and at two years it's 62 percent. Side effects are listed as the major reason. This is a concern because in many cases people aren't adequately informed about side effects; far fewer women stop taking it when they are given more detailed counseling about side effects in advance. Imagine that you are booking a flight from San Francisco to New York but you must change planes in Denver. You see one itinerary that is $500 with a three-hour layover and another that is $200 with a fifty-five-minute layover that the airline says is a legal connection (meaning they think you can make it). So you book the $200 flight because you want to save money and don't want to hang out in an airport for three hours. But then your flight from San Francisco is delayed and you miss the connection. Not good. What if you found out before booking that the flight from San Francisco was late 50 percent of the time? You might still think the risk of missing the connection was worth it to save money, but you'd have made an informed decision. Now if you miss your flight, you will likely be less upset because you knew the risk up front. The same is true for contraception: when people know about side effects in advance and can balance them against the benefits, they tend to be less distressed when a side effect happens, more prepared to manage it, and less likely to quit the method, which could potentially expose them to an unplanned pregnancy.

How to Manage Troublesome Bleeding with Progestins

Irregular bleeding with implants and Depo-Provera can be managed in a variety of ways. These treatments can also be tried for bleeding with progestin-only pills, but there is less data here.

- *NSAIDs:* A dose of 800 mg of ibuprofen three times a day for up to five days, or 500 mg of naproxen sodium twice a day for up to five days. There are other NSAID regimens to consider if these two are not options. Everyone without contraindications should be given this information at insertion/injection and have the pills on hand so they can be started as soon as needed.
- *Tranexamic acid:* Take 650 mg three times a day for up to five days. For more on this medication, see page 217.
- *Any estrogen-containing pill or the contraceptive ring:* Start with one cycle, and if that doesn't work, consider continuing for up to three months. The estrogen may help stabilize the endometrium. This treatment may not be an option for people who are using progestin-only methods because they can't take the dose of estrogen in hormonal contraception.
- *Low-dose estrogen:* For this use, doctors typically prescribe 1.25 mg of conjugated equine estrogen or 2 mg of estradiol, taken orally

once a day for one to two weeks. A transdermal patch could also be used. The lower dose has the same stabilizing effect on the endometrium as birth control pills or the contraceptive ring, but it may be a better option for people who have had side effects with a higher dose.

- *Tamoxifen:* This medication for breast cancer can also reduce bleeding. For this use, the dose is 10 mg twice daily for seven days. It can be used for several months if needed.
- *Mifepristone:* This is one of the medications used for medical abortion. As a treatment for irregular bleeding, there are several dosing regimens to consider.

You might think, "Whoa, that's a lot of medication to try. Why not just switch methods?" This is where it's important to weigh individual benefits and risks. If someone absolutely doesn't want to be pregnant and/or has minimal other side effects and/or enjoys the convenience, they may be willing to do more to improve their experience with the implant or injection. Choices are always good, and having more options to make your choices work for you is even better.

The Progesterone Ring

Although progesterone is not absorbed well across the skin, it's well absorbed from the vagina. A vaginal ring impregnated with progesterone, marketed as Progering, is used to improve the contraceptive effectiveness of breastfeeding (lactational amenorrhea). It works by suppressing ovulation and affecting cervical mucus. The ring is changed every three months for up to one year after delivery. If removed during sex or for another reason, it can only be out of the vagina for two hours before backup contraception is needed. Once the frequency of breastfeeding decreases, another form of contraception should be sought. Progering is available only in some countries in Central and Latin America, but the manufacturer is apparently looking to expand access.

Bottom Line

- Progestin-only contraceptives avoid most of the risks and many of the side effects seen with estrogen-containing contraceptives.
- The biggest disadvantage of progestin-only methods is the risk of irregular bleeding.
- Older progestin-only pills may have had a higher pregnancy rate than estrogen-containing pills; however, the newer pills don't.
- The etonogestrel implant is one of the most effective forms of contraception and is currently approved for three years, but studies show it is effective for five years of use.
- Depo-Provera is also highly effective; the biggest issues are the risk of irregular bleeding and the fact that it may take up to a year for fertility to return.

25

Emergency Contraception

Postcoital contraception is the medical term, but most people know it as emergency contraception (EC) or Plan B, one of the brand names. It can be achieved with oral medications, a copper IUD, or a levonorgestrel IUD. An IUD is more effective but is not typically available emergently and is not an acceptable option for everyone. I mean, who among us hasn't sprinted down the Las Vegas strip at 5 a.m. while on vacation to buy a pack of emergency contraception? But I digress.

Unfortunately, many people are unaware of the existence of emergency contraception and consequently go without it when they need it. Because these options have been mistakenly labeled abortifacients, some medical professionals refuse to discuss them with patients, and when they do, misinformation is sadly common. But emergency contraception is exactly what the name says: contraception, not abortion.

This chapter focuses on oral medications for emergency contraception; IUDs are addressed in Chapter 27.

The History of Emergency Contraception

The first attempts at postcoital contraception involved diethylstilbestrol (DES), a potent synthetic estrogen discovered in 1938. DES was initially approved in 1941 to treat symptoms of menopause, but along the way—as often happens in medicine—doctors started trying it for other conditions related to the reproductive tract. The history of gynecological therapies sometimes seems akin to repeatedly throwing pasta against the wall to see if it will stick. Got a problem and a uterus? Let's try large doses of hormones and see what happens! To be fair, the biology of hormones wasn't well understood at the time, and there were limited therapies for many conditions. Remember, penicillin wasn't available for general use until 1946. DES was eventually abandoned as a candidate because of its risks to a fetus (it causes serious birth defects of the reproductive tract) and the fact that it caused significant nausea and vomiting.

A variety of other synthetic estrogens and progestins were tried for emergency contraception, but none showed impressive results until a paper was published in 1974 with an estradiol-progestin-based regimen from Dr. Albert Yuzpe, a Canadian OB/GYN. (He was my mentor during residency and took great interest in my career. I was floored that *the* Dr. Yuzpe saw something special in me.) The original regimen for emergency contraception even bears his name: the Yuzpe method. The dose was 100 μg of ethinyl estradiol and 1 mg of norgestrel (two tablets of a birth control pill with 50 μg ethinyl estradiol), taken immediately after intercourse and then again twelve hours later. After the encouraging preliminary study, the results of a larger one involving 464 women were published. All of the participants were required to have regular cycles, which was important to determine not only how well the method worked but also *how* it worked. The emergency contraception was started within three days of a single act of unprotected intercourse. The results were impressive. There should have been twelve to thirty pregnancies (depending on how the calculation was performed; there are different ways to look at the question of how many there should be). There was only one.

Norgestrel was soon replaced in estrogen-containing pills with levonorgestrel (a metabolite, so similar in function), and the dose for emergency contraception became 120 μg of ethinyl estradiol and 0.6 mg of levonorgestrel, taken initially and then twelve hours later. There was still no specific emergency contraceptive pill; rather, this regimen was cobbled together by working out how many estrogen-containing pills were needed to get the right dose of ethinyl estradiol and levonorgestrel. It soon became clear that at that dose, the estrogen was causing side effects—for perspective, 120 μg is four pills with 30 μg of ethinyl estradiol, a dose found in many pills today, but together, it is more estrogen than was in mestranol, the first pill. Unsurprisingly, 67 percent of people had nausea and 19 percent had vomiting.

When I was a medical student, I forgot my birth control pills for several days. We worked long hours, often at the hospital for thirty-six hours straight, so it's easy to see how it might happen. When I realized, I took four pills at once to catch up. About an hour later, I was so nauseated that I fainted. I had no idea that a high dose of estradiol could have that effect, as I had just started my OB/GYN rotation and hadn't yet learned about emergency contraception. After I recovered, I sheepishly admitted what I had done to the OB/GYNs who came running when I collapsed. (I wasn't sheepish because it was the pill but because deep down I knew it had been foolish to take four at once.) And that's how I learned to always prescribe a medication for nausea with the Yuzpe method. People shouldn't have to suffer, and if they vomit the medication or don't take the second dose because they feel awful, it makes the whole exercise pointless.

Eventually, research told us that the estrogen wasn't needed—and interestingly, the two hormones together are less effective than levonorgestrel alone—and that the medication could be given all at once instead of divided into two doses, so the Yuzpe method was replaced with a single dose of levonorgestrel. Eliminating the estrogen drastically reduced side effects and improved safety.

The other oral emergency contraceptive is ulipristal acetate, which was developed in the late 1990s and early 2000s. It's a selective progesterone receptor modulator, which is a fancy way of saying that on some tissues it acts like progesterone and on others it blocks the effect of progesterone. The drug was modeled after mifepristone, one of the medications used for abortion, which probably fed the incorrect belief that ulipristal is an abortifacient. It was designed with the goal of addressing a variety of concerns, such as fibroids, endometriosis, contraception, premenstrual mood disorders (PMS and PMDD), and emergency contraception.

How Effective Is Levonorgestrel EC?

The recommended dose is 1.5 mg of levonorgestrel, taken all at once, ideally within three days (72 hours) of unprotected intercourse, but it can be taken up to five days (120 hours) later. We can't calculate pregnancy rates with emergency contraception the same way we do for regular contraception. Instead of looking at pregnancy rates over a year of use, we look at how the medication affects the risk of pregnancy for a given act of unprotected vaginal-penile sex. If no contraception is used, the pregnancy rate on any given day is about

5 to 6 percent. With levonorgestrel emergency contraception taken within 72 hours of unprotected sex, the pregnancy rate is about 2.2 percent. The sooner the medication is taken, the better the effect. There may be some effect on days four and five, so if there are no other options, taking levonorgestrel is still recommended. It isn't wrong to try the Yuzpe method if estrogen-containing contraceptive pills are all you can access, but it is about 50 percent less effective.

Because levonorgestrel emergency contraception is very safe and has minimal side effects, some people wonder about taking it at specific times instead of a daily contraceptive pill. If you have sex four times a month, why not just take 1.5 g of levonorgestrel those four days? This option has been studied, and overall it resulted in a pregnancy rate of 11 to 20 percent, much higher than with a daily progestin-only contraceptive. In addition, it would likely lead to a significant amount of disordered bleeding for many.

How Does Levonorgestrel EC Work?

Sometimes in medicine we must shrug our shoulders, because unraveling the mysteries of how a specific medication works just isn't possible with the technology of the day. Levonorgestrel emergency contraception is not one of those situations, despite what you might hear from right-wing politicians who fancy themselves junior gynecologists. We know exactly how it works, and it has nothing to do with preventing a fertilized ovum from implanting, or disrupting an already implanted embryo. It's not an abortion by *any* definition—it is contraception.

As previously discussed, the LH surge is exquisitely sensitive to progesterone and progestins. When the right dose of levonorgestrel is given two to three days before the LH surge, it can prevent ovulation by stopping, delaying, or blunting the surge; outside of that two- to three-day window, it's either too early or too late to have an effect.

So why do so many people think it's an abortifacient? There are probably several reasons. When Dr. Yuzpe published his initial papers, he did not include a hypothesis about the method of action. I think he knew, because he paid particular attention to the group who were mid-cycle, and he obviously knew about progestins and the LH surge, but he likely couldn't prove it with the technology available at the time. Ultrasound, for example, could not measure follicles with the precision that we can today, so there was no way to know how close someone was to ovulation. In addition, the first study involved taking tissue samples from the lining of the uterus to evaluate the effect of the hormones, and this has somehow—either through a bad game of telephone or willful ignorance—been spun into a hunt for embryos or signs of pregnancy.

A huge factor in perpetuating the myth was undoubtedly information from the FDA and in the packaging. Both stated that the endometrium *might* be affected by levonorgestrel, meaning theoretically it could prevent a fertilized egg from implanting. Although medicine does not consider this an abortion, some people do, based on religious or other personal belief systems. I can see how someone would look at the information and say, "Hey, look, the manufacturer and the FDA say it could be an abortifacient!" But the FDA and package insert always said "may," because there was no data showing an effect on implantation; it was just a hypothesis. It's problematic when politicians misuse an unproven hypothesis, especially in this case, where a lot of data didn't support it. There were studies showing levonorgestrel didn't affect signaling in the endometrium, lab studies showing it didn't affect how embryos attach to the endometrium, and animal studies showing it didn't impact implantation. In addition, many people accidentally take the birth control pill during an early pregnancy when they don't realize they are pregnant, and this doesn't lead to miscarriage, yet these pills have progestins.

We also now have detailed studies where levonorgestrel was taken at different times in the cycle, with close monitoring of hormone levels and ultrasound evaluation of the ovaries. When levonorgestrel is taken at the right time, ovulation and pregnancies are prevented. When it's taken on the day of ovulation—outside its window of effectiveness—ovulation occurs. It is at this time that pregnancies ensue. If levonorgestrel had an effect on anything other than ovulation, it would still work when taken too late in the cycle to prevent ovulation. But it doesn't.

In 2022, the FDA finally caught up with the science and the labeling was changed. The current FDA stance on Plan B and other levonorgestrel methods of postcoital contraception is: "Plan B One-Step prevents pregnancy by acting on ovulation, which occurs well before implantation. Evidence does not support that the drug affects implantation or maintenance of a pregnancy after implantation, therefore it does not terminate a pregnancy."

Just as the science of the 1400s said the world was flat and the science of today says the world is round, the science of the 1970s may have suggested that levonorgestrel could affect the endometrium and prevent implantation of a fertilized egg, but the science of today proves otherwise. As new research methods emerge, what we think we know can change—that's how science works. But when it comes to reproduction, in the United States we live in a post-truth world where politicians, religious leaders, district attorneys, and even the Supreme Court can discard hard science over beliefs about medications. Depending on where you live, you may be exposed to lies about emergency contraception medications. The best defense against disinformation is knowledge, as twisting the truth about how medications work is a common tactic. I might believe I can turn iron into gold, but I should not be able to force everyone else to believe that lie and to change the laws of my country so that iron holds the same value as gold.

Ulipristal Acetate

Ulipristal acetate—trade name ella, with a lowercase *e*—is even better than levonorgestrel at blocking the LH surge before it starts, and it's also pretty good at stopping ovulation even when the LH surge has started. Meaning it provides better protection against pregnancy than levonorgestrel. The pregnancy rate per episode of unprotected sex is about 1 percent. As it's a superior medication, it should be the first choice among the oral medications.

Some people have questioned whether ulipristal acetate is an abortifacient. In this case, the concern is more understandable, as ulipristal acetate blocks the effect of progesterone, and progesterone from the corpus luteum is important in maintaining an early pregnancy. Mifepristone, one of the drugs used for a medication abortion, also blocks progesterone. However, 30 mg of ulipristal acetate, the dose in emergency contraception, has the same impact on the uterine lining as a placebo: none. This isn't surprising, because milligram for milligram, the doses of mifepristone and ulipristal are roughly equivalent, but the dose of mifepristone for an abortion is 600 mg and the dose of ulipristal for emergency contraception is 30 mg. Also, when ulipristal acetate fails and someone gets pregnant, there is no increased risk of miscarriage, and when it is accidentally taken in early pregnancy, an abortion doesn't happen.

The advantage of ulipristal acetate is that it is more effective for longer during the fertile window. The disadvantages are its cost, the need for a prescription in some countries, and the fact that its effectiveness is reduced by some epilepsy medications, the antibiotic rifampin, and St. John's wort. Side effects are a little more common with ulipristal acetate than with levonorg-estrel, with headache and nausea reported most often.

The Impact of Body Weight on Emergency Contraception

The effectiveness of both levonorgestrel and ulipristal acetate may be affected by body weight. The problem is, the data comes from studies that weren't specifically designed to address the impact of weight or BMI on the effective-ness of these medications, so it's not definitive. With levonorgestrel, the efficacy may start to drop with a BMI of 25 to 29.9, and the risk of failure may be four times greater for people with a BMI of 30 or more. This potentially leaves a lot of people at risk. The theory is based on people with obesity having lower levels of levonorgestrel in the blood. To counteract the potential failure, some experts recommended doubling the dose of levonorgestrel (taking 3 mg). However, a study has since shown that doubling the dose didn't improve the effect on ovulation. To get answers, we need a study that compares the regular and higher doses of levonorgestrel and subsequent pregnancy rates. Fortunately, that study is underway as of 2023, but as yet there are no results.

Ulipristal acetate seems to be less impacted by BMI/weight. There may be no change in the pregnancy rate with a BMI under 35. Again, the studies are not definitive, and the fact that we have less data than we need is unaccept-able. Until we have better data, ulipristal acetate is the recommended oral emergency contraception for people with a BMI over 25 or a weight greater than 70 kg (154 pounds).

It's important to mention here that IUDs (see Chapter 27) are the most effective method of emergency contraception, and their efficacy is not impacted by weight or BMI.

If It's Only Effective Right before Ovulation, Why Not Just Take It Then?

This is a great question, and I get asked it a lot. Why take it on day 4 or 23 of the cycle if those days are outside the fertile window? The answer is, ovulation can be unpredictable. While it's true that the window where one can get pregnant is six days, determining that window with accuracy is challenging because there can be cycles where ovulation happens earlier or later than expected. Think of emergency contraception like insurance: you have it not just for the times you think you will need it, but also for the times you can't imagine you will.

Some Final Thoughts

Levonorgestrel is available over the counter (OTC) in many countries, but ulipristal acetate generally requires a prescription. Prices vary greatly, from free (Scotland for all medications, and levonorgestrel in British Columbia) to $50 or more (the United States). In some countries, OTC may be more expensive than prescription. For example, in the United States, the cost of levonorgestrel went up about $20 when it went OTC. This might seem odd, but when a medication goes OTC, insurance companies are no longer negotiating pricing and/or covering part of the cost. Friends in the United Kingdom tell me emergency contraception is free if you can get it from your doctor, but that isn't always an option when it's urgent, so many simply buy it from a chemist (pharmacy).

Even when people have them in their medicine cabinet, emergency contraceptive pills are underused. In one study, 45 percent of people who had them at home did not use them when they had unprotected intercourse. Why isn't known, but I have a few hypotheses. I think people truly forget they have them, and I get it—I continually buy razors thinking I don't have them and am gradually becoming a hoarder of razors. But also, people with emergency contraceptive pills at home may hear misinformation and think the pills aren't effective or are abortifacients. People have even told me they were misinformed about the safety or effectiveness of the pills by a pharmacist! And some people may underestimate their risk of pregnancy.

If you don't want to be pregnant and aren't using a permanent or long-acting reversible method of contraception (an IUD, implant, or injection), consider getting a prescription for emergency contraception filled to keep at home. If traveling, bring it along. Even if you are using a hormonal contraceptive method, you might miss doses of the pill or forget to change a ring or patch; emergency contraception can fill that gap. And condoms can break or slip off. Having to drive to a pharmacy to pick up emergency contraception—or even worse, having to first call a doctor to get a prescription, as many people must do with ulipristal acetate—adds barriers that delay or prevent access.

Consider checking on your emergency contraception supply regularly, as you should be doing for smoke detectors. Given its superior efficacy, ulipristal acetate is the best product to keep on hand, but if it's not an option, then go for levonorgestrel. If Plan A is contraception and Plan B is levonorgestrel emergency contraception, think of ulipristal acetate as Plan B+.

EMERGENCY CONTRACEPTION • 347

Bottom Line

- Hormonal emergency contraception works by inhibiting ovulation.
- A single 1.5 mg dose of levonorgestrel, often called Plan B, can be taken within five days of unprotected intercourse, but taking it within three days is best, and the sooner, the better.
- Ulipristal acetate, in a dose of 30 mg taken within five days of unprotected intercourse, is even more effective than levonorgestrel. Unlike levonorgestrel, it is effective even after the LH surge has started, so it provides better protection for the full five days.
- Levonorgestrel may be less effective for those with a BMI over 25. For those with a BMI over 35, ulipristal acetate may be less effective.
- Emergency contraception is very safe. For perspective, it is safer than many medications that are available over the counter, such as acetaminophen.

26

The History of the Intrauterine Device

The intrauterine device (IUD) is a form of long-acting reversible contraception (LARC). There are currently two types available, based on their active ingredient: hormone or copper. IUDs provide years of highly effective contraception, with failure rates on par with oviduct ligation and vasectomy; they have no limitations based on weight or BMI; and they have a high user satisfaction rate. Unfortunately, like many contraceptives, they are also mired in misinformation and bad press—more so in the United States, it seems, than anywhere else in the world.

The False History of the IUD

There is a very embarrassing medical "history" that used to be recounted about the IUD. I heard it in medical school and residency and have read it since, to my dismay, in several papers. The story is that Bedouins used to insert date pits or stones into the uteruses of camels before long desert treks to prevent pregnancy, because a pregnant camel on a long trek would spell disaster. "And that, my friends," she says, closing the book of fairy tales, "is the story of the very first IUD." This tall tale isn't just 100 percent false, it's an embarrassing display of Western exoticism and a testimony to how lazy people can be, because it's easily disproved. After hearing it repeatedly, I finally, somewhat sheepishly, asked a person with knowledge of camels. They snorted, "Have you ever seen a camel?" Of course: it's ridiculous when you give the idea just a few seconds of thought. How would you get a massive camel to hold still while you thrust not just your hand but your entire arm up its vagina (they have long vaginas; I checked in a textbook of veterinary medicine), then forced a date pit into its uterus by feel? But there's more. Camels have two uterine horns, so you would need to get a date pit into each one by feel alone. Oh, and if you wanted your camel to breed again, you'd have to get the date pits out, and your hand isn't getting into that uterus. The visuals here are . . . remarkable.

Apparently, if you don't want camels to breed, you just keep them apart.

The Real History of the IUD

IUDs took a long time to enter medicine, likely because doctors knew that inserting objects into the uterus caused infection. The forerunners to modern IUDs were devices in the 1800s called stem pessaries, which were typically made of metal or rubber and shaped like a large thumbtack, but without a point at the end of the stem. The stem or rod end was inserted into the cervical canal, and the flat head stuck out, covering the cervix. These devices were abandoned because of infections, and I suspect they caused a great deal of cramping.

The first publication about what we can call a true IUD was in 1909. It was a ring of silkworm gut (made from the silk glands of silkworms; for reference, it looks like fishing wire), with threads hanging out of the cervix for removal. This paper was largely ignored, for reasons unknown, and it wasn't until twenty or so years later that doctors in Germany began playing with different IUD concepts, including adding silver wire to the silk gut so it could be seen on X-rays, then switching to copper and nickel when it became apparent that the body absorbed the silver, staining the gums in the mouth a bluish gray. In the United States, most of the information about these early IUDs would have been passed on by word of mouth, as contraception was largely illegal at the time. Because it was legal in Europe, it isn't surprising that the early work originated there.

In the first wave of IUDs, doctors were basically designing their own, jerry-rigging them from materials at hand. One doctor inserted silkworm gut thread into a gelatin capsule, then inserted the capsule into the uterus.

The capsule dissolved and the thread remained. Kind of ingenious—and yes, the doctor was a woman. A hook-like device could later be inserted through the cervix to snag the thread for removal–and yes, it would have been quite uncomfortable. The big names in American gynecology at the time were vehemently opposed to IUDs, believing they caused infections and cancer of the uterus, and that contraception was a convenience, not a necessity. In addition, laws about contraception made public sales impossible.

Despite the American reluctance to prescribe IUDs, they were used in Europe and Japan, which in the 1950s had thirty-two different devices! Eventually, the data from Japan—a study with thousands of women—broke through the resistance in the United States, and in 1962, the Population Council in New York City convened the first meeting on IUDs, ushering in a second wave. This time, instead of making their own IUDs in the office like making flies for fishing, doctors designed devices and then developed relationships with manufacturers for production and promotion, and sometimes for profit (but not always: Dr. Lippes, of the Lippes loop, did not benefit financially from his device).

The second-wave IUDs were plastic or metal. Plastic was more popular in the United States, in part, I'm guessing, because it could be molded into so many shapes and seemed like cool new tech (there's probably a joke from *The Graduate* in here somewhere). The big issue with plastic devices was that they needed a large surface area to be effective—basically, they had to fill the uterine cavity—and larger devices were more painful to insert and more likely to cause cramping and bleeding and even to be rejected by the uterus.

In 1969 a Chilean physician, Jaime Zipper, discovered that copper is toxic to sperm. I love that his name was Dr. Zipper: a zipper isn't a bad analogy for long-acting reversible contraception, and, like IUDs, zippers can be plastic or metal! Adding copper to an IUD meant the size could be decreased, making them easier to insert and reducing cramping, as well as improving their effectiveness. The first copper device was the Copper-7, with 200 mm² of copper. It had a failure rate of 2 to 3 percent. By the mid-1970s, researchers had found that increasing the amount of copper to 380 mm² dropped the pregnancy rate to less than 1 percent. The Paragard IUD on the market today in the United States has 380 mm² of copper.

The second-wave devices often bore the name of the doctor who invented them: the Tatum-T, the Lippes loop. At one point there were at least twelve commercially important IUDs on the market in the United States, as well as other, less popular devices, but most (probably all) were understudied compared to what we would accept today in terms of product safety. During the 1960s and early 1970s, when the second wave began, medical devices still weren't regulated by the FDA. One of the understudied IUDs was the Dalkon Shield, a small plastic shield-like device (to me it looks more like the spider on Spider-Man's costume) impregnated with copper. It was invented at Johns Hopkins University by Dr. Hugh Davis, an OB/GYN, and Irwin Lerner, an engineer, who sold their design to the A.H. Robins Company. The Dalkon Shield was advertised as a better option for women who had never been pregnant, and it was promoted as having a lower expulsion rate, meaning it was less likely to fall out (a desired quality, as you might imagine). It was on the market from 1970 to 1974. During that time, over two million were inserted in the United States and one million in other countries. However, soon after it went to market, the complications started: over two hundred septic abortions, a very serious complication where an infection develops in the uterus during pregnancy; at least eleven maternal deaths; and thousands of pelvic infections. Many women were left infertile. The rate of uterine infection with the Dalkon Shield was thirteen times higher than with other contemporary IUDs.

There were several issues with the Dalkon Shield. First, it wasn't as effective as claimed, so there were more pregnancies than expected. The original study said the pregnancy rate was 1.1 percent but neglected to mention that women were encouraged to also use spermicide—kind of an important omission. The author of the study also failed to disclose that he was a part-owner of the Dalkon Corporation. The A.H. Robins Company was aware that the pregnancy rates might be higher than expected but did not relay that information to the public. Another major issue was that the string was braided, more like what is used for tampons, so it acted like a wick, drawing bacteria from the vagina up into the uterus. And finally, in the United States the Dalkon Shield was heavily promoted to single women who had never been pregnant, who may have been at higher risk of acquiring sexually transmitted infections (STIs), which would be more problematic given that the string provided a highway for an STI to access the uterus.

A.H. Robins voluntarily removed the Dalkon Shield from the market in 1974, but because IUDs weren't under the purview of the FDA at the time, there was no formal recall, so the company wasn't required to notify women that they were walking around and having sex with a potentially infectious death-stick in their uterus. Infections and complications continued, eventually prompting a class action lawsuit. Domino-like litigation, or fear of litigation, spread to other IUD manufacturers. If one IUD was bad, they all must be. ("And even if they aren't, if we can convince the jury, that's all we need to get a multimillion-dollar class action settlement!") Between 1985 and 1986 the three most popular IUDs were pulled from the market in the United States by their manufacturers to avoid the litigation feeding frenzy, and no new devices were introduced to fill the gap. This left one, the Progestasert, which was only used by 3 percent of the IUD market. Some training programs, major medical centers, and individual providers refused to insert IUDs. Meaning from 1986 to 1988 there was one, albeit significantly less popular, IUD available available in the United States, and finding someone to insert it could be a real challenge. Even after a copper IUD was reintroduced to the market in 1988, it took years for the fears of both medical providers and patients to dissipate.

Although blaming all IUDs for the fault of a single poorly designed, under-tested product was wrong, some of the other devices also had issues (a fact that is frequently ignored). Look at the Majzlin spring. Imagine an accordion made from sewing needles, with a thread hanging down from the eyes of the needles at either end. (I'm picturing a medieval torture device—are you?) The Majzlin spring collapsed to resemble one thick needle and was then pushed through the cervix. Once in the uterus, it would open up and sit in the uterine cavity (I am clenching a bit writing this). But the Majzlin spring didn't fit at all well inside the uterus, and it was sharp, so uterine perforations (bad injuries) and infections occurred. The FDA wanted it off the market, but according to Larry Pilot, the leader of the device regulatory program, there was a gynecologist who was a big proponent of the Majzlin spring and had a stockpile of them in his office that he refused to give up (the only "reason" I can think of is they were paid for, so he wanted to continue to insert them to recoup his costs). Oh, and this doctor was *also* on the FDA's advisory committee for IUDs! He even tried pulling rank, and the FDA had to send U.S. marshals to his office to confiscate his stash of Majzlin springs. I couldn't have made that up if I tried.

Larry Pilot, our man in the FDA who liked to tell it like it is (my kind of person), also told of a woman with a Lippes loop, inserted by Dr. Lippes himself as part of a study. She suffered from severe pain and other issues post-insertion, so she went back to see Lippes, who dismissed her, telling her the IUD had nothing to do with it! Eventually, another gynecologist confirmed that the IUD was at fault and removed it. The only reason the FDA found out about this unreported issue was because the woman worked there! It makes you wonder about the quality of the data on the Lippes loop if the lead investigator felt he needed to gaslight someone who had a complication.

But the issues didn't stop there. One of the doctors who did the initial studies that demonstrated how the string of the Dalkon Shield acted like a wick for bacteria, Howard Tatum, didn't disclose that he was working on a competing IUD, the Tatum-T, when he presented the data about the Dalkon Shield's complications to the FDA. Letting people know about that kind of bias is important, even if your data is correct.

Spurred in part by the Dalkon Shield debacle, plus other shenanigans with cardiac implants, the FDA started regulating devices in 1976 under the Medical Device Amendments. However, IUDs were classified as pharmaceuticals, based on having an active ingredient, so they required, and still do, a higher bar for approval. I've told you these stories not because I get perverse joy out of horrifying you, but because articles bemoaning the lack of IUD options in the United States place some or even all of the blame on the degree of FDA regulation we have now, with statements like: "If only IUDs were regulated like medical devices instead of medications, more companies would introduce their IUDs into the American market!" It is true that many other countries have more IUDs. At my last count, in 2023, there were twenty-two in the United Kingdom and twelve in Canada, so people in those countries have more options for fit and duration of use. In other countries there are smaller IUDs, as well as IUDs that, instead of having the traditional T shape, are U-shaped or even frameless—imagine copper beads on a string that can conform to the shape of the uterus. As of 2023 in the United States, the uterus must be big enough for an IUD that is 6 cm (2.4 inches) in length, but not everyone is built that way.

The FDA has very specific requirements for submissions for IUDs, and doing these studies may not be worth it for manufacturers in other countries. In addition, the United States is more litigious, so even if companies invest the time and effort to conduct studies, they might still need to defend themselves against frivolous lawsuits, which studies don't stop. You can see how the United States ended up with a perhaps overly cautious review process, given the history of American IUDs. When the FDA had to send the EFFING U.S MARSHALS TO COLLECT DANGEROUS IUDS THAT A MEMBER OF ITS ADVISORY COMMITTEE REFUSED TO HAND OVER (yes, I am shouting, because WTF?), understudied Dalkon Shields were killing and maiming women and yet there was no recall, and the inventor of the Lippes loop was apparently ignoring patients enrolled in his study, it tells me that an unregulated system for IUDs didn't exactly benefit women in America. Larry Pilot summed it up this way: "So there was some skepticism, certainly on my part, with regard to this marketplace on intrauterine devices, because folks had their personal interests, competitive interests, financial interests in all of this." I think his skepticism was warranted. Perhaps companies that were selling IUDs in other countries had more scruples, or perhaps their IUD complications were under-reported. But whatever the reason, unfettered American capitalism plus IUDs was not a winning equation for American women in the 1970s.

I'm not convinced that the answer is switching the IUD from a pharma-ceutical to a medical device, with a lower bar for FDA approval. Even today understudied medical devices (not IUDs) enter the market only to be pulled a few years later because they maimed people. The fact that there is a lot of money to be made in the U.S. may play a role, as the markup here on these products is astronomical. A device company that can get approval quickly can make a lot of money, then simply cry "I didn't know!" should issues arise.

The Third Wave of IUDs

The copper IUD, Paragard, so named because it was originally recommended only for parous women (those who had previously had a baby), was approved in the United States in 1988. Paragard ushered in America's third wave of IUDs, meaning they underwent the same rigorous approval process as pharmaceuti-cals. The first modern hormonal IUD, Mirena, was approved in 2000, ten years after it was approved for use in Finland. (Progestasert, also a hormonal IUD, was available until 2001, but it required replacement annually, so as you can imagine, it was never popular.)

A long runway was required for modern IUDs to take off again in the United States. When I moved to the U.S. in 1995, I was shocked by how few health care providers inserted IUDs, because they were worried about infections and infertility. I remember one meeting where the other doctors in my department expressed amazement that I would insert an IUD in someone who had never been pregnant, and that I had inserted so many! One of my partners had never inserted an IUD in her training or afterwards. Not one! The area of the country where she had trained was very litigious, and she and her colleagues had been warned not just about the supposed risks of the IUD, but also about lawsuits. And here I'd been inserting IUDs for five years in Canada during my training and never thought anything of it! It was quite the contrast.

We now know there is no link between modern IUDs and infertility. A large study from Mexico evaluated women with copper IUDs and found no association between the IUD and infertility; the risk for infertility was related to having had a chlamydia infection (an STI). Along the way, one researcher opined that it wasn't the IUDs that caused infections and infertility, it was men. While we do recommend screening for chlamydia and gonorrhea at the time of IUD insertion for people who are at higher risk (those age twenty-five and under or who have multiple partners), if the test is positive, antibiotics can be started after insertion without any increased risk of complications.

It has taken a lot of work from dedicated researchers to undo the disastrous impact of the American IUD misconduct of the 1970s. We also now know it is perfectly safe for people who have not been pregnant to have an IUD, but unfortunately that information has taken a long time to percolate through the medical system. For years after the data showed it was safe, many American doctors continued to refuse to insert IUDs for women who had never been pregnant, so as not to potentially damage their future fertility. One of the best moments in my early blogging career was one young woman's response to my article about why you can have an IUD if you have never been pregnant. Her doctor had told her it was unsafe, so she returned with a print-out of my blog, slammed it on the table, and said, "Well, Dr. Jen Gunter says I can!" And she got her IUD! It shouldn't take that degree of activism to get standard medical care, but at times it does, and that is why I write. Being empowered with facts about your body gives you the tools to take charge.

Modern IUD Mythology

You would think that once American gynecologists realized many countries were inserting IUDs safely, and once safe IUDs and training for insertion became available, the controversy would stop. Well, sorry—American evangelicalism and politicization would like a word.

There is a popular misconception that IUDs work as abortifacients, either by disrupting an implanted embryo or by preventing implantation of a fertilized ovum. This fallacy is based on a rat study from the 1960s that showed silk thread in the uterus (as a proxy for an IUD) prevented implantation. But it turns out that rats are different from humans. In fact, many animals respond to IUDs in markedly different ways. With rats, an IUD prevents implantation of a fertilized embryo; with cows, an IUD impacts the corpus luteum; and with sheep, an IUD creates an inflammatory response that blocks sperm. (No word on what IUDs do to camels.) With humans, both types of IUD damage sperm transport, the sperm itself, and the ovum. In humans, IUDs are not abortifacients.

In studies that have looked at recovering embryos from the uteruses of women with IUDs, no fertilized ovum or embryo has ever been recovered from a woman with a copper IUD. One was recovered from someone with a levonorgestrel IUD, but it was likely due to IUD failure. There have been conflicting results from studies that look at hormone signaling to see if they can identify early pregnancies that subsequently don't implant: fourteen of nineteen showed no evidence of fertilization. Five did, but this technology is unproven. Nowhere else in medicine would we accept this kind of scant data as proof of anything. Imagine if your doctor said, "All the good studies say I should treat your abscess with antibiotics and surgery, but in studies that used technology we don't even know is accurate, five of nineteen suggested that those treatments might be the wrong choice." Would you want to get the antibiotics and surgery based on the good studies, or to go with the unvalidated data?

Sadly, the disinformation about the IUD being an abortifacient is a "valid" reason for some employers in the United States to decline coverage, thanks to the *Burwell v. Hobby Lobby* ruling. Hobby Lobby, for those who don't know, is an arts and crafts store that was reportedly founded on Christian beliefs and that paid the U.S. Government a $3-million fine in 2018 for illegally importing over 5,000 likely stolen artifacts, many labeled as "tile samples," for the Museum of the Bible. They refused to cover IUDs (and some other contraceptives) under their employee health insurance, claiming they were abortifacients, and took their case to court. The Supreme Court ruled in their favor, concluding that believing an IUD is an abortifacient was enough reason for some companies to refuse to cover them.

What is science in the face of belief? It's truly maddening and frightening.

The United States has had a uniquely unfortunate relationship with the IUD thanks to unfettered capitalism, evangelicalism, overzealous medical malpractice litigation, and political exploitation. The modern IUD has not suffered from this combination of reproductive toxicants to the same degree in any other country.

Bottom Line

- Modern IUDs are highly effective contraceptives, and unlike oviduct ligation or vasectomy, they are reversible.
- IUDs were once unregulated in the United States, which led to devices that caused great harm, most notably the Dalkon Shield.
- The legacy of harm from early IUDs created a ripple effect. For a time, IUD insertions dwindled dramatically, given the limited choice, the lack of training for insertion, and fear that IUDs could cause infertility and other complications.
- In the United States, modern IUDs must pass a higher bar for approval than other medical devices; this ensures safety but also limits the number of options, as not all companies want to deal with the cost or regulatory hassle involved with bringing a new IUD to market.
- IUDs are contraceptives. The data does not show that they prevent implantation of a fertilized embryo or cause abortion.

The Modern Intrauterine Device

IUDs can be classified based on their contraceptive component, either the hormone levonorgestrel or copper. IUDs can also be classified based on shape, meaning whether they conform to the inside of the uterus or are frameless (think beads on a string). The previous chapter discussed the history and the science behind IUDs; this one addresses the practicalities you need to know to choose and get the most out of an IUD. Knowing the advantages and disadvantages of both types will help you make the best choice for you.

Even if you know you will never be interested in contraception, this is a still an important chapter because the levonorgestrel IUD isn't just for contraception; it can also treat heavy bleeding, reduce or eliminate periods for those who don't want them, help painful periods and endometriosis, and even be part of menopausal hormone therapy (for more on that, check out *The Menopause Manifesto*). Basically, it's like a Swiss Army knife of gynecology.

Hormonal IUDs

These devices are permeated with the progestin levonorgestrel, which makes the cervical mucus hostile to sperm so it can't get to the ovum. The inflammation generated by the presence of the IUD also damages sperm and ovum, essentially resulting in a missed connection. These IUDs are highly effective, with a pregnancy rate of about 1 percent over the life of the IUD (assuming it's left in for the maximum allowable time). The 52 mg IUD is likely the most effective. The only contraception that performs better is the implant. Although IUDs are very effective at preventing pregnancies in the uterus, they are less effective at preventing ectopic pregnancies, which implant in the oviduct. If someone with an IUD has a positive pregnancy test, it is critical for them to seek medical care immediately so the location of the pregnancy can be identified, as an ectopic pregnancy requires urgent evaluation and specific medical care.

The 52 mg levonorgestrel IUD is also highly effective emergency contraception. When inserted within seventy-two hours after unprotected sex, its pregnancy prevention rate is over 95 percent. The closer to the time of sexual activity, the greater the contraceptive effect.

Other Benefits of a Levonorgestrel IUD

Besides providing worry-free contraception (it's even more effective than the copper IUD), levonorgestrel thins the lining of the uterus and can stop periods or reduce blood loss, because with a high dose of levonorgestrel in the uterus, the endometrium doesn't grow as well (or may not develop at all) from the estradiol produced by the follicles. With the 52 mg IUD, which is the best-studied, the amount of blood lost each menstrual cycle drops significantly: 90 percent of people will have reduced blood loss, and for about 50 percent, menstruation stops altogether.

By decreasing or eliminating the amount of endometrium each cycle, the IUD also significantly reduces or even stops the production of prostaglandins, so it is effective therapy for painful periods as well. The hormone spreads into the pelvic cavity and can have the same effect of opposing growth on endometriosis.

Other advantages of hormonal IUDs include an 80 percent decrease in the risk of endometrial cancers (an effect of the hormone) and a 32 percent reduction in the rate of ovarian cancer. While the mechanism for the latter isn't entirely known, it is believed to be related to the low-grade inflammation caused by the IUD.

Levonorgestrel IUDs vary in the amount of hormone, how much is released daily, the length of contraceptive effectiveness, size (see Table 6, page 361), and (in some parts of the world) price.

The Cons of a Hormonal IUD

The biggest drawback is irregular bleeding, which often goes undertreated. An unacceptably high number of people are shocked when I tell them there is therapy to reduce what is often called "nuisance" bleeding. Look, if irregular bleeding from the penis were a side effect of medications for erectile dysfunction, you can bet every doctor and pharmacist would know about it and everyone would be taking it; in fact, they'd probably sell it in a combo pack. It's important to treat abnormal bleeding when it happens, because (a) you shouldn't have to put up with it, and (b) it might make you want to have your IUD removed. That's why I had mine removed, because after three years I just couldn't take the bleeding bingo anymore. (I didn't try any of the therapies because I thought, "Oh, this will be the last month of this," and then it never was, and life got busy. What I'm saying is, don't suck it up like I did. There are options.)

Bothersome bleeding is common in the first three months after insertion, but if it persists, an ultrasound to confirm that the IUD is in the right position is warranted. The therapies are the same as discussed on page 336 and include NSAIDs, an estradiol patch for a few months, an estrogen-containing contraceptive for two to three months, tamoxifen, and doxycycline.

Overall, other major side effects are uncommon, though some people report headaches, nausea, breast tenderness, and ovarian cysts. There may be an association between the levonorgestrel IUD and depression for a small percentage of people, but the studies are conflicting. Some data suggests that the hormonal IUD may slightly increase the risk of breast cancer (on par with the pill), but this association is far from proven, and it's important to remember that the IUD reduces rates of endometrial and ovarian cancer.

How to Choose a Levonorgestrel IUD

There are four to choose from in the United States (as of 2023) and there are some practical differences between the IUDs (see Table 6). The biggest issue for most people is the duration of use. If you know you don't want to be pregnant in the next eight years, why go through three insertions of a 13.5 mg IUD when a 52 mg IUD will cover you the entire time? When a 52 mg IUD is inserted in someone forty-five or older, it's considered effective until age fifty-five, so that may also be a consideration. For those who are paying for their IUD, cost may also be an issue. Just two of the 13.5 mg IUDs are significantly more expensive than one 52 mg IUD, plus the potential cost of two or three insertions instead of one. Costs may also vary depending on insurance coverage and country; in the United States, the Liletta is typically less expensive for people paying out of pocket.

The risk of bleeding may also factor into IUD choice. Obviously, this is a key point for people who are choosing to use a hormonal IUD for heavy or irregular bleeding (the 52 mg IUD seems best). But many people simply prefer not to have periods and like the idea of a contraceptive that offers this as a bonus. Equally important is the risk of bothersome irregular bleeding, which is more likely with lower hormone doses.

Table 6 • LEVONORGESTREL IUDS

BRAND NAME	TOTAL DOSE	APPROVED DURATION OF USE (U.S.)	RISK OF BOTHER-SOME BLEEDING AT 1 YEAR	OTHER CONSIDERATIONS
Mirena	52 mg	8 years	6%	• Most likely to stop bleeding altogether. • Pregnancy rate over 8 years is 1.09%.
Liletta	52 mg	8 years	6%	• May be less expensive than Mirena, and stops bleeding as effectively. • Pregnancy rate over 8 years is 1.09%.
Kyleena	19.5 mg	5 years	17%	• Insertion may be easier. • Pregnancy rate over 5 years is 1.1%.
Skyla	13.5 mg	3 years	23%	• Lowest chance of stopping periods. • May have fewer hormone-related side effects for those who are susceptible. • Insertion may be easier (it is the smallest IUD). • Pregnancy rate over 3 years is 0.9%.

Levels of levonorgestrel in the blood are highest with a 52 mg IUD, so it is most likely to temporarily impact ovulation, but the effect is short-lived, and by one year ovulation is proceeding as if nothing had happened. If you have been sensitive to the effects of hormones in the past, you may wish to consider a 13.5 mg IUD, although there is no hard data to support this approach. The levonorgestrel in the blood with a 52 mg IUD is about 10 percent of the amount seen with a birth control pill; with the 13.5 mg, it's about 5 percent. It's really a small amount of hormone. In fact, fertility experts can even give hormones to people with a levonorgestrel IUD and do egg retrieval to freeze eggs or embryos! (That's pretty cool when you think about it.)

The Copper IUD

Copper is toxic to sperm, preventing a process called capacitation, which is essential for sperm to penetrate the egg. If you think "Sperm killer!" when you think of copper, you aren't far off. (I like to shout "Sperm killer!" in my head like the fish in *Finding Nemo* scream "Fish killer!" about Darla.) The copper IUD is highly effective, with a failure rate of about 2.5 percent at seven years (to compare it head-to-head with a 52 mg levonorgestrel IUD). It is also the most effective form of emergency contraception, with a pregnancy rate of 1.7 percent.

Only one copper IUD is currently available in the United States: the Paragard TCu380A. There is a dizzying array of copper IUDs of different sizes and shapes in other countries. For example, Canada has nine, which range in duration of use from three to ten years, with a variety of lengths and widths so it doesn't have to be one-size-fits-all. The Paragard is approved for ten years, but studies tell us it's effective for twelve years for women who are twenty-five or older at the time of insertion. When inserted at age thirty-five or older, a Paragard can be relied upon for contraception until menopause, with a negligible risk of pregnancy—a huge upside. In Canada, the closest IUDs are the Liberté TT380 and the Mona Lisa 10, both approved for ten years.

For many people, the appeal of copper IUDs is the lack of hormones. Some people just don't want to take hormones; others prefer having a period, as it reassures them that they aren't pregnant; and some don't like how they feel on hormones. Like the levonorgestrel IUD, copper IUDs reduce the rate of ovarian cancer by about 30 percent, again postulated to be via inflammation. There may also be a decrease in endometrial cancer, but it's not as significant as with the levonorgestrel IUD. Therefore, the copper IUD is not recommended when the goal is to reduce the risk of endometrial cancer.

The main side effects of the copper IUD are heavier periods and more cramps. These drawbacks are sometimes exaggerated by both medical providers and online sources, frightening people away from a good option. Initially, yes, bleeding can be heavier and cramps can be worse, but as with other forms of contraception, both typically improve over the first three months. Estrogen doesn't treat this bleeding, so it's likely due to inflammation. One way to reduce the bleeding and cramping is to take an NSAID every six to eight hours, for five days overlapping with menstruation, during the first three to six menstrual cycles after insertion.

General Considerations

The only medical reason to avoid a levonorgestrel IUD is if you have hormone receptor–positive breast cancer. Avoid a copper IUD if you have Wilson disease, a condition that affects copper metabolism. For both types of IUD, there are some potential challenges regarding the size of the uterus. All of the IUDs in the United States are designed for a uterus that is 6 to 10 cm (2.4 to 4 inches) in length from the outside of the cervix to the top of the inside of the uterus. To measure the uterus, a narrow plastic or metal rod, called a uterine sound, is inserted through the cervix. (Here *sound* refers to depth, as in sounding the depth of a body of water.) Other countries offer alternative IUDs for uteruses smaller than 6 cm (2.4 inches). For example, in Canada there are several copper IUDs designed for a slightly smaller uterus, and some countries have frameless IUDs that may work in this situation.

If fibroids are distorting the uterine cavity, or there are abnormalities in how the uterus developed, such as a septum, then an IUD may not fit or may not cover the uterus as needed for reliable contraception. Such nuances are beyond the scope of this book.

IUDs can be inserted any day of the menstrual cycle, but a pregnancy test should be done first for anyone who could be pregnant. A copper IUD works retroactively to five days before insertion (thus its value as an emergency contraceptive). Unless a levonorgestrel IUD is inserted during the first seven days of the cycle, a backup contraception method is needed for seven days. IUDs can be inserted after an abortion, and after delivery once the placenta has been delivered.

Major complications after IUD insertion are uncommon. The risk of infection is very low (0.14 percent), and antibiotics do not lower it. The risk of perforation (meaning the IUD pierces the uterus, potentially moving into the abdominal cavity) is less than 0.5 percent. The risk of the body expelling the IUD is 3 to 10 percent for anyone who has not been pregnant recently. The expulsion risk is higher in the six months after insertion (which is why we suggest people check the strings for several months), when an IUD is inserted after delivery or a second-trimester abortion, and for people who have never been pregnant, have bad menstrual cramps, or have heavy periods. People who have expelled one IUD may be at higher risk for it happening again; if this has happened to you, make sure to tell your health care provider.

Pain Control with IUD Insertion

There is a wide range of pain experiences with IUD insertion, from minor cramping to excruciating pain. Patients often refuse to consider an IUD because they have heard the insertion is universally awful, but in general, studies tell us that about 50 percent of people have pain scores of 5 or less, meaning they experience some pain but find it tolerable. That doesn't mean we doctors should roll the dice and hope our patients are in that group, but we should let people know that severe pain is not a universal experience.

Pain is uniquely personal. I've had two IUD insertions, and the most I felt was a brief cramp, much less than my menstrual cramps. However, I think bikini waxing is one of the most painful experiences a human can have, so it's not as if I'm immune to pain. My partner at work was in agony during her IUD insertion (I didn't insert it!) but thinks waxing is a walk in the park; she also came back to work early during her cancer therapy because she didn't think chemo was bad at all.

It's a sad truth that pain is undertreated in many areas of medicine. As a medical student, I was horrified when I watched a bone marrow biopsy where the patient seemed to be in significant pain. My eighty-nine-year-old dad screamed through a cystoscopy and was admonished by the staff for his behavior. I've read Twitter threads by people who had root canals with no pain medication. None of this is acceptable. But I also know that women are more likely to have their pain ignored or undertreated. And I am *sure* there have been awful OB/GYNs who thought a punitive IUD insertion might teach a "lesson" about sexual morals.

The first step in getting better access to pain control during an IUD insertion is knowing more about the pain. One thing rarely discussed is that pain control is not as easy here as with other office procedures. There are multiple steps that can be painful, including inserting the speculum, dilating the cervix, grasping the cervix with an instrument to steady it, and inserting the IUD, which may also cause the uterus to cramp. For some people, all these pathways may generate pain; for others, it may be one or a combination. To make things more complex, the pain is not all generated by the same nerves. The vagina and the muscles around it are supplied by one set of nerves and the uterus (including the cervix) by a different set. Neither set can be anesthetized with a simple injection in the office. If they could, treating pain in labor would be much easier and epidurals wouldn't be needed! It is much easier to provide fast, effective numbing medication for stitching a scalp wound, pulling a tooth, or setting a broken wrist than for inserting an IUD.

But we're working on it. There has been quite a lot of research on ways to reduce pain with IUD insertion. On PubMed, an online repository of published medical articles, as of April 2022 there were 157 clinical trials in this area, more than 40 of them published in the past four to five years. We also know that certain factors are linked to increased pain with IUD insertion, including pain with sex and/or pelvic exams, previous sexual trauma, and anticipated pain (so it's possible being exposed repeatedly to horror stories about insertions may make things worse). If any of these factors apply to you, discuss them with your medical provider in advance so you can review the options and come up with the best plan. The evidence-based pain-control options include:

- *NSAIDs:* The consensus from the studies is that these drugs, such as ibuprofen, are worth taking thirty minutes before the insertion.
- *A support person:* In one study, a support person was more effective than opioids.
- *Wearing a TENS unit during the procedure:* Although this hasn't been studied for IUD insertion, TENS (see page 260) does help with pain during other procedures on the uterus, so it might be worth a try.
- *Anxiety medication:* These drugs, such as lorazepam (Ativan), have no effect on pain scores, which is not surprising as they don't treat pain. However, they can be helpful to reduce anxiety before a procedure, which might improve the experience.

- *Numbing medication, such as lidocaine:* A paracervical nerve block (an injection) can help with pain from the cervix. Applying topical numbing medication to the cervix doesn't seem to be very effective, and neither is injecting liquid numbing medication into the uterus to try to numb it from the inside.

It is important to know that manipulating the cervix can overstimulate the vagal nerve for some people, causing a vasovagal reaction, where heart rate and blood pressure drop. It can cause nausea, dizziness, a wave of heat, sweating, yawning, ringing in the ears, and even fainting. If you can catch it as soon as it starts, contract your arms and hands (like making a fist) to pump blood back to the center of your body, ask for a cool cloth on your forehead, smell an alcohol swab (a simple version of smelling salts), and, if possible, elevate your legs above your heart. Your provider should be looking out for a vasovagal reaction and be able to offer all of these options, and ideally, they should be warning you about it in advance.

Many people wonder why every doctor doesn't just provide sedation in the office. In some places, there are specific credentialling issues for sedation that are related to the building, so it may not be an option owing to a higher-up administrative decision. These issues aside, some physicians can offer moderate sedation to make you sleepy without losing consciousness, but they must have the training, equipment, and personnel to do so safely, and not every doctor does. Most people who get IUDs are young and healthy, so complications from sedation are uncommon, but they can happen, and when they do, they can go from bad to catastrophic in a minute. It's in handling these complications where special training is critical. If your medical provider offers moderate sedation, ask if they do it regularly. If they provide abortions in their clinic, for example, they are more likely to have appropriate training, equipment, and personnel. Some doctors bring in a specialist dedicated to managing anesthesia and arrange procedures that need sedation on that day. A final option is going to a surgery center or operating room with a trained anesthesia provider; this also allows deeper sedation, which some people may need, especially if they experience pain with pelvic exams, have had previous trauma, have had pain with previous IUD insertions, or are anxious about pain.

A word on therapies for pain that *don't* work well for IUD insertions, because I often see comments online from people who are upset that they weren't offered the following:

- *Misoprostol:* This medication can soften the cervix, but paradoxically it increases pain with IUD insertion, as well as the risk that it will later be expelled (not ideal, to say the least). It can be helpful, however, if your doctor previously tried to insert an IUD and couldn't dilate your cervix.
- *Nitrous oxide:* Laughing gas offered no benefit for IUD insertion in one study, and studies on it for other procedures on the uterus show no reduction in pain scores.
- *Oral opioids:* Many people assume opioids are the "best" pain medications, but no study comparing them head-to-head with NSAIDs shows them to be superior for the kind of pain we manage in the office.

For approaching pain with IUD insertion, discuss your fears upfront, consider if there are any reasons that might make the procedure more painful for you, and ask your provider what the options are for pain control. Many of the office-based options previously mentioned work quite well. But you also need the pain control you need, and so if you need more anesthesia than can happen in your provider's office, then that's what you need. Also, I always remind people that we can stop at any time and book the procedure with an anesthesiologist.

IUD Removal

Pulling on the string causes the IUD arms to collapse, and it almost always comes out easily and nearly instantaneously. Most people find that if there is significant pain it is very short-lived. It's rare to need pain control here, but everyone is different. If inserting the IUD was painful, it's worth discussing options for pain control for removal.

What about self-removal, since it's literally just grabbing the strings and pulling? Some data suggests it is a safe option, and it might save you the cost of removal and a trip to the doctor. If it doesn't come out easily, then you need to see a health care provider. Examine the IUD to make sure it all came out (you can find an image of your IUD online and compare it to what you removed). If you think you might want to remove your own IUD, tell your doctor before insertion, and they can leave the strings on the longer side.

String Issues

There are a couple of string-related issues to consider. If you can't feel the strings with your fingers, it's important to see your health care provider to make sure the IUD hasn't moved in the uterus, hasn't perforated the uterus, or hasn't come out. Typically, an ultrasound is needed. If the IUD is in the right place and it's just that the strings are no longer visible, nothing needs to be done, though your doctor should have a plan for removal, as special equipment may be needed. An IUD that has moved and a perforated uterus require care that is beyond the scope of this book.

During sex, a partner may say they feel the IUD. The most likely situation is that a string is hanging straight down, like a barb. In this situation, your doctor can trim the string so it's just inside the cervix but still visible. They should check to make sure the IUD itself hasn't slid down so that the end is sticking out the cervix (a partial expulsion); in that case, it should be removed.

Bottom Line

- IUDs are a highly effective, reversible contraception method that provides years of protection.
- Levonorgestrel IUDs work by making cervical mucus hostile to sperm. Copper IUDs damage sperm so they can't fertilize an egg (and may also damage eggs).
- Levonorgestrel IUDs significantly reduce menstrual bleeding, which is a bonus for many people, but they can be associated with bothersome irregular bleeding, especially in the first three months after insertion.
- Copper IUDs may initially increase menstrual bleeding and cramping, but these side effects improve over time, and taking NSAIDs for five days each menstrual cycle may help.
- Pain with IUD insertion is a concern for about 50 percent of people. Discuss pain control with your doctor prior to insertion, because there are options.

28

Abortion

You might be wondering why there's a chapter on abortion in a book on menstruation. Abortion is a way to restore your menstrual cycle. In fact, over the years when it was illegal, doctors who circumvented the law often used the euphemisms *menstrual extraction* or *menstrual regulation* as code. As in, "Oh, your period is three weeks late? Well, we better do a menstrual extraction, so no toxins accumulate and your cycle gets back on track." At the time, ultrasound had yet to be invented, and the lack of easily available, fast, and accurate pregnancy tests meant that it wasn't always known whether someone was pregnant, especially early on. If no specimen was sent to the lab, there was no way for law enforcement to know if the menstrual extraction was a way to treat irregular periods or an abortion, assuming no one said anything. In addition, older medical teaching suggested that dilation and curettage, a procedure to remove tissue from the lining of the uterus, which is very similar to an abortion, might kick-start periods. If everyone in the clinic and the woman having the abortion were sworn to secrecy, it would be easy to fob off an early abortion as a menstrual extraction. This type of hush-hush abortion was typically available only for those with money and connections.

Education about abortion is important, because it's suboptimal to learn how to access one only when you need it, especially if you live in a place with limited or unequal access to abortion or where it is illegal. Even where it is legal, people can be disenfranchised by the medical system and/or society and still encounter roadblocks to medical care. When I was a resident, several women who had traveled for abortion care told me they had no idea abortion was not only legal but also covered by the Canadian health care system. Once they found out they were pregnant, it took them weeks to find out the truth and get an appointment. These women had been lied to about the legality and availability of abortion by health care providers. It was pre-Internet, so getting access to quality information about a private matter, especially in smaller communities, was hard. If you don't want anyone to know, how do you find out the truth if it's never mentioned in magazines or books and not discussed in school or at home? Even now, disinformation about abortion is common, so my hope is that the information here will help people who eventually need an abortion or have a friend or family member who needs one. And that is a lot of people: almost one out of every four women and 4 percent of trans and nonbinary people with a uterus will need an abortion. We have less data for trans and nonbinary people, but while their rates of abortion may be lower, they may be even more likely to have difficulty accessing care.

Even if you think a chapter on abortion could never apply to you, I urge you to read on. First, changing laws can affect you even if you have no desire to have an abortion. For example, medications to help manage miscarriage are the same as those for medication abortion, and there are stories of pharmacists refusing to dispense these medications for fear they're for abortion and not miscarriage. As someone who performed abortions for fifteen or so years, I have met many women who thought they would never have an abortion, but because situations change in ways that can't be anticipated, now they needed one. Sometimes a serious complication develops in a pregnancy, necessitating an abortion, and if the pregnant person lives in a U.S. state where abortion is illegal, they must arrange transportation to another state; if they're not well enough to do so, they simply must hope for the best. And pregnant people are getting suboptimal cancer care in situations where an abortion is recommended because doctors are delaying chemotherapy and/or radiation because of the potential toxicity to the fetus. Experts estimate that, each year, about 1,500 people who live in a state that restricts access to abortion will develop cancer during their pregnancy, and 135 to 420 of them will get subpar therapy because they can't get the abortion they need to start treatment. Some of them will die as a result.

The Case for Abortion

The risk of dying from a legal abortion in the United States is 0.41 in 100,000 pregnancies. It is much safer to have an abortion at any gestational age than to be pregnant, especially in the United States, which has an egregiously high rate of maternal mortality. The risk of death during pregnancy includes up to one year after birth, and in the United States it is a shocking 23.8/100,000 pregnancies—19.1/100,000 for non-Hispanic White people, 18.2/100,000 for Hispanic people, and a devastating 55.5/100,000 for non-Hispanic Black people. On average, the risk of death during pregnancy is fifty-eight times greater than the risk of dying from a legal abortion. Given these statistics, there can be no "pro-life" stance about abortion that is not hypocritical, unless the life of the pregnant person is inconsequential. It is always safer to have an abortion than to be pregnant, even in countries with lower maternal mortality. For example, maternal mortality is 3.2/100,000 in Germany. It's absurd that there are laws in some countries restricting abortion but no laws anywhere against impregnating someone. People who seek to deny access to abortion are not pro-life, they are forced-birthers.

Maternal mortality is only the most extreme negative outcome of pregnancy. People who suffer a blood clot and survive may be very sick for some time or have long-term consequences from a stroke caused by the clot. A vaginal delivery can result in injury that causes fecal incontinence, urinary incontinence, and/or chronic pain. A cesarean section is a major surgery with its own risks. And then there is postpartum depression. A pregnancy can go sideways in myriad ways, altering life for the person—sometimes irrevocably. Gestating and delivering a human has physical and emotional consequences. Autonomy demands that people get to choose whether they want to bear those risks.

Personally, I think every politician who votes against abortion access should have their anus cut and repaired to create the equivalent of a fourth-degree laceration (the largest tear that can happen during delivery). In the best of situations, a fourth-degree laceration heals well over an excruciating several weeks; at worst, it is painful for years and causes fecal incontinence. When these politicians are three months out from the procedure and are still sitting on a donut to take the pressure off their anus, crying with each bowel movement, leaking stool in public in the most unpredictable ways, and still unable to have sex because of the pain, they can explain why the medical ramifications of pregnancy are inconsequential and abortion is unnecessary.

Before abortion was legalized in the United States in 1973, with the landmark *Roe v. Wade* decision, there were about eight hundred thousand clandestine abortions every year. But that number is likely grossly underestimated, because it's not as if you are going to report your illegal abortion, you know? In Canada, deaths from illegal abortions were common until the 1960s, when the chief coroner of Ontario, Dr. Morton Shulman, became so sickened by the bodies of desperate women in his autopsy suite that he decided to hold a public inquest into each death. He wanted the public to witness these tragedies. His actions eventually became a catalyst for changing the law in Canada, and in 1969 abortion became legal, but only in hospital, with the approval of a three-doctor committee. Not great, but far better than its being illegal. In 1988, the abortion law was struck down. Abortion is no longer in Canada's Criminal Code and is simply considered a medical procedure. There are still access issues, but decriminalization was an essential step.

In countries where abortion is illegal, the rate of clandestine abortions among unintended pregnancies can be as high as 50 percent. In the United States, a country with many laws limiting access, the abortion rate for unintended pregnancies was 34 percent before the reversal of *Roe v. Wade* in 2022. In Canada over a similar time frame, 37 percent of unintended pregnancies ended in abortion. It's clear that laws don't affect how many people have abortions; what they do is hinder or delay abortion and lead to unsafe procedures.

Worldwide there are 21.6 million unsafe abortions every year, resulting in at least 47,000 deaths—a staggering 13 percent of maternal deaths. In some parts of the world, 49 percent of maternal deaths are due to clandestine abortions. Yes, you read that correctly: 49 percent. An estimated 5 million women are hospitalized because of complications from these procedures, and many others who suffer serious complications don't seek care. Legalization has a major impact on abortion's safety. For example, in South Africa in 1994, when abortion was largely illegal, the rate of death from an abortion was almost 38 in 1,000 After legalization, it fell to .59 in 1,000.

Lack of access to abortion has other consequences. In the landmark Turnaway Study, which enrolled women seeking abortion and then compared those who received one to those who were turned away because they had just passed the gestational age limit, women who did not get an abortion and subsequently gave birth were more likely to live in poverty and suffer domestic violence. If they already had children, their children were more likely to have developmental milestone delays. Two women in the study died from complications related to pregnancy.

Economics are also a factor in who needs an abortion and who gets one—especially who gets one safely. Financial security affects access to health care and hence contraception. We know that when offered all methods of contraception for free, women in the United States are more likely to choose long-acting reversible contraception (LARC), the methods with the lowest failure rate, and that among teens, using LARC is associated with a reduction in the rate of abortion. When a generic oral contraceptive is $5 and an IUD is $800 out of pocket and requires time off work for the insertion, only some can access the most reliable forms of contraception.

People need abortions for many reasons. Rape, incest, fetal malformations, and the health of the pregnant person are often seen as "good" reasons; contraceptive failure, economic concerns, bad timing, and not wanting to be pregnant are viewed as "bad" reasons. That thinking is inaccurate and, quite frankly, unacceptable. If you need an abortion, you should have access to one that is safe, affordable, and free of legal ramifications. There are no "good" or "bad" abortions; there are only abortions. This is about body autonomy. In many parts of the United States, you have more say over your body if you are dead than if you are alive and have a uterus. If you don't sign an organ donor card, your organs cannot be harvested against your wishes; if you want an abortion where it is illegal, you can be arrested and jailed for having one.

Abortion Myths

Forced-birth advocacy groups constantly spread disinformation about the consequences of abortion, often under the guise of looking out for the health of the pregnant person. Abortion is not associated with breast cancer, depression, or infertility. What is associated with a negative effect on mental health is being denied a wanted abortion.

Many people ask how they can be sure their medical provider isn't a forced-birther. While you can't always know, if they are a member of the American Association of Pro-Life OB/GYNs (AAPLOG), they belong to an extremist group that spreads disinformation about abortion.

Medication Abortion

Also known as a medical abortion, medication abortion is a relatively new method, but it is rapidly increasing in use and has revolutionized safety and access to this procedure. There are two drugs used for medication abortion: mifepristone and misoprostol. Some may know mifepristone by its older name, RU-486. It blocks progesterone receptors in the endometrium, affecting the decidua, the endometrial changes that are essential for implantation and the early success of a pregnancy. It causes the placental tissue to detach from the endometrium, which decreases production of the pregnancy hormone human chorionic gonadotropin (hCG), causing progesterone levels to fall. It also softens the cervix and makes the uterus more sensitive to chemical signaling that can cause contractions. Taking both mifepristone and misoprostol is the most effective method of medical abortion. Together, these two medications can also be used to complete some miscarriages.

Misoprostol, often known by its trade name, Cytotec, acts like prostaglandins, which are important signaling hormones for the uterus. It also softens the cervix, helps it dilate, and stimulates uterine contractions. Misoprostol can be used for a medical abortion by itself, albeit with slightly lower success rates. It is also used to induce labor and prevent stomach ulcers that can develop from taking NSAIDs.

Both mifepristone and misoprostol, or misoprostol alone, can be used to induce abortion up to twenty-four weeks, but the success rate decreases slightly as the pregnancy advances (see Table 7). For abortions up to ten weeks, 200 mg of mifepristone is taken orally, and twenty-four to forty-eight hours later, 800 µg of misoprostol can be placed vaginally or put under the tongue (sublingual administration) or between the cheek and the gum (buccal administration) and left to dissolve; thirty minutes later, you swallow any remnants. When mifepristone isn't available, the recommended dose of misoprostol is 800 µg every three hours for up to three doses. The risk of a serious complication in the first trimester with mifepristone and misoprostol, the preferred regimen, is 0.3 percent. After 10 weeks the regimens are slightly different.

Table 7 • SUCCESS RATES WITH MEDICATION ABORTION*

WEEKS INTO THE PREGNANCY	MIFEPRISTONE AND MISOPROSTOL	MISOPROSTOL ALONE
≤ 10 weeks	97%	84%–87%
10–12 weeks	95%	75%–93%
12–24 weeks	93%	77%

* Abortion completed and no other intervention needed.

In determining how far along you are, you can go by the date of your last menstrual period; the precise dating provided by ultrasound isn't needed. Unfortunately, in the United States, many states require a transvaginal ultrasound as part of routine abortion care, even though it is medically unnecessary—it's a way to increase the cost and discomfort of the procedure. In fact, even a visit with a medical provider is unneeded. Medical abortion can be provided safely and remotely with a telehealth visit. An ultrasound is necessary if you don't know the date of your last period or if there is concern about an ectopic pregnancy, which is indicated by pain in the abdomen or pelvis, as that requires either different medications or surgery. Ectopic pregnancy is a potential emergency. Anyone who is pregnant with an IUD in place should have an ultrasound, as about 50 percent of the time the pregnancy is ectopic.

Medical abortion is *not* recommended when someone has an allergy to the medications or when an IUD is in place, even after an ectopic pregnancy has been ruled out. It may be contraindicated for people with a blood disorder; those who are taking certain medications, such as blood thinners (anticoagulants); or those who have been on steroids for a long time.

A medical abortion will induce bleeding, like a heavy period or even heavier. Bleeding requiring more than two maxi pads an hour for two hours is a concern, and you should speak with a medical provider. There will also be cramping, and while it is often described as a "crampy period," pain is a significant issue for many, with 50 to 60 percent of people reporting severe pain (typically 7 or higher on an 11-point scale). Those who oppose abortion often use the bleeding and pain as a reason why medication abortion is "bad"; however, no pregnancy ends without pain and bleeding. It's one of those sucky evolutionary bargains. One therapy to help reduce pain, besides medications like ibuprofen and acetaminophen, is a TENS unit (see page 260). It can reduce the pain by 2 points on an 11-point scale. Other side effects of a medication abortion include nausea, vomiting, diarrhea, headache, dizziness, and feeling either hot and flushed or cold. These are all temporary and are almost all related to the misoprostol.

Some advantages of a medical abortion include avoiding surgery, a greater degree of autonomy, and no risk of surgical injury to the uterus. In addition, a medication abortion very early on in the pregnancy (at four or five weeks) is more likely to be effective than a procedure abortion, which can sometimes miss a very small embryo. A medication abortion may also be preferred late in the second trimester (when it's often called induction of labor) for pregnancies that have genetic abnormalities or birth defects. It allows the pathologist to do a detailed evaluation, which might yield information for subsequent pregnancies. The disadvantages of medication abortions are the failure rate (for a small percentage of people, the medications don't work and they will need a procedure), the bleeding, cramping, and diarrhea, and the time involved. For those in the second trimester, a medical abortion can sometimes take several days, as it is essentially inducing labor.

Self-Managed Abortion

Abortion has changed a lot over my lifetime. In the United States, it has gone from being illegal nationwide to legal nationwide to illegal in some states. It has moved from dirty rooms and back alleys to hospitals to clinics to the home. It's gone from a procedure to either a procedure or medication. The residents training today in the United States have not known a time when medical abortion didn't exist.

A self-managed medical abortion is the next step in the evolution of abortion care. It may mean using online telemedicine, where you provide some basic information and then receive pills in the mail, or obtaining the pills yourself and using them without online support. It may sound unsafe, but if a miscarriage is something people can have at home, then a self-managed abortion is equally safe. In fact, it appears to be as safe as an abortion under the guidance of a health care provider. With some general information, provided on many websites, people can manage it on their own if they so choose or if it is their only option. If we can trust people to read the instructions on a bottle of acetaminophen, which can cause liver failure and even death if taken incorrectly, we can trust them with a self-managed abortion. If we can trust people to drive a car . . . well, you get the point.

As we fight for reproductive justice, it's important to be mindful of the symbols we use. While the coat hanger—a nod to a tool sometimes used for clandestine abortions—was once used as a rally symbol for safe, legal abortion, today we should be using pills. We don't want to give people the idea that a coat hanger is an option. Given the wealth of safety data for medication abortion, pills symbolize both a safe option and the right of self-determination.

Whether you get abortion pills from a medical provider or choose a self-managed route, no doctor or nurse can tell by your cramping or bleeding, or by an exam, if you are having a miscarriage or a medical abortion. The only way they would know would be if they found remnants of misoprostol pills in your vagina. That's easy to avoid by putting them under your tongue or against your cheek, as previously described. I want to emphasize this point: there is no physical sign or complication unique to a medical abortion, so if a doctor or nurse or anyone in the hospital tells you they need to know if you took pills before they can help you, they don't. There are, unfortunately, cases of people telling their health care providers they took medication for abortion and being turned over to the police. And if anyone suggests that they can test your blood to tell if you had a medical abortion, as of 2023 there is no commercially available blood test to detect mifepristone. Misoprostol is cleared quickly from the blood, so all traces should be gone by several hours after a single dose; for those who used it every three hours for three doses (the regimen for a misoprostol-only abortion), it should be gone by twelve hours after the last dose. Also, the test to detect misoprostol is typically not readily available.

If you may be interested in a self-managed abortion, some organizations that can provide information on the process and on how to get safe medications include Women on Web; Women Help Women; Safe2Choose; and Plan C. There are also many excellent local abortion advocacy groups; you can find the closest one to you at abortionfunds.org. These groups may also be able to help in other ways, such as helping you get funds and safe access to abortion procedures. They have the boots on the ground and are truly your advocates. If you have a little money to donate, a local abortion advocacy group is a great choice, as your money will be going to help someone in need.

Abortion Procedures

Most abortion procedures occur in the first trimester, meaning before thirteen weeks, but about 10 percent happen at thirteen weeks or later. Safety-wise, these procedures are on par with medication abortion. The risk of a major complication with a first-trimester procedure is 0.16 percent, and it is 0.41 percent with a second-trimester procedure. For perspective, the major complication rate with a screening colonoscopy for cancer is 0.28 percent, and I've seen no political campaigns to regulate those for safety.

Procedure abortions are often called surgical abortions, but we are trying to move away from that terminology. They are as safe as a colonoscopy or wisdom tooth removal, and we manage to refer to those as procedures and not surgery. Also, referring to abortion as surgery can frighten some people and makes the procedure sound riskier than it is. Disinformation here is already an issue, as lies about abortion safety are used to enact legislation to restrict access.

Techniques and procedures vary not just by gestational age but also based on the available facilities and pain control options. Most procedure abortions are done with devices that create suction. For those who are about fourteen weeks or later, the cervix typically needs to be prepared a day in advance so it can be dilated enough to remove the tissue. Dilation will be done either with vaginal misoprostol or by small rods in the cervix that expand gradually over twelve hours or so. When rods need to be inserted, an additional office visit is required. In general, the farther along the pregnancy, the more uncomfortable the procedure, and so different pain medications or anesthesia will be used.

A procedure abortion is recommended if it is your preference; where there are contraindications to a medication abortion; and when sterilization is also desired (the two procedures can happen at the same time, with the same anesthetic). The disadvantages of a procedure abortion are pain from the procedure, expense, and the need for anesthesia or sedation for pregnancies that are past thirteen to fourteen weeks (this varies by practitioner).

Emmenagogues and Abortifacients

The use of emmenagogues, which are plants or extracts that bring on a period (historically often code for *abortion*), and outright abortifacients has been recorded throughout human history. In the United States, there has been a potentially deadly resurgence of interest in the subject due to the erosion of access to safe abortion, and sadly these products are used around the world where abortion is illegal or restricted. People who take herbal abortifacients are highly likely to be hesitant to seek care afterward, for fear of repercussions, further increasing their risks. Sometimes these products are discussed by well-meaning but uninformed activists, but I've also seen dangerous messaging about them on Instagram from people who are capitalizing on fear and desperation.

There are several issues with accepting "ancient" recipes for abortion. A major one is that it isn't possible to know if they were actually abortifacients. Euphemisms were often used, and the terminology is open to interpretation. Many recipes that some claim are emmenagogues or abortifacients have been interpreted by other scholars as aphrodisiacs or fertility enhancers. In addition, because early pregnancy couldn't be diagnosed precisely in ancient times, the results of an abortifacient couldn't truly be known, given the high rate of early miscarriage. And depending on the culture, the time of the menstrual cycle when conception occurred and when someone was considered pregnant varied from today's definition. For example, the Ancient Greeks thought conception happened over several months, and the "diagnosis" of pregnancy was left up to the woman. Many of the products recommended as abortifacients cause vomiting, diarrhea, or both. It's possible that people thought purging might trigger an abortion (although there is no evidence it does), or that they mistook the dramatic purging as signs the product was working. Clearly, translating all these variables into medical care for someone today is problematic.

The idea that herbal abortifacients were common knowledge and widely used doesn't fit with historical birth and infant mortality rates. If people were routinely controlling pregnancies on a grand scale, the population would likely have dwindled. There is also a glaring contradiction, noted by Helen King, a renowned scholar and expert in ancient gynecology, in her book *Hippocrates' Women*: if effective herbal abortion was known to our ancestors and their midwives, why were there so many unwanted pregnancies outside of marriage? Today there are 21.6 million unsafe abortions worldwide every year, and millions more result in serious complications. If there were safe, effective herbal abortion alternatives passed down by elders, how did they get lost in every culture? How did women forget about these methods but not about ginger for nausea in pregnancy or heat for menstrual cramps?

There is obviously very little research on these substances, with most of the data coming from poison control centers and reports of injury. Because these products are often taken where abortion is illegal or restricted, it's understandable that people might not be forthcoming about what they took, so the scope of the problem isn't known. Most of the proposed botanicals don't have a mechanism of action that relates specifically to abortion, meaning we can't say there is a medical reason to suspect they can cause an abortion. But many of them are literally poisons, and while some poisons may indeed damage the placenta and/or fetus or make the pregnant person so ill that oxygen delivery to the fetus drops, leading to an abortion, the poison can also harm the person who ingested it.

For some of these products, it isn't the plant itself that's concerning, but rather the extract or concentrate that is used. A plant that is benign to eat can be far more potent and problematic as an extract. Toxicologists are fond of saying the dose makes the poison. And it's typically not even possible to know the dose of these products. It is a dangerous game of buyer beware, and sadly, when people are desperate, they may be willing to take the risk.

The following herbal products are among the most often proposed emmenagogues or abortifacients. There is no evidence they work, and all are toxic and should be avoided.

- **Pennyroyal** *(Mentha pulegium)***:** Of all the abortifacients, pennyroyal is probably mentioned the most often, and it's one of the most dangerous, toxic to the liver and the central nervous system. Deaths have been reported. It is toxic even in very small amounts and should never be taken.
- **Rue** *(Ruta graveolens)***:** This plant contains several toxic compounds and can cause vomiting, bleeding, abdominal pain, multisystem organ failure, and death.
- **Parsley** *(Petroselinum crispum)***:** Yes, the herb. Parsley contains myristicin and apiol, which are both toxic. When we eat it, we are not consuming a pharmacological dose, so it's safe, but extracts and oils are associated with hemorrhage, liver damage, and death. Some sources recommend inserting sprigs of parsley in the vagina, changing them every three days. This could cause a serious infection that could trigger a septic abortion, a potentially fatal complication. A woman in Argentina died from an infection caused by this practice.

- **Cola de quirquincho** *(Lycopodium saururus)*: Also known as club-moss, this plant contains multiple concerning chemicals. Extracts can cause vomiting, diarrhea, convulsions, and death.
- **Savin oil** *(Juniperus sabina)*: Well known as a poison for humans, animals, and even bees (the pollen is toxic), oil of savin can cause vomiting, stomach pain, coma, liver damage, kidney failure, and death.
- **Blue cohosh** *(Caulophyllum thalictroides)*: The N-methylcytosine and anagyrine in blue cohosh can cause blood vessels in the heart to constrict (not a good thing) and can induce nausea, vomiting, and tremors.
- **Cantharides** *(Lytta vesicatoria)*: Also known as cantharidin powder, cantharides is made from the powdered dried bodies of Spanish fly, a blister beetle that uses cantharidin as a defense mechanism. It is highly caustic and causes blistering on contact. When taken orally, it can cause blisters and burns in the mouth and gastrointestinal tract and can damage the kidneys. It is lethal at a low dose. A fisherman who got some on his finger died when he accidentally stuck himself with a hook. Cantharidin powder has been implicated in at least one abortion-related death.
- **Hellebore:** This is actually a genus of approximately twenty different plants, and whether a hellebore concoction is dangerous or not depends on the species. Black and white hellebore are both toxic and can cause death.
- **Castor oil:** Prepared from the seeds of the *Ricinus communis* plant, commercial castor oil isn't toxic and has been used for thousands of years as medicine, as an emollient for the skin, and as oil for lamps. But the seeds contain ricin, which is one of the most toxic substances found in plants and can cause organ failure and death. Ricin is water-soluble and becomes a waste product during the processing of properly prepared commercial oil. Castor oil can cause dramatic vomiting and diarrhea and has been used historically to stimulate labor, but there is no good evidence that it works. It's likely the false belief that it is effective at triggering labor that has led some people to think it could be an abortifacient. Crushing the seeds releases the ricin, so trying to make castor oil at home without

commercial equipment is highly dangerous. Ingesting as little as two seeds is often enough to kill someone.

- **Queen Anne's lace** (*Daucus carota*), which you might know as wild carrot, and the seeds or unripe fruit of papaya are also often used as abortifacients. There is no evidence to show they work, but they are likely benign.

Bottom Line

- Abortion is safer than pregnancy.
- Medication abortion with mifepristone and misoprostol is very effective in the first trimester and can be used in all trimesters.
- When mifepristone isn't available, misoprostol can be used on its own.
- Medical abortion is safer than acetaminophen, and in the first trimester, a procedure abortion is as safe as a colonoscopy.
- Despite historical writings, there is no safe, effective method of herbal abortion. Misoprostol is far safer and more effective.

29

Surgical Sterilization, Barrier Contraception, and Fertility Awareness Methods

Surgical sterilization, barrier contraception, and fertility awareness methods have no impact on the menstrual cycle beyond preventing a pregnancy from stopping menstruation. They are the oldest forms of contraception, and like every method, they have pros and cons. They range from the easiest to use (surgical sterilization, you're done and dusted!) to the most user-intensive (fertility awareness methods).

The Background on Surgical Sterilization

If you want this surgery, you should have it. That's really the gist of it. There are far too many stories of women who have begged for years, going from OB/GYN to OB/GYN trying to get their tubes tied or removed. It's just unacceptable. Men are not asked to write a letter in blood for a vasectomy. It says so much about society when access to permanent sterilization is often easier for the person who will not be physically harmed by pregnancy and who typically provides less childcare than for the one who risks physical harm and is more likely to be financially affected by children.

Denying women permanent sterilization is patriarchy in action. It is a manifestation of the belief that they are breeders and are damaged and selfish for not wanting to be pregnant. Clearly, they have not thought it through and don't know their own minds and desires, so a savior OB/GYN must make the decision for them. Coming home from the hospital with a baby is irreversible, yet society imposes no burdens to "make sure" this is "really" what a woman wants. Do some people change their minds after surgical sterilization? Sure, but adults get to make their own decisions—that is autonomy, and it's not my job or your job to interfere with it (also, it's less common than most people think). By some reports, one in seven men regrets having a vasectomy, yet somehow that doesn't lead to draconian measures to "protect" other men from it.

In the United States, people with Medicaid, a publicly funded health insurance, may have additional barriers to surgical sterilization. In some states, you must be twenty-one to get the procedure, and there is a form that must be signed and dated more than 30 days beforehand but not more than 180 days (in some cases, the wait can be reduced to 72 hours). This measure was implemented in the 1970s to reduced forced and coerced sterilization. If the rules are not followed, the surgeon, anesthesia provider, and hospital don't get paid, and in the case of postpartum sterilization, none of the pregnancy care is reimbursed by Medicaid. The policy prevents some people from getting the procedure, and the delays can lead to unplanned pregnancies. It also adds to the incorrect belief that a waiting period is medically important.

We have new data on how effective oviduct removal is for prevention of ovarian cancer, and some expert groups are recommending that everyone consider it. The data is compelling. Many ovarian cancers start in the oviducts, and removing them is expected to prevent about 80 percent of these cancers. The lifetime risk of ovarian cancer is 1.4 percent, and it is almost impossible to diagnose early, when it is most likely to be curable, so the risk of dying is about 50 percent. Only in a patriarchal society would it take cancer prevention to potentially make surgical sterilizations easier.

Surgical Sterilization

Female permanent contraception is the most common contraception method worldwide, used by almost 24 percent of those who use contraception. The failure rate over ten years is about 1 to 2 percent, which is on par with a copper IUD. The implant and the levonorgestrel IUD have slightly lower pregnancy rates. If a pregnancy happens after sterilization, it is very important to seek care immediately, as about 33 percent are ectopic pregnancies, which are potentially lethal if inappropriately treated.

Common options for sterilization are to remove both oviducts (a bilateral salpingectomy); to burn (cauterize) the oviducts, or obstruct them with a clip via laparoscopic (keyhole) surgery; or to remove sections of the oviducts after delivery with a small incision below the belly button (the uterus is still very large for a few days after delivery, so the oviducts are higher up, close to the belly button, rather than lower down in the pelvis). This latter procedure is called postpartum sterilization and can also be performed immediately after a cesarian section. The best procedure for cancer reduction is the bilateral salpingectomy.

The risk of a major complication from the anesthetic or injury from the surgery itself, such as severe bleeding, infection, and/or damage to other organs, is about 1 percent. From a surgery standpoint, this is low risk. Some women report hot flashes after surgical sterilization, but research suggests it is correlation, not causation: interestingly, those who are more likely to have hot flashes are also more likely to have a tubal ligation. In addition, multiple high-quality studies show that surgical sterilization has no effect on hormone levels or the age of menopause, and it doesn't itself cause irregular bleeding. However, the risk of irregular bleeding increases with age, and overall, people tend to be older when they get a surgical sterilization, so it might seem that the surgery caused bleeding issues when it was really correlation. Social media grifters used to say surgical sterilization would wreck your hormones. Ah, the good old days. But seriously, hormone grifting is like whack-a-mole. Sweeping statements are made about a form of contraception based on little to no data, research disproves the fearmongering, and then it's on to the next one.

Finally, what about regret? Five years after surgical sterilization about 7 percent of women regret their procedure, but in that same study, 6 percent also regretted their husband's vasectomy. It's also important to know that regretting a procedure and wanting it reversed are different things, and the number of people who seek a reversal is quite low (about 1-2 percent). In my experience, when someone requests surgical sterilization, they have typically already thought about it a lot and know what they want. Informed consent should be on par with every other surgery, meaning a discussion of the risks and benefits of the procedure as well as information about other options.

Condoms

Condoms are a barrier method of contraception, meaning they block sperm. They appear in Greek mythology in the story of King Minos (son of Zeus, and the king of Crete), who apparently ejaculated "serpents and scorpions," which sounds terribly painful for Minos and was apparently so potent that it killed several of his mistresses. The answer was an animal gallbladder or bladder that went in his wife's vagina or on the scorpion-spewing penis itself, depending on the version of the story.

Early condoms made of animal membranes seem to have emerged in the Middle Ages. Their exact origin is unknown, but they likely existed mostly for disease protection, probably against syphilis. As previously discussed, one of the first known clinical trials was conducted by Gabriele Falloppio in the 1500s, using linen sheaths on the penis to prevent syphilis. Sometime in the eighteenth century, condoms' value as contraceptives became appreciated. Eventually, rubber condoms became available, and then latex. Today, condoms can be external, to cover a penis, or internal, to be inserted into a vagina or rectum. External condoms are made of latex, polyurethane, or lamb intestine (often called sheepskin or lambskin); internal condoms are made of polyurethane.

The clear advantage of condoms is that they provide protection from many STIs as well as contraception. And they're used only on demand, so to speak, which appeals to some people. However, they aren't always on hand. With perfect use—meaning the condom is on the entire time during penetration—over a one-year period, 2 percent of people using external condoms will get pregnant. With typical use, the pregnancy rate for external condoms is much higher, 13 percent, and for internal condoms, it is 21 percent. It's also important to recognize that some people are afraid to ask their partners to wear a condom because of an implied threat of violence.

External condoms should be used with a lubricant, as they create more friction against the vaginal or rectal mucosa, increasing the risk of condom failure as well as causing discomfort. Oil-based lubricants can weaken latex, so that combination should be avoided, but water-based and silicone-based lubricants are fine. Polyurethane condoms have a slightly higher failure rate, primarily due to their fit not being as snug as it is with latex, given latex's ability to stretch. (There are countless videos online of people putting a latex condom over their arm or another item of ridiculous size to demonstrate the miracle of latex. No penis is too big.) Lambskin condoms are less effective for STIs, as viruses can pass through the lambskin; they also might not appeal to vegans or vegetarians.

With internal condoms, it takes about three tries to get comfortable with correct insertion. Trying it without the pressure of sex might be helpful. Internal condoms are more expensive than external ones.

As an aside, condoms are one of the greatest health interventions to protect the vaginal microbiome. Condom use is associated with a significant reduction in vaginal infections like bacterial vaginosis, in addition to their protection against STIs. Avoid condoms with spermicide, as they are impregnated with nonoxynol-9, which does not improve their effectiveness, shortens their shelf life, and paradoxically increases the risk of sexually transmitted disease if exposed, as it damages the vaginal microbiome. For info on lube selection for vaginal health, see my book *The Vagina Bible*, which has an entire chapter on the subject!

Diaphragms and Cervical Caps

These are also barrier methods of contraception. A diaphragm is a flexible, soft disc that sits in the vagina, and a cervical cap fits over the cervix (and looks a little like a hat). Diaphragms and cervical caps are meant to be used with spermicide, although how much it contributes to their contraceptive efficacy isn't known. Pregnancy rates with diaphragms and caps over a one-year period are about 6 percent with perfect use and 17 percent with typical use. Both a cervical cap and a diaphragm must be left in for at least six hours after sex so any viable sperm dies. (You don't want some rogue sperm making a dash for your uterus if the device is removed too soon.) A diaphragm can be left in for up to twenty-four hours, and a cervical cap for up to forty-eight hours, but always check the manufacturer's instructions, as with new data, recommendations may change. If you want to have sex again before removal, insert more spermicide. Always follow the manufacturer's instructions for use and cleaning.

Not everyone finds diaphragms and caps comfortable, and they can be associated with an increased risk of urinary tract infections. The upsides are that they are within your control, they are reusable, and you can put them in up to two hours before sex. There are four main options, as of 2023:

- *FemCap:* A cervical cap that comes in three sizes. It doesn't require fitting, and the website explains how to find the size that's best for you. A prescription is required.
- *Caya:* A diaphragm that's one-size-fits-most, so an exam isn't typically needed for fitting. If you feel like it's not in correctly, tell your medical provider so they can check. Caya has a unique shape that some people might find easier for insertion and removal.
- *Singa:* A diaphragm that comes in seven sizes and requires a prescription and a fitting by a medical provider. Singa is available in the United Kingdom, France, Germany, and several other countries but is not available in North America.
- *Milex Wide-Seal:* A diaphragm that comes in eight sizes and needs to be fitted by a medical practitioner. It's widely available in many countries.

A diaphragm is inserted by squeezing it together and pushing it, ideally, deep into the vagina, aiming for behind the cervix, then guiding it up behind the pubic bone, just like a menstrual disc (which, if you remember, was based on the design for a diaphragm; head back to page 172 to see the diagram for fit). It shouldn't fall out when you get up or be uncomfortable, and you should be able to empty your bladder. It's removed by hooking it with a finger and pulling; it collapses during removal. A cervical cap can be more mechanically challenging to fit, and some people with a long vagina and/or short fingers may not be able to make it work, because you must be able to touch your cervix. Cervical caps have a loop to grab for removal.

There are a few diaphragm and cervical cap don'ts: they can't be used within six weeks of delivery, miscarriage, or abortion, and they shouldn't be used by anyone with a history of toxic shock syndrome.

Spermicides and Contraceptive Gels

Spermicides can be directly toxic to sperm or can create an environment where sperm can't swim. They come in the form of vaginal gels, suppositories, and films. At one point there was a disposable vaginal sponge impregnated with spermicide (made infamous by an episode of *Seinfeld*), but it has since been discontinued because of its high failure rate and an association with toxic shock syndrome. Spermicides and contraceptive gels can be used alone or in conjunction with condoms or a diaphragm or cervical cap. In the United States, there are prescription and nonprescription products.

Nonoxynol-9, a spermicide many people are familiar with, is no longer recommended for people at risk of HIV exposure or with recurrent vaginal infections, as it can damage vaginal bacteria. The typical failure rate over one year is 21 percent. Other spermicidal gels are typically made of cellulose and lactic acid and don't harm the vaginal ecosystem. The cellulose provides a mechanical barrier (the sperm get stuck in the gel) and lactic acid helps keep the vagina acidic, which also damages sperm. Two brands are Contragel and Caya.

A prescription option is Phexxi, a vaginal acidifier that contains lactic acid, citric acid, and potassium bitartrate. It was initially developed as a lubricant but never went to market for that use. It is expensive—as of 2023 a box of twelve doses is approximately US$267.50. The company advertises a failure rate of around 13 percent, which sounds better than for other spermicides . . . except that it is 13 percent over seven months. Converting that rate to one year, assuming people will continue to get pregnant at the same rate, gives a pregnancy rate of 27 percent, according to both *The Medical Letter* and the MPR (Medical Professionals' Reference).

Fertility Awareness Methods

Fertility awareness methods (FAMs), formerly known as the rhythm method and sometimes called natural family planning, use biological variables to determine the "fertile window," meaning the days when intercourse could theoretically lead to conception. Sex is avoided during this time, or a backup method of contraception is used. There is a lot of misinformation online about these methods. The way some people promote them on social media makes it sound like FAMs are a contraceptive magic wand, and they are most definitely not. There is more effort involved than with any other method of contraception. That's okay for some but not for others, as with many things in life. Some people want to nourish their own sourdough starter, some people bake bread with yeast, and some just want to buy a loaf from the store.

It's not uncommon for me to be tagged in posts that simultaneously criticize hormonal contraception and promote FAMs, with a meme of a woman staring off into space and some version of "Mind blown wondering why women take a hormonal contraception pill daily, when they can only get pregnant one or two days each cycle." Sigh. It's hard to say whether this is willful ignorance or a tragic illustration of the lack of education about basic human biology. Although the lifespan of an egg after ovulation is twelve to twenty-four hours, sperm can live up to five days, so the fertile window is six days. This type of comment is a good example of why facts matter and how pervasive misinformation is with all forms of contraception.

To determine the fertile window, you need to track biological variables such as dates of menstruation, basal body temperature (temperature first thing in the morning), cervical mucus, position of the cervix, and levels of some hormones in the urine. App-based methods use one or more of these variables, combined with a computer algorithm, to decide the fertile window.

There are many different FAMs, and it's not possible to review them all here. Pregnancy rates are often reported as 24 percent, but that data is from older, calendar-based methods that likely came with little to no education. Some newer methods add extra checks for more protection. However, it's important to know that most of the studies looking at these methods are of mediocre quality. For this reason, even though the pregnancy rates in some studies are below 18 percent, the CDC still classifies FAMs in the higher-pregnancy-rate category.

The basic types of fertility awareness methods include:

- *Calendar tracking:* You track your cycle and avoid sex on fertile days, typically days 8 to 19. Some apps that use this method claim their computer algorithm improves the effectiveness, although, as discussed in Chapter 11, many get the fertile window wrong. Calendar-only methods are not appropriate for anyone with irregular cycles. The Standard Days Method is a calendar method and has a pregnancy rate of 11 to 14 percent.
- *Basal body temperature charting:* You track cycles with a calendar *and* measure your temperature first thing every morning. You can chart your cycle on your own or use an app, such as Natural Cycles. The app's algorithm is supposed to improve the effectiveness. With Natural Cycles, you also have the option of adding in urine testing to detect the rise in luteinizing hormone (the LH surge) twenty-four to forty-eight hours before ovulation. The pregnancy rate if you chart your cycle on your own is 9 to 10 percent; with Natural Cycles, it's 6.5 percent.
- *Cervical mucus testing:* You chart cervical mucus every day. Cervical mucus changes consistency during the menstrual cycle. It's minimal

during the first part of the follicular phase, but as estrogen levels rise, it becomes thicker and sticky, signaling that ovulation is approaching. When you observe a change in cervical mucus, you assume you are in the fertile window. With the two-day method, you check cervical mucus daily, then ask yourself two questions: Did I note cervical secretions today? and Did I note secretions yesterday? If the answer to either question is yes, you could get pregnant. There are a fair number of rules with cervical mucus methods. For example, with the Billings Method, during the first part of the cycle, right after menstruation ends, you can only have sex every other evening. Because the mucus is sampled at the vaginal opening, detection depends on your being up and moving for a few hours; if you have sex every day, leftover ejaculate can impede evaluation of your mucus. Vaginal infections and vaginal medications can also affect discharge and your ability to assess the mucus. One advantage of cervical mucus methods is that they can be used even with irregular cycles. The pregnancy rate is typically reported at 14 percent.

- *Symptothermal method:* You perform either a single check, using change in cervical mucus and temperature charting, or a double check, which includes cervical mucus, temperature, calendar tracking, and sometimes the position of the cervix. The pregnancy rate for the single-check method is 13 percent; for the double-check method Thyma, it's 11 to 33 percent; and for the double-check method Sensiplan, it's reported to be as low as 2 to 3 percent.

- *Hormone monitoring:* You monitor hormone levels in your urine and may also check cervical mucus and use calendar tracking. Hormone monitoring on its own has a pregnancy rate of 2 to 7 percent. The monitor-plus method, which includes checking cervical mucus, has a rate of 6 to 7 percent. The Marquette Method is one option for hormone monitoring.

You may be thinking, "Wow, pregnancy rates appear quite low with some FAMs," but unlike with hormonal contraceptives, failures aren't typically reported and tracked after the study ends, as they are with pharmaceuticals, and there are fewer studies to go by. Where studies do exist, the participants tend to have a high level of motivation that may not reflect that of the general population. In addition, people with irregular cycles may not be well represented, so the data may not apply to everyone. In 2018, the Swedish public broadcaster SVT reported that over a four-month period, 37 of 668 women who sought an abortion at one hospital had been using Natural Cycles for contraception. That doesn't mean the failure rate of Natural Cycles is higher or lower than reported, but it is certainly plausible that the general population may have higher pregnancy rates than what is published.

Valley Electronics, a company that makes a fertility tracker (thermometer, algorithm, and an app called Daysy), published flawed data about their product in a medical journal and, according to the Stanford Law Review (June 2023), used these findings to advertise 99.4% effectiveness at preventing pregnancy on social media, even though this product did not have FDA clearance to be marketed as a contraceptive. I say the data was flawed because Dr. Chelsea Polis, a reproductive health epidemiologist with expertise in calculation of contraception effectiveness, wrote about this serious issue, including publishing a commentary laying out the methodological concerns with their study. Her commentary led to the retraction of Valley's paper. Polis also filed an allegation of regulatory misconduct to the U.S. Food and Drug Administration (FDA), and the agency ultimately required the company to change their marketing language. What was Valley Electronics' response? First, they dismissed Dr. Polis (who had attempted to contact the company privately and directly with her concerns, before writing her commentary or taking any public-facing actions), and then when she spoke out publicly, they sued her. Fortunately, science prevailed, and the case was dismissed. This kind of legal action sends a chilling message to researchers, especially those who want to inform the public about their concerns. For this reason, I recommend against using Daysy.

With all these issues in mind, if you want to use a fertility awareness method associated with an app, as of 2023 there are two apps cleared by the FDA as medical devices: Natural Cycles and Clue. Natural Cycles reported to the FDA a 1.8 percent perfect-use failure rate and a 6.5 percent typical-use failure rate; Clue reported a 3 percent perfect-use failure rate and an 8 percent typical-use failure rate. Both apps use a proprietary algorithm based on menstrual cycle data and basal body temperature. With Natural Cycles, you can use an Oura Ring (a wearable biomonitoring ring) to measure basal body temperature, instead of an oral thermometer.

FAMs appeal to people for a variety of reasons. For example, some religions forbid using formal contraception, some people don't want to use pharmaceuticals, and some find the idea of being more intimately involved with their menstrual cycle appealing.

When thinking about whether a FAM is right for you, consider whether your cycle is regular, which can affect the effectiveness of some methods; which backup methods you can use if you do wish to have sex during the fertile window; and what biological variables you are willing and able to track. Remember, FAMs can be a lot of work.

There are two other considerations with FAMs. Some of the sites where people go to learn about them more have religious leanings and some provide incorrect information about menstrual cycles and hormonal contraception. What you read is often designed subtly or not so subtly to keep you on that method of FAM. Remember, fertility awareness methods that are based on apps, and websites that require registration or that have any cost associated with them, are not friends helping you to track your periods and get contraception, they are companies and should be scrutinized in the same way you scrutinize pharmaceutical companies. Please be wary of them as a source of health information. And as we discussed in Chapter 11, the data that the company receives about you could potentially have legal ramifications.

Bottom Line

- Anyone who is eighteen years or older who wants a surgical sterilization procedure should be able to have one.
- Condoms should be used with lubricant. Don't forget about internal condoms as an option.
- Spermicides have the highest failure rate of any form of contraception.
- There is a wide range of fertility awareness methods for contraception, and they vary in their effectiveness. Natural Cycles and Clue have been cleared by the FDA for this purpose.
- When choosing a method of contraception with a higher failure rate, such as condoms, diaphragms, and FAMs, consider how a pregnancy will impact you, including how you will access abortion if you choose to have one.

30

Contraception Potpourri

The case for contraception is clear. The ability to reliably prevent and plan pregnancies, if desired, is one of the greatest modern medical achievements, along with sanitation and vaccines. It allows women and trans men and non-binary people with a uterus to have sex for pleasure, unencumbered by the ramifications of pregnancy. The pill is responsible for incredible economic gains achieved by women since 1960. Reliable contraception helps people stay out of poverty and improves pregnancy outcomes through spacing of pregnancies or allowing time to improve medical health. Planning pregnancy also means people can take a supplement with folic acid before conception to lower the risk of neural tube defects, a serious type of birth defect. The risk of maternal mortality is always much greater than the risk of contraception, and if you live somewhere that abortion isn't readily available or is illegal, or you simply don't want to be faced with that decision, you are less likely to need an abortion if you have access to reliable contraception. Simply put, contraception serves the person who doesn't want to get pregnant, the person who does want to get pregnant, a potential fetus, and even society. It does not, however, serve those who seek to control people who can get pregnant.

As the previous chapters have discussed in detail, many methods of contraception also offer a myriad of health benefits, from controlling heavy periods to treating polycystic ovarian syndrome to preventing cancer.

What Is the Best Method of Contraception?

This is a common question, and in many ways it's like asking "What's the best meal for dinner?" It depends. How hungry are you? Do you have time to eat now, or can you wait? Do you want to cook or do takeout? Do you have special dietary needs? Vegan? Lactose intolerant? What foods do you like? Is it dinner for two or ten? And so on.

Just as there is no best dinner, there is no best contraception among the many options. Even for a given person, the "best" option may change over time. For me, over my reproductive years, there were four best options. When I was in my twenties and thirties, I needed to reduce heavy periods and cramps, so the contraceptive pill was optimal (hormonal IUDs weren't yet available). After my delivery, I chose a levonorgestrel IUD, but I was in the small subgroup who spotted all the time (like, all the time). That form of contraception was the best only until it was clear the bleeding wasn't going to stop. Then I switched to the copper IUD, and as this was at the same time as my menopause transition . . . well, I thought my periods in my teens were a crime scene, but these were a massacre. Since I didn't know whether the IUD was making it worse or it was just the menstrual mayhem of menopause, I had it pulled. Sadly, reader, it made no difference. But by then I had a new partner who'd had a vasectomy, so I was good to go. Four methods for four different times in my life.

Finding the right contraception is key, as almost 50 percent of pregnancies worldwide are unplanned, the result of either lack of access to contraception or contraception failure. In fact, 48 percent of people with an unplanned pregnancy were using contraception when they conceived, but they may have been unable to use the method correctly or consistently, and of course, all methods have an inherent failure rate. Those who wish to reduce the rate of abortion should expend their efforts on contraception, because abortion laws don't affect the rate.

When deciding on the best method of contraception for you, the first consideration is how important it is to not be pregnant. Some people never want to be pregnant, and others are okay with a contraceptive failure. If you were to get pregnant, would you want an abortion, and if so, do you live where accessing one is a possibility? Not being pregnant may also be crucial from a health perspective—either your own or the health of a potential child. For example, if you have a significant heart condition, pregnancy may carry greater risks. Or if you are taking isotretinoin for acne, avoiding pregnancy is very important, as that medication causes birth defects.

In the previous chapters, regarding failure rates I've discussed what happens in an ideal study setting and with typical use of contraception. It's important to remember that with studies there are usually nurses or research assistants who check up on use and/or provide reminders. People who enroll in studies often have a different motivation and may even be screened in advance to see if they can follow the requirements of the study. And participants are unlikely to run out of pills or condoms or be late getting a Depo-Provera shot. If we could replicate study conditions, we could reduce a lot of unplanned pregnancies. Meaning it's best to consider the typical use from a failure-rate perspective.

If you absolutely don't want to get pregnant, long-acting reversible contraception (IUDs and implants) and surgical sterilization have the lowest pregnancy rates. These methods are highly effective not only because they work so well, but also because there is no pill to forget or condom to break or prescription that can't be obtained.

Here are some other considerations when choosing a method of contraception:

- Do you have menstrual symptoms you'd like to control?
- Do you mind putting in some effort?
- Can you safely use estrogen?
- Can you tolerate irregular bleeding?
- Do you prefer a nonhormonal method?
- Are you looking for contraception that also reduces the risk of ovarian cancer and/or endometrial cancer?

The Origin of the Home Pregnancy Test

The ability to learn whether or not you are pregnant in the privacy of your own home has also contributed greatly to reproductive self-determination. The earlier you know you are pregnant, the earlier you can seek an abortion or prenatal care. Early pregnancy tests are an interesting side note that I am loath to leave out, so although they're not strictly contraception related, I am shoehorning them into this chapter in honor of the two women who made them possible.

It wasn't until 1928 that the hormone that is now the basis of all pregnancy tests, human chorionic gonadotropin (hCG), was identified. Initially, it was believed to come from the pituitary, but in the late 1930s, Dr. Georgeanna Jones proved it was produced by the placenta. Large amounts of hCG are found in the urine during pregnancy, so early tests involved injecting urine from women who thought they were pregnant into mice, toads, or rabbits. If there was hCG in the urine, it would cause the animal to ovulate—and the only way to know was to sacrifice the animal and look at the ovaries under the microscope. That is the basis for an old joke often made by women: when asked "How did your tests go?" the answer was "Well, the rabbit died." It's not accurate, medically speaking, as the rabbit always died, but I wonder if the dark humor was an acknowledgement of the hazards of an unplanned pregnancy in the era of clandestine abortions.

Other early pregnancy tests involved taking hormones (very similar to those in oral contraceptive pills) for several days and then stopping. If a person was pregnant, nothing would happen. If they weren't, they would bleed. This is an essential backstory, considering that some American politicians want to make hormonal contraception methods illegal under the guise that they work by being covert abortifacients. This early use of the hormones tells us they can't be.

Eventually, blood-based and urine-based tests that could identify hCG were introduced, sparing the lives of countless mice, toads, and rabbits. Initially, the tests were sent off to a lab, but then Margaret Crane, a twenty-six-year-old product designer at Organon Pharmaceuticals, had the idea to create a test that could be done at home. Her superiors balked; nevertheless, she persisted. Her test was quickly approved for home use in Canada, but approval in the United States took several years. Opponents feared that women were too emotionally fragile to find out they were pregnant without the guidance of a physician. My eyes did a 360-degree roll when I learned that nugget. I mean . . . too emotionally fragile to find out you are pregnant on your own, but not too emotionally fragile to *be* pregnant? Make it make sense.

The Business of Hating on Birth Control

It's important to acknowledge that, like many medications, hormonal contraception has very real side effects and some serious complications (discussed in previous chapters, and fortunately rare). Moreover, many women have had their side effects or concerns dismissed by the medical profession, and some have felt they had hormonal contraception "pushed" on them, but these are errors of medication counseling, not of the medications themselves.

Instead of helping to fill that gap, an active chorus of people who are against hormonal contraception spouts disinformation online, especially on Instagram and TikTok, driven by naturopaths, functional medicine doctors, medical malpractice lawyers, filmmakers, religious proselytizers, and a variety of health coaches and health-adjacent "professionals" (I'm not sure what to call a male influencer who worries about the size of women's taints, and yes, such a person exists). All appear to profit in one way or another from their fearmongering. You can't coach someone to a "better" period. In addition to encouraging people to waste money on untested and unregulated supplements, coaching services, and unnecessary tests, these disinformers create confusion and fear that can scare people away from options that may be a better choice, either for contraception or to treat medical conditions. There are more posts on the subject than one could read in one lifetime, but so far, I've yet to read one that presents the facts about hormonal contraception in an unbiased, ethical way. They also invariably cherry-pick information and misrepresent data and feature fear-inducing headlines.

Providing disinformation about contraception is not feminism; it is misogyny.

Most of these accounts default to a belief in the superiority of natural family planning or a copper IUD. But for many people, these are not acceptable or medically appropriate options. I think of my own situation: if I had not been on hormonal contraception, I couldn't have done a five-year OB/GYN residency, given my heavy periods and cramps. Without the pill, I'd have had to scrub out of some surgeries to change, or simply soak myself and try not to be distracted by the blood running down my leg.

Many people around the world struggle for access to contraception. According to the Global Burden of Disease study, more than 160 million women and adolescents need contraception but can't get it. We should not forget that access to contraception remains a privilege for many when it should be a right. This point is especially salient right now in the United States. It's imperative that people have access to several types of contraception so they can choose what is right for them. What may be a suitable choice for one person is entirely unsuitable for another, and a wholesale dismissal of hormonal contraception significantly narrows the availability of highly effective options.

It is true that inadequate counseling about contraception, especially hormonal contraception, is a major concern. It makes people feel dismissed or even coerced into therapy, and it can also lead to unplanned pregnancies when contraception is stopped because of side effects. Good counseling reduces concerns about side effects. If you know irregular bleeding is common in the first three months after starting a method, you can decide in advance if that is acceptable, and if it happens, you are generally less concerned. I often compare it to when a pilot warns about turbulence ahead of time, versus an unexpected mid-air jolt that leads me to spill Diet Coke all over my open laptop. When I'm warned about turbulence, I guzzle my beverage and close my laptop.

It's unacceptable for a doctor to listen to someone talk about their irregular periods and excess facial hair and simply say, "Here, take the pill"; instead, they should be listening to all of the patient's symptoms, explaining that they might have polycystic ovarian syndrome and what that is, and reviewing all the treatment options, which include estrogen-containing contraception for those who aren't trying to get pregnant. If you feel dismissed by a health care provider, find another one if you can.

It's also true that studies have failed for years to answer many questions and concerns about hormonal contraception. For example, quality studies about whether there might be a relationship between depression and contraception are relatively new. And while it's right to be angry about not having the needed data, the gaps in our knowledge don't mean hormonal contraception is bad. They simply prove that the systems that fund health research overwhelmingly ignore the needs of women, trans men, and nonbinary people.

Medicine is starting to do better. In the past twenty years, we have seen an explosion of quality studies on hormonal contraception, as well as on new methods. We now have contraception specialists, which we did not have thirty years ago. These doctors, who complete fellowships in complex family planning after residency, are driving contraception research to deliver better care and more precise medicine. Many questions are now being answered. Others will always be difficult to answer because we can't do randomized double-blind studies with hormonal contraception—it would be unethical to withhold contraception for a control group, to provide a less effective method, or to require that someone use a method that doesn't appeal to them.

Are We All in Big Pharma's Pocket?

While some doctors make money doing talks or consulting for Pharma, most don't. Doctors in the United States must disclose these connections, whereas there is no such requirement of naturopaths, chiropractors, nutritionists, and period coaches.

The reimbursement doctors get for contraception counseling is low compared to other things they could be doing, such as surgical sterilizations and procedures for managing irregular bleeding. Of course, many doctors are on salary, so they get paid the same regardless. But if a doctor who isn't on salary gives you the pill and your bleeding stops, there is no income for them from endometrial biopsies and ultrasounds or procedures to stop the bleeding. It's also more profitable to run a high-volume obstetric practice than to prescribe hormonal contraception. Basically, the pill is a money loser. The reimbursement for putting in an IUD is also quite low.

The fact that doctors are paid very little for contraception counseling and putting in IUDs is damning evidence of a system that doesn't value this vital practice or the people who need these services.

Do I Need Cervical Cancer Screening to Get the Pill?

For years contraception counseling was often contraception lecturing and shaming about sexual activity. In addition, many providers tied contraception prescriptions to annual Pap smears (which is how often we did them back in the day). No Pap, no pill! That's offensive and, quite frankly, stupid. Contraception and cervical cancer are unrelated, but by linking the two, doctors ensured they were paid for prescriptions instead of refilling them for free. There is a valid argument about what work doctors should and shouldn't be paid for, but refilling contraception is such a little thing, I personally feel it's just part of the gig and shouldn't require payment.

The patriarchy also thought women couldn't be trusted to come in for Pap smears (the implication being they're too stupid to understand the importance of cervical cancer screening), so the idea was to lasso them with contraception. If you deny someone contraception because they haven't had cervical cancer screening, how is an unplanned pregnancy going to help? Is the goal to "teach them a lesson"? If so, what is the lesson? That it's better to be pregnant and have cervical cancer than to just have cervical cancer?

No, you don't need cervical cancer screening to get contraception.

Can Some Medications Interfere with Hormonal Contraception?

Many people think that common antibiotics, such as penicillin or doxycycline, interfere with hormonal contraception, but they don't. However, there are medications that can increase the rate at which the hormones in hormonal contraceptives (except for Depo-Provera) are broken down by the body, effectively reducing hormone levels and potentially compromising their efficacy. These include certain medications for epilepsy, the antibiotic rifampin, some medications used as anesthesia, and the botanical St. John's wort.

Do I Need a Break from the Pill/Patch/Ring?

There's an old myth that people need to go off the pill for a cycle or longer to let their body "reset," but I've never heard it explained in any greater detail. At one point in time it may have been a strategy to deal with irregular bleeding on the pill, but it's not an effective approach if the long-term plan is to stay on the medication. There are only two reasons to stop oral contraception or any hormonal contraception: if the side effects aren't worth the benefit the product is giving you, or if you no longer want to be on contraception.

What about before surgery? It's true that major surgery can increase the risk of blood clots. With short surgeries, like surgical sterilization, there is generally no clotting concern. While there's currently no recommendation to stop estrogen-containing contraception before major surgery, it's worth discussing with your surgeon, because some people are at higher risk than others and risk also varies by surgery. In those situations, a medication to reduce the risk of clots might be considered, or stopping an ECC with enough lead time to have a benefit. It can take four to six weeks for the elevated blood clot risk from an ECC to resolve, so it would need to be stopped at least six weeks before surgery. For some, that could increase the risk of an unplanned pregnancy.

Are Synthetic Hormones Bad?

Synthetic does not mean a Frankenhormone; it's simply a chemistry term that means "not found in nature." And natural chemicals aren't necessarily safe. Botulinum toxin, one of the deadliest substances on earth, is natural. Lidocaine, the anesthetic we inject so you don't feel pain from a biopsy or dental work, is synthetic. Some natural hormones can cause cancer, and some synthetic hormones can prevent cancer. A chemical's risks and benefits are simply due to its properties, not whether it's synthetic or natural.

As discussed previously, the hormones in contraceptives are made from steroid-like compounds found in some yams and soybeans, by a process of semi-synthesis called the Marker degradation (yes, it does sound like the title of a *Big Bang Theory* episode). These hormones were originally chosen for the contraceptive pill because natural ones didn't work and the technology to make them work didn't exist at the time. But synthetic compounds offered other advantages over natural hormones. For example, progestins were chosen over progesterone because they were better absorbed from the gastrointestinal tract, didn't cause sedation, and had a more favorable bleeding profile.

Is the Pill a Group 1 Carcinogen, and Does It Cause Cancer?

Alarmist posts about cancer are the medical hydra of Instagram—knock one down and two more seem to take its place. Sometimes they're amped up a notch with a headline such as "The WHO classifies the pill as a Class 1 carcinogen."

Yes, estrogen can be carcinogenic. Perhaps the best example is endometrial cancer. Estrogen made by the body can cause endometrial cancer, but so can pharmaceutical estrogen. This is a property of all estrogens, not some dirty little secret. But it's not as if the World Health Organization can slap a black box on your ovaries, so of course their warning applies only to estrogens made in a lab. The WHO has a whole guide about who can or can't take hormonal contraception. Funnily enough, they don't have a similar guide for smoking. They obviously think hormonal contraception is fine, though; in fact, they list it as an essential medicine.

Estrogen signals cells to grow and divide. It's during cell division that DNA mutations can occur, and sometimes these mutations can be cancerous. Estrogen can also cause cancer by releasing certain molecules when it's broken down by the body for removal. Because we make a lot of estrogen over a life-time, the body has checks and balances. One is that the progesterone released after ovulation counteracts the effect of estrogen on the endometrium. Another is the BRCA1 gene, which codes for a protein that fixes DNA. People with a BRCA1 mutation don't make enough of the protein, which is why they have a higher risk of some cancers.

The risk of breast cancer is elevated by 8 to 24 percent with hormonal contraception, and while that may sound scary, the baseline rate for most women is very low; increasing a very low number even by 24 percent still gives you a very low number. Overall, if 7,690 women take the pill for one year, an additional one person will get invasive breast cancer. For women thirty-five years or younger, the risk is 1 in 50,000 women for each year on the pill. When women stop taking the pill after being on it for several years, there is conflicting data on whether the risk quickly returns to baseline or persists for several years before dropping back down. The birth control pill is believed to cause breast cancer by triggering a small, undetectable cancer to grow. Basically, estrogen or the progestin provides fertilizer for a cluster of abnormal cells that may or may not otherwise have grown into a cancer. That is why the rate drops when you stop taking the pill.

I want to highlight that this is likely the same mechanism by which pregnancy causes breast cancer. As with oral contraception, the risk is low—about a 5 percent increased risk—and it stays elevated for five years. You might have heard stories, especially now in the United States, about pregnant women with breast cancer who have their cancer care delayed because of draconian forced-birth laws. These are pregnancy-related breast cancers. The fact that pregnancy can cause breast cancer is always neglected by the anti-pill brigade. If their concern were really about breast cancer, they'd mention it. But they don't.

You may have heard that pregnancy reduces the risk of breast cancer. It does. So how is that possible? How can it both increase and decrease the risk? The increased risk is in the short term, meaning in the five years afterward. The decrease is in the long term, so twenty years after pregnancy, the risk of breast cancer is lower.

Another fact that the anti-pill advocates who profess to care for your health conveniently ignore is that hormonal contraception reduces the risk of endometrial and ovarian cancers. Considering that there is no screening test for ovarian cancer, this is a very important benefit.

Does Hormonal Contraception Cause Depression?

In the past ten years, quite a few studies have tried to assess whether there's a link between hormonal contraception and depression. Our ability to definitively answer this question is hampered by the fact that the research is typically done with large databases, meaning researchers look at groups of people—those who are taking hormonal contraception and those who aren't—and then try to ascertain if one group is more likely to be diagnosed with depression or to take medications for depression. However, with these studies, the subjects' reasons for starting a specific method of contraception aren't clear. Did they choose a hormonal method because they were hoping it would help their mood? Might people who choose hormonal contraception have a higher baseline risk of depression? Might they be more likely to be in a relationship with intimate partner violence, a risk factor for depression? Might they have polycystic ovarian syndrome, which is associated with a higher risk of depression?

Studies evaluating depression and hormonal contraception are inconsistent. It's possible that, for a small percentage of people, these medications could trigger depression, but the data is conflicting. For example, one study suggests that 1 in 200 people develop depression while on hormonal contraception, and the risk may be highest for teens, but another similar study does not show that effect. Interestingly, those who develop depression on the pill may then later be more likely to develop postpartum depression. This doesn't mean the pill causes postpartum depression, rather some people may have an underlying biological vulnerability to hormone transitions that is unmasked or revealed by hormonal contraception.

It is possible that hormonal contraception could trigger depression for a small percentage of people, but this needs to be balanced against the fact that some people find this medication beneficial for mood and other symptoms, such as heavy periods, painful periods, and menstrual diarrhea to name but a few. And of course, pregnancy is associated with postpartum depression, so preventing pregnancy or allowing people to time their pregnancy when they have optimized their health and have more support could be a net benefit for mental health for many. It's also important to remember that younger mothers are also at a higher risk for postpartum depression. These are all factors to consider in contraception counseling and in follow up.

What about people who feel unwell on hormonal contraception? Current studies may not capture symptoms that aren't severe enough to qualify for a diagnosis of depression. But any medication can affect how people feel. I like to think holistically here and ask people what else is going on in their life, because sometimes starting a new contraception is associated with other changes that might affect mood. At the end of the day, some people feel awful during pregnancy, some people feel amazing, and others feel no change at all. In the absence of conclusive data, it is logical to assume that the same could be true with hormonal medications.

Does the Pill Kill Libido?

Libido, a spontaneous desire for sex, is complex and related to many factors. Some people have a high libido; others have receptive desire, meaning it kicks in when sex is initiated by a trusted partner. It is not uncommon to experience both, not just over the course of a lifetime but over the course of a single relationship. It is also normal for desire to kick in after sexual arousal has started. Relationship status and concerns about pregnancy can affect desire, as can bleeding and medical conditions. I've spoken with patients who can't link a decrease in libido with any factor except starting the pill, and I've spoken with people who are on the pill because their partner of twenty years, with whom they have three children, is refusing to get a vasectomy, and now they find their interest in sex waning. Obviously, in the latter situation, there may be factors other than the pill to explore.

Some people do report a decrease in libido with hormonal contraception, but many others find that it improves libido, perhaps because their heavy periods or PMS is being treated, or because their fear of pregnancy is reduced. Or maybe even because of the hormones. Many factors play a role in sexuality. People are complicated, and reasons to start contraception are varied. Because of this complexity, studies have been unable to definitively link lower libido with oral contraception. Some people have suggested that the pill reduces libido by lowering androgens (due to estrogen's effect on sex hormone binding globulin), but we have good data that shows testosterone levels are not predictive of libido. On the other hand, side effects of hormonal contraception such as irregular bleeding and bloating do appear to decrease libido, and it does make sense that feeling unwell can reduce desire.

When it comes to libido, many people have significant misconceptions about what is normal or typical. There is a whole school of thought on how women's sexual desire is impacted by narrow gender roles for women, gender norms about initiating sex, and the presumption of a nurturing role for women, which often leads to an overlap between being a lover and being a mother. If you are worried about your libido, I recommend learning more about the subject, whether or not you decide to switch contraception methods. An excellent resource is *Better Sex Through Mindfulness,* by Dr. Lori Brotto.

Here are some options if you have libido-related concerns while on an estrogen-containing contraceptive pill:

- Switch to a pill with a lower dose of estrogen (a 10 or 20 µg pill).
- Try a pill with drospirenone as the progestin.
- Consider a pill with one of the newer estrogens.
- Try a transdermal method, such as the patch or ring.
- Switch to a progestin-only method.
- Consider a copper IUD.

Does the Pill Deplete Nutrients?

While it's true that hormones impact the gut microbiome, which could theoretically affect the absorption of some nutrients, there is no evidence to suggest that nutrient depletion is a concern with the pill. Given how high the doses of hormones were in the original pill, a negative impact on the microbiome should have been obvious. And we would almost certainly have seen worse outcomes among those who had recently taken the pill and were now pregnant, but we didn't.

Some low-quality data shows reduced folate levels for those on the pill, but it's unclear if this is a measurement artifact (meaning the hormones in the pill slightly affect the test) or a true phenomenon. Most of the literature suggests it's not a true finding. Regardless, complications of low folate, such as anemia, aren't linked with contraception, and taking the pill isn't a risk factor for a pregnancy with a neural tube defect (something associated with lower levels of folate), so if there are changes in folate, they are minimal and not medically significant.

There is data linking lower levels of vitamin B_{12} with the pill. However, the studies are conflicting and may simply represent shifts in vitamin B_{12} within the body due to the pill. People who get little to no vitamin B_{12} in their diet (meaning vegetarians or vegans) or who are at risk of vitamin B_{12} deficiency due to medical conditions may want to have their levels checked and consider a supplement. But they should do so whether they are on the pill or not.

Some data suggests that reduced levels of vitamin B_6 may be linked with the pill. Again, the results are mixed, and the studies are not great, but some have wondered if this could be a mechanism for pill-related mood changes, specifically depression. A few small studies have found that a vitamin B_6 supplement can help PMS. However, the pill also treats PMS. If the pill were depleting vitamin B_6, causing PMS, then it wouldn't be able to treat PMS. There's no harm in trying a vitamin B_6 supplement if you develop low mood on the pill, but again, the evidence that it will help isn't great.

Hormonal contraception reduces blood loss with menstruation, preventing iron loss and anemia, which can have serious health consequences. Preventing blood loss with the pill could even save someone from needing a hysterectomy. Higher levels of vitamin D are also seen with oral contraception. In addition, contraception of course prevents pregnancy, which is taxing on the body nutritionally. It's always a tell when the people who raise concerns about nutritional deficiencies related to the pill ignore the nutritional advantages.

Is There a Post–Birth Control Pill Syndrome?

There is no evidence that such a thing exists. It's not even possible to describe it, because it is not a medical condition or a defined syndrome. It appears to have been invented by naturopaths who conveniently sell supplements to treat it. I asked Dr. Lucky Sekhon, a board-certified reproductive endocrinologist, what she thought of the claims. After all, she sees many women who are hoping to get pregnant after recently stopping contraception, and she often puts people on the pill to time fertility protocol. She told me there "is no scientific evidence to support the idea that a 'post birth control' syndrome exists." Think about how high the doses of hormones were in the first pill. If post–birth control pill syndrome existed, it should have been far worse in the 1960s and 1970s, not something just appearing now, when doses are significantly lower.

Many women go on contraception for a health reason, perhaps PMS, PCOS, or painful periods. And those conditions can make them feel unwell. When they stop taking the pill, their original symptoms may well return. The pill wasn't masking those symptoms; it was treating them. People are sometimes on contraception for so long they may not remember what they felt like before they started. In addition, many young women start contraception before they are ovulating regularly—in other words, before primary dysmenorrhea, PMS, and symptoms related to PCOS emerge. Going on contraception doesn't prevent these issues, it just puts them on ice until ovulation restarts.

Birth control pills suppress ovulation, and this effect reverses as soon as they are stopped. The hormones are out of the blood within seven days at the latest. There is no delay in starting the next cycle, which is only further evidence of the pill's temporary effect. The concept of post–birth control pill syndrome is an extraordinary claim. Instead of publishing data investigating this brand-new syndrome so we can all learn about it, those who invented it spend most of their time selling supplements to treat it. Enough said.

Does the Pill Cause Polycystic Ovarian Syndrome?

No. We have excellent data showing that the estrogen-containing contraceptive pill is the most effective treatment for several symptoms of PCOS, and we know that PCOS existed for thousands of years before hormonal contraception was invented. Biologically, there is no mechanism by which contraception could cause PCOS. However, if someone starts estrogen-containing contraception when they are sixteen or seventeen, before they know they are going to develop PCOS, the ECC treats the symptoms of PCOS they would otherwise have experienced. When they decide to stop the ECC, the symptoms emerge.

In addition, many people gain weight over time—it is just part of being human. Although weight does not cause PCOS, it can make some symptoms worse. So after five or ten years on the pill, someone who gained weight while on it might have worse symptoms when they stop taking it than they did before they started.

Does Hormonal Contraception Affect Metabolism?

Hormones can affect different aspects of metabolism, but not in the way you might think. The most common impact is on lipid profiles, but the net effect depends upon the contraception's potency and estrogen/progestin doses, as well as on the route (oral, transdermal, or injection). For example, when estrogen is taken by mouth, it can decrease LDL (often called "bad cholesterol") and increase HDL ("good cholesterol"), but it can also increase triglycerides and total cholesterol, which are markers for heart disease. There is no specific recommendation for lipid screening before starting hormonal contraception, but it's recommended that all women have a lipid screening and cholesterol test at age twenty and then every four to five years. If changes over time raise concerns, then you might consider a different contraception. The ring appears to have the least impact of all the ECCs, and no impact is seen with the levonorgestrel IUD.

Several studies have evaluated the pill's impact on weight. The average weight gain is about 2 to 3 kg (4.5 to 6.5 pounds), but it's not necessarily hormone related. Researchers didn't just compare people who started the pill to those who didn't; they also compared people who started the pill to those who had a copper IUD inserted. This is important, because people choose contraception for a reason, and those reasons might be associated with other factors that affect weight gain. As it turns out, people who chose the copper IUD gained the same amount of weight as people who chose the pill. Weight gain from Depo-Provera is discussed in Chapter 24.

Hormonal contraception does not cause diabetes. According to the CDC's guidelines on contraception, among women with insulin-dependent or non-insulin-dependent diabetes, contraception with estrogen has "limited effect" on insulin requirements, and over the long term it does not impact control of diabetes or increase the risk of developing complications related to diabetes. People who have vascular disease or neuropathy related to their diabetes may not be candidates for an ECC, but they can absolutely use hormonal contraception without estrogen.

Does Hormonal Contraception Cause Hair Loss?

Androgens such as testosterone can cause hair loss, and estrogen can support hair growth and counteract the effect of testosterone. Some of the progestins in hormonal contraception can act like androgens on hair follicles, but thanks to the lower doses and types of progestins now used and the impact of estrogen, there is no good data showing a link between the estrogen-containing pill and hair loss. Progestin-only methods, like some IUDs, the implant, and Depo-Provera, can cause hair loss for some people, likely because of the androgenic effect of the progestins with no counteracting estrogen. The risk varies by the method: with the implant and the shot, it ranges from 1 to 10 percent; with the IUDs, it's 0.33 percent.

The estrogen-containing contraceptive pill is effective therapy for one kind of hair loss, androgenetic alopecia (AGA), which is related to increased androgens and commonly occurs with PCOS. Iron deficiency is another cause of hair loss, and because hormonal contraception reduces blood loss from menstruation, it raises iron levels.

A temporary hair loss that is linked with both estrogen-containing contraception and pregnancy is called telogen effluvium (TE). Hair goes through a cycle of being active and growing, called anagen, and then through a rest phase, called telogen. Hair falls out during telogen, the hair follicle rests, and then it wakes up and starts to grow again. Medications, pregnancy, and even stress can trigger more hairs than usual to go into telogen, meaning all the hair loss that might be expected over a few months happens all at once. As we typically lose fifty to a hundred hairs a day, this increased hair loss can be dramatic and distressing. People can lose up to 50 percent of their hair. TE may be particularly pronounced after someone stops taking an estrogen-containing pill, versus stopping other drugs, because estrogen triggers anagen. So when estrogen is taken away, more hair may be biologically ready to enter telogen. TE doesn't happen when a progestin-only method is stopped, which is further evidence that it's due to withdrawal of the growth-promoting effect of the estrogen. This isn't some kind of hormonal shock; it's like stopping fertilizer and letting the hair follicle finally go into its rest period. TE can be very distressing, but it's a hormonal phenomenon, not a pill-specific one.

If you have hair loss, see a dermatologist, not a gynecologist.

Does the Pill Alter Your Brain or Behavior?

Many experiences alter your brain. MRI scans show that contraception changes the brain in some ways, but so do pregnancy, breastfeeding, the menstrual cycle, nutrition, stress, and menopause. The question is, does hormonal contraception alter the brain in a concerning way? This topic is discussed frequently on social media and podcasts alike, leaving some women terrified. Experts who recently wrote on the subject for the journal *Nature Neuroscience* offered a striking reproof of those who fan the flames: "there is a fine line between empowerment through knowledge and power gained from the premature and inaccurate wielding of that knowledge (intentional or not) to potentially threaten access to hormonal contraception." Currently, there are no MRI or other neuroimaging studies that tell us hormonal contraception is harming the brain.

Research has looked at partner attractiveness on and off the pill, and the possible impact of stopping the pill on marital relationships. The hypothesis is that people look for different traits when they are fertile. But the studies yielded conflicting results from which no meaningful conclusions can be drawn. Interestingly, although there is a study showing that women's preferences for a masculine versus a less masculine face change from pregnancy to postpartum, I have yet to see a headline positing that women will leave their men because they no longer find them attractive postpartum. In contrast, the conflicting data on the pill has been spun into clickbait headlines that it leads people to choose the "wrong" partner. And then, apparently, they wake up one day after stopping the pill and decide they no longer find their partner attractive. I was discussing this with a friend who had never used hormonal contraception, and she laughed and said, "So what do I blame my divorce on?" I don't mean to make fun of the research, but humans are very complex, and drawing sweeping conclusions from the data isn't possible.

The pill treats painful periods and PMS—how might that affect partner choice versus not having them treated? Might partner choice be affected by an unplanned pregnancy, which increases the likelihood of poverty? The pill may factor into earning potential—how does a study account for that? As someone who met a partner while on the pill and left him after stopping it, I can confidently say my decision had nothing to do with no longer finding him attractive because I had stopped the pill. I stopped taking the pill because I was not going to be sexually active with someone I wanted to divorce. I made the decision to divorce, and then I stopped taking the pill.

We need more data on the effects of hormonal contraception on the brain. But in the meantime, we must not cherry-pick from inconclusive preliminary studies to guide medical care. The good news is that this is an active area of research, and I, for one, am excited to learn more.

Does Mirena Crash Syndrome Exist?

Mirena crash syndrome is purported to be a collection of varied symptoms caused by the "crash" when hormones are removed from circulation after an IUD is removed. The extensive list of symptoms includes acne, anxiety, breast pain and swelling, depression, fatigue, fertility issues, hair loss, headaches and migraines, lowered libido, mood swings, nausea, and weight gain.

It's always hard to explain something that doesn't exist in the medical literature but is surprisingly well described both on alternative medicine sites and by medical malpractice lawyers. I have removed plenty of IUDs and never once had anyone report these symptoms. Does that mean no one ever has them? No. But my unpublished anecdotal information is as medically valid as the proof that Mirena crash syndrome exists (spoiler alert: there is none).

Before going further, I want to emphasize that when people are having symptoms, the symptoms are real. I am not saying people aren't nauseated or aren't suffering from breast tenderness, just that the preponderance of evidence suggests that their symptoms are caused by other factors and not the removal of their IUD.

We can dismiss the claims of fertility issues, because ample data from multiple studies shows that fertility returns to normal within two cycles after a hormonal IUD is removed. Might some people who have an IUD removed find out they have infertility? Yes, but that would be because they already had infertility; they just didn't know it because they weren't trying to get pregnant. We also know that stopping a progestin isn't associated with hair loss.

Many of the side effects listed as part of Mirena crash syndrome are known side effects of levonorgestrel IUDs; not only is this awfully suspiscious, but it seems biologically implausible that they would get worse after removal. In addition, hormone levels are quite low with the levonorgestrel IUDs, so removing one simply cannot cause a "crash" in hormones. And finally, the hormones in the IUD don't interfere with ovulation. You can even take the hormones for in vitro fertilization and do an egg retrieval while you have a hormonal IUD!

Extraordinary claims require extraordinary evidence, and in the case of Mirena crash syndrome, that evidence simply doesn't exist. I'd encourage people to look for other causes for their symptoms and, of course, to pursue therapy for them.

Is the Movie *The Business of Birth Control* Worth Watching?

This movie, from Ricki Lake and Abby Epstein, is promoted as a documentary about the birth control pill, but it's anything but. The information is cherry picked and features some people who I don't consider to be experts in hormonal contraception, some of whom seem to profit from stoking fears about these products. An Instagram post supporting the movie made a claim about the pill inducing a "menopause-like state"—I'd be disappointed if a third-year medical student told me that. There are also some concerning conflicts of interest. For example, there is a masterclass associated with the film . . . for a price. I guess to become more uninformed about hormonal contraception.

And, as pointed out by *Rolling Stone* in their review, some of the companies promoted in the movie are also backers, "a relationship that's only revealed in the closing credits and separate promotional materials."

If that weren't enough, the movie was funded in part by Valley Electronics, the makers of the fertility awareness method Daysy, also featured in the film. It was Valley Electronics that sued a researcher who raised concerns about flaws in one of their studies. This really bothers me.

In my opinion, the movie is peak patriarchy disguised as a feminist venture.

Bottom Line

- When it comes to frightening information about the pill, always consider the source. Do they profit from it by selling supplements, coaching services, or an app?
- Pill panics are often the result of cherry-picked information or inconclusive data presented as gospel or as something "they" don't want you to know.
- There is no data to support the existence of post-birth control pill syndrome or Mirena crash syndrome. That doesn't mean people don't have symptoms, just that they are caused by something else.
- The pill doesn't wreck metabolism or cause diabetes, polycystic ovarian syndrome, or weight gain.
- There is conflicting data on whether hormonal contraception plays a role in depression, but it may be a factor for a minority of teens.

Final Thoughts

There are so many more things to learn and questions to answer, but eventually a book must end. My goal was to provide you with a solid background to help you better understand what is happening with your body and why. I find it unacceptable that people aren't given vital information about how the body works. With knowledge comes a better ability to advocate for the right medical care and to make the choices that work for you. Without knowledge, there can be no informed consent.

I worry that science is at an alarming inflection point. Misinformation and lies have gained a dangerous foothold, and distinguishing between science and pseudoscience is becoming harder and harder. There are many gaps in medicine that pseudoscience seeks to exploit, and both the traditional media and social media have played a big role. Look, when the press covers "health advice" from sites like GOOP, they legitimize them as sources of information. People are predisposed to conflate repetition and accuracy; this is called the illusory truth effect. It is believed to be related in part to processing fluency, which is the ease with which humans can digest a piece of information. If we have heard or read something before, it's easier to process when we are exposed to it again. Researchers have studied the illusory truth effect in five-year-olds, ten-year-olds, and adults, and they found the same results across all age groups. The illusory truth effect has the greatest impact over shorter periods of time, and social media have mastered short-term repetition with their 24/7 content and the algorithmic beast that feeds you what it has calculated you will consume, based on your history. Think about how social media content goes viral: you see something once, and if it hits, then it's everywhere.

(Hello, Sbagliato! If you know, you know.) But even when the misinformation is spaced out, it can have an effect.

Social cues can also make information more persuasive. For example, a source seen as credible (such as a medical professional or an influencer), or one who is attractive or powerful (celebrities, influencers, and politicians), can sway us more easily. When we see health care professionals or celebrities spreading incorrect information, the information is stickier. I'm reminded of a recent video clip with the actress Ricki Lake, one of the forces behind the infomercial *The Business of Birth Control*, opining about the birth control pill affecting pheromones, which she held up as a reason not to take them. I can see how someone might hear that and think, "Oh, maybe I should be concerned." Most of us have heard of pheromones, so it sounds truthy. Fear is planted that the birth control pill interferes with something natural, and the damage is done. Except, as we've already discussed, humans don't have a vomeronasal organ, the body part needed to detect pheromones. To someone like me, Lake's comment is akin to saying the birth control pill interferes with our ability to breathe underwater.

What's even more concerning is that the illusory truth effect works with blatantly false statements. While most people don't know the science behind the vomeronasal organ, they do know the earth is not a perfect square. And yet researchers got people to start giving credence to the square earth theory after five exposures. Basically, propaganda works.

So how can you protect yourself against the illusory truth effect? Fact-check. Every single time. Which is scary when you consider how social media algorithms work. Instead of watching and scrolling, you need to disengage and research. I understand that it's hard. I think misinformation creates a sort of health FOMO (fear of missing out), and people worry that if they don't keep following a celebrity or influencer, they may miss some vital information. The situation only worsens if you wade into the comments, where you find people replying, "I told you so!" or "That diet changed my life." Comment after comment repeats the misinformation as gospel. You might even start to think, "Hey, those people are just like me." Which makes you more vulnerable to the illusory truth effect. By then, the opportunity to fact-check has almost certainly passed.

Even if you say, "Okay, this is bullshit—there is no way I'm paying $69.99 a month for an untested supplement based on the color of my menstrual blood," or "I know the titanium dioxide in tampon strings isn't concerning," when you pause to read something or watch a few seconds of a video, whether to hate-watch or with genuine curiosity, Instagram or TikTok assumes you must like it, finds something similar, and then feeds that to you. Also, the more you watch a video, the more engagement it gets and the more likely the algorithm will boost that content, potentially spreading the contagion further.

Curate Your Social Media Feed

In surgery, we say the solution to pollution is dilution, referring to irrigating a wound to remove as many bacteria as possible. You can't take a hose to Instagram or TikTok (too bad, eh?), but you can limit your exposure. Be intentional about your use of social media, which I know is hard! I've been sucked into video after video before stopping to think, "Why *am* I watching stories about people who have been killed by sharks?" (That is one of my deepest fears, and somehow the algorithm knows.) Don't let the algorithm be the driver; be in charge. If you know information is false, block the account. Don't give them a second chance. Don't worry about FOMO. If they are spreading obvious misinformation—for example, that you should consider trying seed cycling—they are not worth following, no matter how amazing their makeup tips or yoga poses or novels or podcasts. If they cared about accuracy, they would have fact-checked with a reliable source. Remember, these influencers are looking for provocative posts that scare people, to boost views and likes and work the algorithm. That is why we see all those videos of men shouting about birth control pills damaging your brain (nope) or tampons causing menstrual blood to flow backward (sigh). When you block a post, you are telling the algorithm you want less of that type of content.

What if you aren't sure whether the content is false? Disengage and check. Hopefully this book will help, as will my Substack called *The Vajenda*, where I am continuing to add content that I regrettably couldn't include here because a book can only be so long. Good information can also be found at the American College of Obstetricians and Gynecologists (ACOG), the American Academy of Family Physicians (AAFP), the Society of Obstetricians and Gynaecologists of Canada (SOGC), the Endocrine Society, and the Royal College of Obstetricians and Gynaecologists (RCOG), for starters. Put your question into a search engine, then type the name of one of these organizations, and that will help the search engine bring quality information to the top. One thing the hormone scammers are experts at is manipulating the search engine, and often their content comes up first.

OB-GYNs to follow on social media are Dr. Karen Tang, Dr. Jennifer Lincoln, Dr. Heather Irobunda, Dr. Danielle Jones, Dr. Staci Tanouye, Dr. Lucky Sekhon (also a fertility expert), and Dr. Shannon Clark (also a specialist in high-risk pregnancy). I also follow Dr. Alyssa Olenick, PhD, who is an expert in exercise, metabolism, and female physiology. There are obviously many more, but following these experts can help elevate the medical content you see.

Anyone who recommends testing for MTHFR, a genetic variant, should be an automatic block. The MTHFR gene produces the enzyme methylenetetrahydrofolate reductase, and we inherit two MTHFR genes, one from each parent. There are two variations in the MTHFR gene that can result in reduced activity of the MTHFR enzyme, and an estimated 30 to 40 percent of people in the United States have at least one (the incidence varies a little depending on where you live). Having a MTHFR variant means nothing medically; real experts don't recommend testing. It's about as useful as testing to see if someone has brown eyes or blue eyes. But many naturopaths and functional providers do the test because it means they can sell unneeded supplements and diets to the 30 to 40 percent who test positive.

Naturopaths Are Not Hormone Experts

A stunning amount of misinformation comes from naturopaths, so let's discuss. I get a lot of pushback about this, but I think people deserve to know about the training of those who are passing along medical information or treating them. A naturopath goes to naturopathic school for four years. (By comparison, I did four years of medical school, a five-year residency, and then a year-long fellowship.) The four years of naturopathic school comes to, on average, 5,900 hours of training, and then they can practice independently (depending on the state or province; many don't recognize naturopathic training). Residencies are not required. Medical school is about 11,700 hours of training, but even after graduating we can't practice. A board-certified family physician in the United States or Canada (to whom naturopaths often compare themselves) must do a three-year residency after medical school to be able to practice independently. Before they can touch a patient without supervision, a family medicine doctor has spent about 21,000 hours in training. And the quality of the training is vastly different. I've read through one of the main naturopathic textbooks, and it is abysmal what passes for knowledge. For example, naturopaths are taught that homeopathy is real, but it's a scam. Of the training, Britt Hermes, a former naturopath, wrote: "The basic science courses taught in naturopathic schools are entry-level courses and not on-par with the rigorous science-based courses taught in medical schools."

Consider it another way. You can pick one of two pilots. One spent 21,000 hours at a nationally accredited flight school; the other spent 5,900 hours at a flight school with lower-quality education that allows them to fly planes in only some states and provinces, and they were taught that magic carpets can fly. Which pilot do you want flying your plane?

I understand that medicine has so many gaps they are really craters. People's health concerns are dismissed, we don't have adequate research in many areas, and people sometimes have symptoms we can't explain. But the answer isn't to capitalize on those gaps by selling supplements and incorrect narratives about evidence-based medical therapy, leaving people less informed about their bodies. The answer is to demand that medicine do better.

What About Supplements?

Here's a solid recommendation: don't take advice from health care providers or coaches who are selling supplements. When you sell a product, you have become part of Pharma. Imagine a new hormonal contraceptive pill with a brand-new estrogen called Estrawesome. We'll call the pill Contraceptique, and it's made by Ginorma Pharmaceuticals. Your doctor is a partner in Ginorma, carries Contraceptique in their office, and recommends it to you as the best option. You would probably quite rightly pause and think, "You are recommending this pill because you literally profit from it!" You would probably consider that practice unethical. Yet this happens all the time with a variety of providers. They sell or recommend supplements with names like "Birth Control Detox" or "Period Repair" and they profit from the sales. These supplements have never been appropriately studied, yet hypocritically, the people selling them often claim that medicine is profit driven.

Supplements are simply unregulated pharmaceuticals. Because no testing is required, the profit margins are massive. Many people who push supplements pass them off as "natural," but being found in nature doesn't make a product safe. I've seen people recommending one castor seed a month as a natural contraceptive, but castor seeds contain ricin, one of the most toxic substances we know of—deaths from ingesting just two seeds have been reported!

But aren't doctors paid for writing prescriptions? No, we're not. That is a lie perpetuated by those who want to denigrate evidence-based care. It is true that doctors can get paid to give talks about products and to give advice to pharmaceutical companies, and you should know whether your doctor does that, especially if they recommend specific medications. In the United States, you can research your doctor on at OpenPaymentsData.CMS.gov/search to see what money they have made from Pharma. But there is no database for naturopaths, chiropractors, or nutritionists, so you can't research how they're profiting from supplements.

Are All Supplements Bad?

According to the Food and Drug Administration, "supplements are intended to add to or supplement the diet" and should be considered drugs. Supplements can be extracts, like curcumin; the actual botanical or herb, like ginger; probiotics; vitamins, like vitamin B_6; or minerals, like calcium. They can be an individual ingredient, such as vitamin B_6, or they can contain multiple ingredients, like a multivitamin. It's helpful to think of supplements in three categories: single-ingredient supplements; regular multivitamins; and special blends like so-called period repair or liver shield supplements.

We have some good data on some single-ingredient supplements. For example, folic acid prevents neural tube defects during pregnancy, and iron treats iron-deficiency anemia. Multivitamins can be helpful for people who have difficulty absorbing nutrients (for example, after bariatric surgery), but otherwise, for people who are getting a nutritionally complete diet, multivitamins have not been shown to be beneficial.

In this book, I mention a few single-ingredient supplements, such as vitamin B_6 for premenstrual syndrome, making it clear that the data supporting their use is usually lower-quality. I have yet to recommend a special blend because these multi-ingredient supplements are rarely if ever tested in a meaningful way. If they were and they worked, we'd recommend them! And the fact that they aren't tested is concerning, because together, the ingredients could have a more detrimental effect than each one on its own. Supplements are a growing cause of liver failure. Many of the products contain "proprietary blends," and you literally have no idea what you are getting. The data is dismal, and often nonexistent, for multi-ingredient special blends, yet that important piece of information is typically lacking in the language used by those who recommend them.

The Myth of Ancient Wisdom

One myth that many people who spread disinformation tie into is the idea of secret female knowledge: that ancient women had great herbal lore that could cure everything and induce abortion. There are some serious flaws here. The first, which I have addressed a few times in the book, is that plucking an ancient recipe out of a time and/or culture where medicine and spirituality were almost certainly intertwined—and before key medical concepts, like germ theory and how we reproduce, had been determined—doesn't translate to treating conditions such as endometriosis or polycystic ovarian syndrome, diagnoses that did not exist in ancient times. If an herbalist of today recommends a recipe for an abortifacient from the Ancient Greeks, then they must also accept that the uterus wanders the body or that women have wetter flesh than men, because that recipe was created around those beliefs.

It's important to recognize that almost nothing written in ancient texts comes from women, so we know very little about what they thought. All we know is what men of the day claimed these women thought. We should also consider that any ancient therapies that actually worked as medicine have stuck around in one form or another: ginger is still used for nausea; willow bark, used for pain, became aspirin; and ergot became ergotamine, a drug still sometimes used today in obstetrics.

It's also crucial to be aware that offering a traditional practice may be cultural appropriation. There is a big difference between using a traditional healing method from your own culture within the context of that culture, which is something medicine should support, and the commodification of these practices as trendy or edgy or alternative therapies.

And So . . .

The menstrual cycle is a unique mechanism that supports humanity. It provides resource curation to ensure the healthiest pregnancy outcome, but at the expense of the person who menstruates. What's more, a patriarchal society punishes you for it, via employment discrimination, the cost of menstrual products, the inability to get contraception and abortion, the cost of medications, neglect from uncaring medical providers, and insufficient funding for research. And many people try to capitalize on these very real issues.

The best offense I can give you against these massive gaps is knowledge.

Acknowledgements

First, I want to acknowledge me. Women don't pat themselves on the back enough for a job well done, but we should. It was a lot of work to wrestle such a large topic into a cohesive structure and retain enough of the science without (hopefully) being a snoozefest. But it was important to me, because I see so many people who suffer from bad care or ineffective therapies or who spend thousands of dollars on useless tests and supplements, and I wonder, what if they had known what I know? Bad care and charlatans aside, shouldn't you know how your body works and your options when it isn't working how you wish it would? It shouldn't be such a mystery; after all, it's your body.

A big thank you to Amanda Betts, Denise Silvestro, and the amazing teams at Penguin Random House Canada and Kensington Publishing. You are all rock stars. Your questions, guidance, and patience were so important. Especially your patience. (Deadlines? What deadlines?) Thank you for helping me to deliver (ha ha) the best outcome. Thank you to Sue Sumeraj for her incredibly thorough copy edit. Shout-out to my superb publicists, Sharon Klein and Ann Pryor. And thank you to Clara Diaz and the amazing team at Little, Brown in the United Kingdom.

To my agent, Jill Marr, thank you for being a relentless cheerleader.

Thank you, Dr. Lucky Sekhon, for the fact-checking. And you are amazing; keep doing what you are doing. Thank you to Dr. Chelsea Polis, Dr. Alyssa Olenick, Dr. Kevin Folta, Kim Rosas, Dr. Alan Levinovitz, Dr. Mike Armour, and Damian Hall for answering my questions and being so generous with your time.

To everyone who asks me questions online, thank you! Really. I may not always reply, but I tuck it away for later. A lot of what you have asked over the years informed this book.

Oliver and Victor, my two boys . . . okay, you are men, but that sounds weird to me. I know I was busy writing. A lot. So thank you for rolling with the punches and keeping me honest, as only you two know how to do. I am so lucky to be your mom.

And finally, to the love of my life, Todd, for always believing in me, standing by my side, listening to me complain, and pushing me to be better. You are my sun, my moon, and my stars. I truly am the luckiest woman alive to have you in my life.

References

Introduction

Dunsworth HM, Warrener AG, Deacon T, et al. Metabolic hypothesis for human altriciality. *PNAS* 2012; 109 (38): 15212–216.

Ernster VL. Letter: "Menstrual toxin." *Lancet* 1974; 1 (7870): 1347.

Evans Reid H. The brass-ring sign. *Lancet* 1974; 303 (7864): 988.

National Institutes of Health. History of women's participation in clinical research. https://orwh.od.nih.gov/toolkit/recruitment/history. Accessed April 5, 2023.

Thurber C, Dugas LR, Ocobock C, et al. Extreme events reveal an alimentary limit on sustained maximal human energy expenditure. *Sci Adv* 2019; 5 (6): eaaw0341.

Chapter 1: Why Menstruation?

Brosens JJ, Parker MG, McIndoe A, et al. A role for menstruation in preconditioning the uterus for successful pregnancy. *Am J Obstet Gynecol* 2009; 200 (6): 615.e1–e6.

Catalini L, Fedder J. Characteristics of the endometrium in menstruating species: Lessons learned from the animal kingdom. *Biol Reprod* 2020; 102 (6): 1160–69.

Critchley HOD, Babayev E, Bulun SE. Menstruation: Science and society. *Am J Obstet Gynecol* 2020; 223 (5): 624–64.

Dean-Jones L. Menstrual bleeding according to the Hippocratics and Aristotle. *Trans Am Philol Assoc* 1989; 119: 177–92.

Diedrich K, Fauser BCJM, Devroey P, Griesinger G; Evian Annual Reproduction (EVAR) Workshop Group. The role of the endometrium and embryo in human implantation. *Human Reprod Update* 2007; 13 (4): 365–77.

Emera D, Romero R, Wagner G. The evolution of menstruation: A new model for genetic assimilation: Explaining molecular origins of maternal responses to fetal invasiveness. *Bioessays* 2012; 34 (1): 26–35.

Gellersen B, Brosens JJ. Cyclic decidualization of the human endometrium in reproductive health and failure. *Endocr Rev* 2014; 35 (6): 851–905.

Haeusler M, Grunstra NDS, Martin RD, et al. The obstetrical dilemma hypothesis: There's life in the old dog yet. *Biol Rev Camb Philos Soc* 2021; 96 (5): 2031–57.

Muter J, Brosens JJ. Decidua. In MK Skinner, ed. *Encyclopedia of Reproduction*, vol. 2, 2nd ed. Cambridge, MA: Academic Press; 2018: 424–30.

Schatz F, Guzeloglu-Kayisli O, Earlier S, et al. The role of decidual cells in uterine hemostasis, menstruation, inflammation, adverse pregnancy outcomes and abnormal uterine bleeding. *Hum Reprod Update* 2016; 22 (4): 497–515.

Thomas VG. The link between human menstruation and placental delivery: A novel evolutionary interpretation: Menstruation and fetal placental detachment share common evolved physiological processes dependent on progesterone withdrawal. *BioEssays* 2019; 41 (6): e1800232.

Top euphemisms for "period" by language. Clue, March 10, 2016. https://helloclue.com /articles/culture/top-euphemisms-for-period-by-language. Accessed April 5, 2023.

Chapter 2: Menstrual Cycle 101

American College of Obstetricians and Gynecologists. ACOG committee opinion no. 651: Menstruation in girls and adolescents: Using the menstrual cycle as a vital sign. *Obstet Gynecol* 2015; 126 (6): e143–46.

American College of Obstetricians and Gynecologists. Committee opinion no. 700: Methods for estimating the due date. *Obstet Gynecol* 2017; 129 (5): e150–54.

Bull JR, Rowland SP, Berglund Scherwitzl E, et al. Real-world menstrual cycle characteristics of more than 600,000 menstrual cycles. *NPJ Digit Med* 2019; 2: 83.

Dean-Jones L. Menstrual bleeding according to the Hippocratics and Aristotle. *Trans Am Philol Assoc* 1989; 119: 177–92.

Ecochard R, Gougeon A. Side of ovulation and cycle characteristics in normally fertile women. *Hum Reprod* 2000; 15 (4): 752–55.

Hampson E. A brief guide to the menstrual cycle and oral contraceptive use for researchers in behavioral endocrinology. *Horm Behav* 2020; 119: 104655.

Herbison AE. The gonadotropin-releasing hormone pulse generator. *Endocrinology* 2018; 159 (11): 3723–36.

Lessey BA, Young SL. Chapter 9: Structure, function, and evaluation of the female reproductive tract. In JF Strauss III, RL Barbieri, eds. *Yen & Jaffe's Reproductive Endocrinology: Physiology, Pathophysiology, and Clinical Management*, 8th ed. Philadelphia: Elsevier; 2019: 206–47.

Lew R. Natural history of ovarian function including assessment of ovarian reserve and premature ovarian failure. *Best Pract Res Clin Obstet Gynaecol* 2019; 55: 2–13.

McGee EA, Hsueh AJW. Initial and cyclic recruitment of ovarian follicles. *Endocr Rev* 2000; 21 (2): 200–214.

Mihm M, Gangooly S, Muttukrishna S. The normal menstrual cycle in women. *Anim Reprod Sci* 2011; 124 (3–4): 229–36.

O'Herlihy C, Robinson HP, de Crespigny LJ. Mittelschmerz is a preovulatory symptom. *Br Med J* 1980; 280 (6219): 986.

Ross JA, Davison AZ, Sana Y, et al. Ovum transmigration after salpingectomy for ectopic pregnancy. *Hum Reprod* 2013; 28 (4): 937–41.

Sharpe J. *The Midwives Book*, 1671.

Strauss JF, Williams CJ. Chapter 8: Ovarian life cycle. In JF Strauss III, RL Barbieri, eds. *Yen & Jaffe's Reproductive Endocrinology: Physiology, Pathophysiology, and Clinical Management*, 8th ed. Philadelphia: Elsevier; 2019: 167–205.

Treloar AE, Boynton RE, Behn BG, Brown BW. Variation of the human menstrual cycle through reproductive life. *Int J Fertil* 1967; 12 (1 Pt 2): 77–126.

Vanden Brink H, Chizen D, Hale G, Baerwald A. Age-related changes in major ovarian follicular wave dynamics during the human menstrual cycle. *Menopause* 2013; 20 (12): 1243–54.

Ziel HK, Paulson RJ. Contralateral corpus luteum in ectopic pregnancy: What does it tell us about ovum pickup? *Fertil Steril* 2002; 77 (4): 850–51.

Chapter 3: The Brain-Brain-Ovary Connection

Barbieri RL. Chapter 10: Breast. In JF Strauss III, RL Barbieri, eds. *Yen & Jaffe's Reproductive Endocrinology: Physiology, Pathophysiology, and Clinical Management*, 8th ed. Philadelphia: Elsevier; 2019: 248–55.

COVID-19 vaccines and menstrual cycles. Apple Women's Health Study. https://www .hsph.harvard.edu/applewomenshealthstudy/updates/covid-19-vaccines-and -menstrual-cycles/. Accessed April 6, 2023.

Edelman A, Boniface ER, Benhar E, et al. Association between menstrual cycle length and coronavirus disease 2019 (COVID-19) vaccination. A U.S. cohort. *Obstet Gynecol* 2022; 139 (4): 481–89.

Edelman A, Boniface ER, Male V, et al. Association between menstrual cycle length and covid-19 vaccination: Global, retrospective cohort study of prospectively collected data. *BMJ Med* 2022; 1 (1): e000297.

Gunter J. Heavy menstrual bleeding and COVID-19 vaccines. *The Vajenda*, October 30, 2022. https://vajenda.substack.com/p/heavy-menstrual-bleeding-and-covid. Accessed April 6, 2023

Herbison AE. The gonadotropin-releasing hormone pulse generator. *Endocrinology* 2018; 159 (11): 3723–36

Kennedy KI, Goldsmith C. Chapter 17: Contraception after pregnancy. In RA Hatcher, AL Nelson, J Trussell, et al, eds. *Contraceptive Technology*, 21st ed. New York: Ayer; 2018: 511–42.

McCartney CR, Marshall JC. Chapter 1: Neuroendocrinology of reproduction. In JF Strauss III, RL Barbieri, eds. *Yen & Jaffe's Reproductive Endocrinology: Physiology, Pathophysiology, and Clinical Management*, 8th ed. Philadelphia: Elsevier; 2019: 1–24.

Mihm M, Gangooly S, Muttukrishna S. The normal menstrual cycle in women. *Anim Reprod Sci* 2011; 124 (3–4): 229–36.

Moravek MB, Kinnear HM, George J, et al. Impact of exogenous testosterone on reproduction in transgender men. *Endocrinology* 2020; 161 (3): bqaa014.

Narayan P, Ulloa-Aguirre A, Dias JA. Chapter 2: Gonadotropin hormones and their receptors. In JF Strauss III, RL Barbieri, eds. *Yen & Jaffe's Reproductive Endocrinology: Physiology, Pathophysiology, and Clinical Management*, 8th ed. Philadelphia: Elsevier; 2019: 25–57.

Suzuki S, Hosono A. No association between HPV vaccine and reported post-vaccination symptoms in Japanese young women: Results of the Nagoya study. *Papillomavirus Res* 2018; 5: 96–103.

Taub RL, Ellis SA, Neal-Perry G, et al. The effect of testosterone on ovulatory function in transmasculine individuals. *Am J Obstet Gynecol* 2020; 223 (3): 229.e1–e8.

Thurber C, Dugas LR, Ocobock C, at al. Extreme events reveal an alimentary limit on sustained maximal human energy expenditure. *Sci Adv* 2019; 5 (6): eaaw0341.

Chapter 4: The Basics of Bleeding

Bremmer RH, de Bruin DM, de Joode M, et al. Biphasic oxidation of oxy-hemoglobin in bloodstains. *PLoS ONE* 2011; 6 (7): e21845.

Critchley HOD, Babayev E, Bulun SE. Menstruation: Science and society. *Am J Obstet Gynecol* 2020; 223 (5): 624–64.

Kuijsters NPM, Methorst WG, Kortenhorst MSQ, et al. Uterine peristalsis and fertility: Current knowledge and future perspectives: A review and meta-analysis. *Reprod Biomed Online* 2017; 35 (1): 50–71.

Lessey BA, Young SL. Chapter 9: Structure, function, and evaluation of the female reproductive tract. In JF Strauss III, RL Barbieri, eds. *Yen & Jaffe's Reproductive Endocrinology: Physiology, Pathophysiology, and Clinical Management*, 8th ed. Philadelphia: Elsevier; 2019: 206–47.

Magnay JL, Nevatte TM, Dhingra V, O'Brien S. Menstrual blood loss measurement: Validation of the alkaline hematin technique for feminine hygiene products containing superabsorbent polymers. *Fertil Steril* 2010; 94 (7): 2742–46.

Magnay JL, O'Brien S, Gerlinger C, Seitz C. Pictorial methods to assess heavy menstrual bleeding in research and clinical practice: A systematic literature review. *BMC Women's Health* 2022; 20 (1): 24.

Maybin JA, Critchley HOD. Menstrual physiology: Implications for endometrial pathology and beyond. *Hem Reprod Update* 2015; 21 (6): 748–61.

McGann JP. Poor human olfaction is a 19th-century myth. *Science* 2017; 356 (6338): eaam7263.

Mihm M, Gangooly S, Muttukrishna S. The normal menstrual cycle in women. *Anim Reprod Sci* 2011; 124 (3–4): 229–36.

Porter MB, Goldstein S. Chapter 35: Pelvic imaging in reproductive endocrinology. In JF Strauss III, RL Barbieri, eds. *Yen & Jaffe's Reproductive Endocrinology: Physiology, Pathophysiology, and Clinical Management*, 8th ed. Philadelphia: Elsevier; 2019: 916–61.

Varsha J, Chodankar RR, Maybin JA, Critchley HOD. Uterine bleeding: How under-standing endometrial physiology underpins menstrual health. *Nat Rev Endocrinol* 2022; 18 (5): 290–308.

Warner PE, Critchley HOD, Lumsden MA, et al. Menorrhagia I: Measured blood loss, clinical features, and outcome in women with heavy periods: A survey with follow-up data. *Am J Obstet Gynecol* 2004; 190 (5): 1216–23.

Chapter 5: Reproductive Hormones: A Handbook

American College of Obstetricians and Gynecologists. ACOG committee opinion no. 773: The use of antimüllerian hormone in women not seeking fertility care. *Obstet Gynecol* 2019; 133 (4): 840–41.

Christenson LK, Devoto L. Cholesterol transport and steroidogenesis by the corpus luteum. *Reprod Biol Endocrinol* 2003; 1: 90.

Dawood MY. Primary dysmenorrhea: Advances in pathogenesis and management. *Obstet Gynecol* 2006; 108 (2): 428–41.

Goldin BR, Adlercreutz H, Gorbach SL, et al. Estrogen excretion patterns and plasma levels in vegetarian and omnivorous women. *N Engl J Med* 1982; 307 (25): 1542–47.

Gruber CJ, Tschugguel W, Schneeberger C, Huber JC. Production and actions of estrogens. *N Eng J Med* 2002; 346 (5): 340–52.

Gunter J. MTHFR testing and estrogen. *The Vajenda*, March 21, 2021. https://vajenda. substack.com/p/mthfr-testing-and-estrogen. Accessed April 7, 2023.

Hickey SE, Curry CJ, Toriello HV. ACMG Practice Guideline: Lack of evidence for MTHFR polymorphism testing. *Genet Med* 2013; 15 (2): 153–56.

Matyas RA, Mumford SL, Sliep KC, et al. Effects of over-the-counter analgesic use on reproductive hormones and ovulation in healthy, premenopausal women. *Hum Reprod* 2015; 30 (7): 1714–23.

McCartney CR, Marshall JC. Chapter 1: Neuroendocrinology of reproduction. In JF Strauss III, RL Barbieri, eds. *Yen & Jaffe's Reproductive Endocrinology: Physiology, Pathophysiology, and Clinical Management*, 8th ed. Philadelphia: Elsevier; 2019: 1–24.

National Academies of Sciences, Engineering, and Medicine. *The Clinical Utility of Compounded Bioidentical Hormone Therapy: A Review of Safety, Effectiveness, and Use.* Washington, DC: National Academies Press; 2020.

Santen RJ, Simpson E. History of estrogen: Its purification, structure, synthesis, biologic actions, and clinical implications. *Endocrinology* 2019; 160 (3): 605–25.

Stefanick ML. Estrogens and progestins: Background and history, trends in use, and guidelines and regimens approved by the US Food and Drug Administration. *Am J Med* 2005 (Suppl 12B); 118: 64–73.

Strauss JF, FitzGerald JA. Chapter 4: Steroid hormones and other lipid molecules involved in human reproduction. In JF Strauss III, RL Barbieri, eds. *Yen & Jaffe's Reproductive Endocrinology: Physiology, Pathophysiology, and Clinical Management*, 8th ed. Philadelphia: Elsevier; 2019: 75–114.

Stuenkel CA, Gompel A. Primary ovarian insufficiency. *N Eng J Med* 2023; 388 (2): 154–63.

Synthetic. *Cambridge Dictionary*. https://dictionary.cambridge.org/us/dictionary/ english/synthetic. Accessed April 7, 2023.

Tsuchiya Y, Nakajima M, Yokoi T. Cytochrome P450-mediated metabolism of estrogens and its regulation in human. *Cancer Lett* 2005; 227 (2): 115–24.

Udoff LC. Overview of androgen deficiency and therapy in women. UpToDate. https://www.uptodate.com/contents/overview-of-androgen-deficiency-and -therapy-in-women. Accessed February 4, 2023.

Chapter 6: Menarche: Journey to the First Period

den Tonkelaar I, Oddens BJ. Preferred frequency and characteristics of menstrual bleeding in relation to reproductive status, oral contraceptive use, and hormone replacement therapy use. *Contraception* 1999; 59 (6): 357–62.

De Silva, NK. Abnormal uterine bleeding in adolescents: Evaluation and approach to diagnosis. UpToDate. https://www.uptodate.com/contents/abnormal-uterine -bleeding-in-adolescents-evaluation-and-approach-to-diagnosis. Accessed February 3, 2023.

Fitzpatrick KH. Foraging and menstruation in the Hadza of Tanzania. PhD dissertation, University of Cambridge, 2018.

Greenspan LC, Lee MM. Endocrine disruptors and pubertal timing. *Curr Opin Endocrinol Diabetes Obes* 2018; 25 (1): 49–54.

Lin PC, Bhatnagar KP, Nettleton GS, Nakajima ST. Female genital tract anomalies affecting reproduction. *Fertil Steril* 2002; 78 (5): 899–915.

National Research Council (US) and Institute of Medicine (US) Forum on Adolescence; Kipke MD, ed. *Adolescent Development and the Biology of Puberty: Summary of a Workshop on New Research*. Washington, DC: National Academies Press; 1999.

Robboy SJ, Kurita T, Baskin L, Cunha GR. New insights into human female reproductive tract development. *Differentiation* 2017; 97: 9–22.

Strauss JF, Williams CJ. Chapter 8: Ovarian life cycle. In JF Strauss III, RL Barbieri, eds. *Yen & Jaffe's Reproductive Endocrinology: Physiology, Pathophysiology, and Clinical Management*, 8th ed. Philadelphia: Elsevier; 2019: 167–205.

Warholm L, Petersen KR, Ravn P. Combined oral contraceptives' influence on weight, body composition, height, and bone mineral density in girls younger than 18 years: A systematic review. *Eur J Contracept Reprod Health Care* 2012; 17 (4): 245–53

Witchel SF, Topaloglu AK. Chapter 17: Puberty: Gonadarche and adrenarche. In JF Strauss III, RL Barbieri, eds. *Yen & Jaffe's Reproductive Endocrinology: Physiology, Pathophysiology, and Clinical Management*, 8th ed. Philadelphia: Elsevier; 2019: 394–446.

Yoshihara M, Wagner M, Damdimopoulos A, et al. The continued absence of functional germline stem cells in adult ovaries. *Stem Cells* 2023; 41 (2): 105–10.

Chapter 7: Menopause: The Afterparty

American College of Obstetricians and Gynecologists. ACOG committee opinion no. 773: The use of antimüllerian hormone in women not seeking fertility care. *Obstet Gynecol* 2019; 133 (4): 840–41.

Burger HG, Hale GE, Dennerstein L, Robertson DM. Cycle and hormone changes during perimenopause: The key role of ovarian function. *Menopause* 2008; 15 (4 Pt 1): 603–12.

Crandall CJ, ed. *Menopause Practice: A Clinician's Guide*, 6th ed. Pepper Pike, OH: North American Menopause Society; 2019.

Croft DP, Johnstone RA, Ellis S, et al. Reproductive conflict and the evolution of menopause in killer whales. *Curr Biol* 2017; 27 (2): 298–304

El Khoudary SR, Greendale G, Crawford SL, et al. The menopause transition and women's health at midlife: A progress report from the Study of Women's Health Across the Nation (SWAN). *Menopause* 2019; 26 (10): 1213–27.

Gurven MD, Gomes CM. Mortality, senescence, and life span. In MN Muller, RW Wrangham, DR Pilbeam, eds. *Chimpanzees and Human Evolution*. Cambridge, MA: Belknap Press of Harvard University Press; 2017: 181–216.

Hale GE, Hughes CL, Burger HG, et al. Atypical estradiol secretion and ovulation patterns caused by luteal out-of-phase (LOOP) events underlying irregular ovulatory menstrual cycles in the menopause transition. *Menopause* 2009; 16 (1): 50–59.

Harlow SD, Gass M, Hall JE, et al. Executive summary of the Stages of Reproductive Aging Workshop + 10: Addressing the unfinished agenda of staging reproductive aging. *Menopause* 2012; 19 (4): 387–95.

Hawkes K, O'Connell JF, Blurton Jones NG. Hadza women's time allocation, offspring provisioning, and the evolution of long postmenopausal life spans. *Curr Anthropol* 1997; 38 (4): 551–77.

Lobo RA. Chapter 14: Menopause and aging. In JF Strauss III, RL Barbieri, eds. *Yen & Jaffe's Reproductive Endocrinology: Physiology, Pathophysiology, and Clinical Management*, 8th ed. Philadelphia: Elsevier; 2019: 322–56.

Shanley DP, Kirkwood TB. Evolution of the human menopause. *BioEssays* 2001; 23 (3): 282–87.

Tepper PG, Randolph Jr JF, McConnell DS, et al. Trajectory clustering of estradiol and follicle-stimulating hormone during the menopausal transition among women in the Study of Women's Health across the Nation (SWAN). *J Clin Endocrinol Metab* 2012; 97 (8): 2872–80.

Thompson ME. Comparative reproductive energetics of human and nonhuman primates. *Annu Rev Anthropol* 2013; 42 (1): 287–304.

Vanden Brink H, Chizen D, Hale G, Baerwald A. Age-related changes in major ovarian follicular wave dynamics during the human menstrual cycle. *Menopause* 2013; 20 (12): 1243–54.

Chapter 8: The Pelvic Exam

Ameer MA, Fagan SE, Sosa-Stanley JN, et al. Anatomy, abdomen and pelvis: Uterus. *StatPearls*, updated December 6, 2022. https://www.ncbi.nlm.nih.gov/books/NBK470297/. Accessed April 8, 2023.

American College of Obstetricians and Gynecologists. Committee opinion no. 754: The utility of and indications for routine pelvic examination. *Obstet Gynecol* 2018; 132 (4): e174–80.

American College of Obstetricians and Gynecologists. Updated cervical cancer screening guidelines. Practice Advisory, 2021. https://www.acog.org/clinical/clinical-guidance/practice-advisory/articles/2021/04/updated-cervical-cancer-screening-guidelines. Accessed April 8, 2023.

Ferry G. Marie Boivin: From midwife to gynaecologist. *Lancet* 2019; 393 (10187): 2192–93.

O'Laughlin DJ, Strelow B, Fellows N, et al. Addressing anxiety and fear during the female pelvic examination. *J Prim Care Community Health* 2021; 12.

Schiffman M, Doorbar J, Wentzensen N, et al. Carcinogenic human papillomavirus infection. *Nat Rev Dis Primers* 2016; 2.

US Preventive Services Task Force; Bibbins-Domingo K, Grossman DC, Curry SJ, et al. Screening for gynecologic conditions with pelvic examination: US Preventive Services Task Force recommendation statement. *JAMA* 2017; 317 (9): 947–53.

US Preventive Services Task Force; Davidson KW, Barry MJ, Mangione CM, et al. Screening for chlamydia and gonorrhea: US Preventive Services Task Force recommendation statement. *JAMA* 2021; 326 (10): 949–56.

Well-woman annual health assessment. In *Guidelines for Women's Health Care: A Resource Manual*, 4th ed. Washington, DC: American College of Obstetricians and Gynecologists; 2014: 217–32.

WHO Guideline for Screening and Treatment of Cervical Pre-cancer Lesions for Cervical Cancer Prevention, 2nd ed. Geneva: World Health Organization; 2021. License: CC BY-NC-SA 3.0 IGO.

Williams AA, Williams M. A guide to performing pelvic speculum exams: A patient-centered approach to reducing iatrogenic effects. *Teach Learn Med* 2013; 25 (4): 383–91.

Wong K, Lawton V. The vaginal speculum: A review of literature focusing on specula redesigns and improvements to the pelvic exam. *Columbia Undergraduate Research Journal* 2021; 5 (1).

Wright D, Fenwick J, Stephenson P, Monterosso N. Speculum "self-insertion": A pilot study. *J Clin Nurs* 2005: 14 (9): 1098–111.

Chapter 9: Premenstrual Symptoms: PMS, PMDD, and Breast Pain

Appleton SM. Premenstrual syndrome: Evidence-based evaluation and treatment. *Clin Obstet Gynecol* 2018; 61 (1): 52–61.

Barbieri RL. Chapter 10: Breast. In JF Strauss III, RL Barbieri, eds. *Yen & Jaffe's Reproductive Endocrinology: Physiology, Pathophysiology, and Clinical Management*, 8th ed. Philadelphia: Elsevier; 2019: 248–55.

Hofmeister S, Bodden S. Premenstrual syndrome and premenstrual dysphoric disorder. *Am Fam Physician* 2016; 94 (3): 236–40.

Osborn E, Wittkowski A, Brooks J, et al. Women's experiences of receiving a diagnosis of premenstrual dysphoric disorder: A qualitative investigation. *BMC Women's Health* 2020; 20 (1): 242.

Richardson JT. The premenstrual syndrome: A brief history. *Soc Sci Med* 1995; 41 (6): 761–67.

Srivastava A, Mansel RE, Arvind N, et al. Evidence-based management of mastalgia: A meta-analysis of randomised trials. *Breast* 2007; 16 (5): 503–12.

Verkaik S, Kamperman AM, van Westrhenen R, Schulte PFJ. The treatment of premenstrual syndrome with preparations of *Vitex agnus castus*: A systematic review and meta-analysis. *Am J Obstet Gynecol* 2017; 217 (2): 150–66.

Yonkers KA, Simoni MK. Premenstrual disorders. *Am J Obstet Gynecol* 2018; 218 (1): 68–74.

Chapter 10: Beyond the Uterus: Hormones and Your Health

Baker FC, Lee KA. Menstrual cycle effects on sleep. *Sleep Med Clin* 2018; 13 (3): 283–94.

Benton MJ, Hutchins AM, Dawes JJ. Effect of menstrual cycle on resting metabolism: A systematic review and meta-analysis. *PLoS ONE* 2020; 15 (7): e0236025.

Campochiaro C, Host LV, Ong VH, Denton CP. Development of systemic sclerosis in transgender females: A case series and review of the literature. *Clin Exp Rheumatol* 2018; 36 Suppl 113 (4): 50–52.

Desai MK, Brinton RD. Autoimmune disease in women: Endocrine transition and risk across the lifespan. *Front Endocrinol* (Lausanne) 2019; 10: 265.

Fenster L, Waller K, Chen J, et al. Psychological stress in the workplace and menstrual function. *Am J Epidemiol* 1999; 149 (2): 127–34.

Gorczyca AM, Sjaarda LA, Mitchell EM, et al. Changes in macronutrient, micronutrient, and food group intakes throughout the menstrual cycle in healthy, premenopausal women. *Eur J Nutr* 2016; 55 (3): 1181–88.

Hannoun AB, Nassar AH, Usta IM, et al. Effect of war on the menstrual cycle. *Obstet Gynecol* 2007; 109 (4): 929–32.

Joffe H, Hayes FJ. Menstrual cycle dysfunction associated with neurological and psychiatric disorders: Their treatment in adolescents. *Ann NY Acad Sci* 2008; 1135: 219–29.

Klein SL, Flanagan KL. Sex differences in immune responses. *Nat Rev Immunol* 2016; 16 (10): 626–38.

McCartney CR, Marshall JC. Chapter 1: Neuroendocrinology of reproduction. In JF Strauss III, RL Barbieri, eds. *Yen & Jaffe's Reproductive Endocrinology: Physiology, Pathophysiology, and Clinical Management,* 8th ed. Philadelphia: Elsevier; 2019: 1–24.

McNulty LK, Elliott-Sale KJ, Dolan E, et al. The effects of menstrual cycle phase on exercise performance in eumenorrheic women: A systematic review and meta-analysis. *Sports Med* 2020; 50 (10): 1813–27.

Natri H, Garcia AR, Buetow KH, et al. The pregnancy pickle: Evolved immune compensation due to pregnancy underlies sex difference in human diseases. *Trends Genet* 2019; 35 (7): 478–88.

Nguyen BT, Pang RD, Nelson AL, et al. Detecting variations in ovulation and menstruation during the COVID-19 pandemic, using real-world mobile app data. *PLoS ONE* 2021; 16 (10): e0258314.

Oertelt-Prigione S. Immunity and the menstrual cycle. *Autoimmun Rev* 2012; 11 (6–7): A486–92.

O'Neal MA. Estrogen-associated migraine, including menstrual migraine. UpToDate. https://www.uptodate.com/contents/estrogen-associated-migraine-including -menstrual-migraine. Accessed April 8, 2023.

Pinkerton JV, Guico-Pabia CJ, Taylor HS. Menstrual cycle–related exacerbation of disease. *Am J Obstet Gynecol* 2010; 202 (3): 221–31.

Roeder HJ, Leira EC. Effects of the menstrual cycle on neurological disorders. *Curr Neur Neurosci Rep* 2021; 21 (7): 34.

Rothstein S. Instagram post, May 6, 2019. https://www.instagram.com/p/BxJHMWinf9n /?img_index=1 Accessed April 10, 2023.

Whitacre FE, Barrera B, Briones TN, et al. War amenorrhea: A clinical and laboratory study. *JAMA* 1944; 124 (7): 399–403.

Chapter 11: Menstrual Tracking

A day in the life of your data: A father-daughter day at the playground. April 2021. Apple, Inc. https://www.apple.com/privacy/docs/A_Day_in_the_Life_of_Your _Data.pdf. Accessed April 8, 2023.

Duane M, Contreras A, Jensen ET, White A. The performance of fertility awareness–based method apps marketed to avoid pregnancy. *J Am Board Fam Med* 2016; 29 (4): 508–11.

Liao S. Do seed oils make you sick? Consumer Reports, May 31, 2022. https://www .consumerreports.org/healthy-eating/do-seed-oils-make-you-sick-a1363483895/. Accessed April 11, 2023.

Setton R, Tierney C, Tsai T. The accuracy of web sites and cellular phone applications in predicting the fertile window. *Obstet Gynecol* 2016; 128 (1): 58–63.

Toler S. Seed cycling: I tried it. (And dug into the research on whether it works.) Clue, January 28, 2020. https://helloclue.com/articles/culture/seed-cycling-i-tried-it -and-dug-into-the-research-on-whether-it-works. Accessed April 10, 2023.

Chapter 12: The History and Safety of Menstrual Products

Berger S, Kunerl A, Wasmuth S, et al. Menstrual toxic shock syndrome: Case report and systematic review of the literature. *Lancet Infect Dis* 2019; 19 (9): e313–21.

Branch F, Woodruff TJ, Mitro SD, Zota AR. Vaginal douching and racial/ethnic disparities in phthalates exposures among reproductive-aged women: National Health and Nutrition Examination Survey 2001–2004. *Environ Health* 2015; 14: 57.

DeVries AS, Lesher L, Schlievert PM, et al. Staphylococcal toxic shock syndrome 2000–2006: Epidemiology, clinical features, and molecular characteristics. *PLoS ONE* 2011; 6 (8): e22997.

Ding N, Lin N, Batterman S, Park SK. Feminine hygiene products and volatile organic compounds in reproductive-aged women across the menstrual cycle: A longitudinal pilot study. *J Women's Health* (Larchmt) 2022; 31 (2): 210–18.

Dudley S, Nassar S, Hartman E, Wang S. Tampon safety. National Center for Health Research. https://www.center4research.org/tampon-safety/. Accessed April 10, 2023.

Early commercial tampons. Museum of Menstruation and Women's Health. http://www.mum.org/fibs.htm. Accessed April 10, 2023.

European Parliament. Exemption from VAT for menstrual hygiene products. Parliamentary Question E-003636/2021. https://www.europarl.europa.eu/doceo/document/E-9-2021-003636_EN.html. Accessed April 10, 2023.

Fitzpatrick KH. Foraging and menstruation in the Hadza of Tanzania. PhD dissertation, University of Cambridge, 2018.

Goldberg B. New York state's "tampon tax" targeted in class action suit. Reuters, March 3, 2016. https://www.reuters.com/article/us-new-york-menstruation-idUSKCN0W52NE. Accessed April 10, 2023.

Hallett V. What Kenya can teach the U.S. about menstrual pads. NPR, May 10, 2016. https://www.npr.org/sections/goatsandsoda/2016/05/10/476741805/what-kenya-can-teach-the-u-s-about-menstrual-pads. Accessed April 10, 2023.

Hill DR, Brunner ME, Schmitz DC, et al. In vivo assessment of human vaginal oxygen and carbon dioxide levels during and post menses. *J Appl Physiol* (1985) 2005; 99 (4): 1582–91.

Horwitz R. Menstrual tampon. *Embryo Project Encyclopedia*, May 25, 2020. ISSN: 1940-5030. http://embryo.asu.edu/handle/10776/13151.

Kidd, L. Menstrual technology in the United States, 1854 to 1921. Theses and Dissertations, Iowa State University, 1994. https://lib.dr.iastate.edu/rtd/10617.

Kim HY, Lee JD, Kim J-Y, et al. Risk assessment of volatile organic compounds (VOCs) detected in sanitary pads. *J Toxicol Environ Health A* 2019; 82 (11): 678–95.

Kohen JM. The history of the regulation of menstrual tampons. Third-year paper, Harvard University; 2001. http://nrs.harvard.edu/urn-3:HUL.InstRepos:8852185.

Lin N, Ding N, Meza-Wilson E, et al. Volatile organic compounds in feminine hygiene products sold in the US market: A survey of products and health risks. *Environ Int* 2020; 144: 105740.

Nonfoux L, Chiaruzzi M, Badiou C, et al. Impact of currently marketed tampons and menstrual cups on *Staphylococcus aureus* growth and toxic shock syndrome toxin 1 production in vitro. *Appl Environ Microbiol* 2018; 84 (12): e00351–18.

Old Bailey Proceedings Online. February 1733, trial of Sarah Malcolm, alias Mallcombe (t17330221-52). www.oldbaileyonline.org, version 8.0, April 11, 2023.

Read S. *Menstruation and the Female Body in Early Modern England*. New York: St. Martin's Press; 2013.

Sadlier A. New research reveals how much the average woman spends per month

on menstrual products. SWNS Digital, September 6, 2021. https://swnsdigital.com
/us/2019/11/new-research-reveals-how-much-the-average-woman-spends-per
-month-on-menstrual-products/. Accessed April 10, 2023.

Schlievert PM, Davis CC. Device-associated menstrual toxic shock syndrome. *Clin Microbiol Rev* 2020; 33 (3): e00032-19.

Trussell J, Aiken ARA, Micks E, Guthrie KA. Chapter 3: Efficacy, safety, and personal considerations. In RA Hatcher, AL Nelson, J Trussell, et al, eds. *Contraceptive Technology*, 21st ed. New York: Ayer; 2018: 95–128.

Upson K, Shearston JA, Kioumourtzoglou M-A. Menstrual products as a source of environmental chemical exposure: A review from the epidemiologic perspective. *Curr Environ Health Rep* 2022; 9 (1): 38–52.

U.S. Food and Drug Administration. Menstrual tampons and pads: Information for premarket notification submissions (510(k)s)—Guidance for Industry and FDA Staff. July 2005. https://www.fda.gov/regulatory-information/search-fda-guidance
-documents/menstrual-tampons-and-pads-information-premarket-notification
-submissions-510ks-guidance-industry. Accessed April 5, 2023.

U.S. Patent Office. Catamenial appliance. Leona W Chalmers. https://patents.google
.com/patent/US2089113. Accessed April 10, 2023.

Vostral SL. Rely and toxic shock syndrome: A technological health crisis. *Yale J Biol Med* 2011; 84 (4): 447–59.

Vostral SL. *Under Wraps: A History of Menstrual Hygiene Technology*. Plymouth UK: Lexington Books; 2008.

Chapter 13: Modern Menstrual Products

Beksinska ME, Smit J, Greener R, et al. Acceptability and performance of the menstrual cup in South Africa: A randomized crossover trial comparing the menstrual cup to tampons or sanitary pads. *J Women's Health* (Larchmt) 2015; 24 (2): 151–58.

Boronow KE, Brody JG, Schaider LA, et al. Serum concentrations of PFASs and exposure-related behaviors in African American and non-Hispanic white women. *J Expo Sci Environ Epidemiol* 2019; 29 (2): 206–17.

Farage MA. A behind-the-scenes look at the safety assessment of feminine hygiene pads. *Ann NY Acad Sci* 2006; 1092: 66–77.

Fenton SE, Ducatman A, Boobis A, et al. Per- and polyfluoroalkyl substance toxicity and human health review: Current state of knowledge and strategies for informing future research. *Environ Toxicol Chem* 2021; 40 (3): 606–30.

Glüge J, Scheringer M, Cousins IT, et al. An overview of the uses of per- and poly-fluoroalkyl substances (PFAS). *Environ Sci Process Impacts* 2020; 22 (12): 2345–73.

Loria K. Should you be concerned about PFAS chemicals? Consumer Reports, April 8, 2019. https://www.consumerreports.org/toxic-chemicals-substances/pfas
-chemicals-should-you-be-concerned-a2708998896/.

Mitchell MA, Bisch S, Arntfield S, Hosseini-Moghaddam SM. A confirmed case of toxic shock syndrome associated with the use of a menstrual cup. *Can J Infect Dis Med Microbiol* 2015; 26 (4): 218–20.

National Academies of Science, Medicine and Engineering. *Guidance on PFAS Exposure, Testing, and Clinical Follow-Up*. Washington, DC: National Academies Press; 2022.

Nonfoux L, Chiaruzzi M, Badiou C, et al. Impact of currently marketed tampons and menstrual cups on *Staphylococcus aureus* growth and toxic shock syndrome toxin 1 production in vitro. *Appl Environ Microbiol* 2018; 84 (12): e00351–18.

Ragnarsdóttir O, Abdallah MA, Harrad S. Dermal uptake: An important pathway of human exposure to perfluoroalkyl substances? *Environ Pollut* 2022; 307: 119478.

Reame NK. Chapter 51: Toxic shock syndrome and tampons: The birth of a movement and a research "vagenda." In C Bobel, IT Winkler, B Fahs, et al, eds. *The Palgrave Handbook of Critical Menstrual Studies*. Singapore: Palgrave Macmillan; 2020: 687–704.

Schnyer AN, Jensen JT, Edelman A, Han L. Do menstrual cups increase risk of IUD expulsion? A survey of self-reported IUD and menstrual hygiene product use in the United States. *Eur J Contracept Reprod Health Care* 2019; 24 (5): 368–72.

Seale R, Powers L, Guiahi M, Coleman-Minahan K. Unintentional IUD expulsion with concomitant menstrual cup use: A case series. *Contraception* 2019; 100 (1): 85–87.

U.S. Food and Drug Administration. Per and polyfluoroalkyl substances (PFAS) in cosmetics. Updated February 25, 2022. https://www.fda.gov/cosmetics/cosmetic -ingredients/and-polyfluoroalkyl-substances-pfas-cosmetics. Accessed April 23 2023.

U.S. Food and Drug Administration. Title 21—Food and Drugs, Chapter I: FDA Department of Health and Human Services. Subpart H—Special Requirements for Specific Devices. Sec. 801.430 User labeling for menstrual tampons. https://www .accessdata.fda.gov/scripts/cdrh/cfdocs/cfCFR/CFRSearch.cfm?fr=801.430. Accessed April 10, 2023.

van Eijk AM, Zulaika G, Lenchner M, et al. Menstrual cup use, leakage, acceptability, safety, and availability: A systematic review and meta-analysis. *Lancet Public Health* 2019; 4 (8): e376–93.

van der Veen I, Schellenberger S, Hanning A-C, et al. Fate of per- and polyfluoroalkyl substances from durable water-repellent clothing during use. *Environ Sci Technol* 2022; 56 (9): 5886–97.

Woeller KE, Hochwalt AE. Safety assessment of sanitary pads with a polymeric foam absorbent core. *Regul Toxicol Pharmacol* 2015; 73 (1): 419–24.

Chapter 14: Menstrual Product Myths

Archer JC, Mabry-Smith R, Shojaee S, et al. Dioxin and furan levels found in tampons. *J Women's Health* (Larchmt) 2005; 14 (4): 311–15.

DeVito MJ, Schecter A. Exposure assessment to dioxins from the use of tampons and diapers. *Environ Health Perspect* 2002; 110 (1): 23–28.

Dudley S, Nassar S, Hartman E, Wang S. Tampon safety. National Center for Health Research. https://www.center4research.org/tampon-safety/. Accessed April 10, 2023.

Gunter J. Can a menstrual cup cause uterine prolapse? *The Vajenda*, September 15, 2022. https://vajenda.substack.com/p/can-a-menstrual-cup-cause-uterine.

Han H-Y, Yang M-J, Yoon C, et al. Toxicity of orally administered food-grade titanium dioxide nanoparticles. *J Appl Toxicol* 2021; 41 (7): 1127–47.

Health Canada. Titanium dioxide (TiO_2) as a food additive: Current science report. https://www.canada.ca/en/health-canada/services/food-nutrition

/reports-publications/titanium-dioxide-food-additive-science-report.html. Accessed March 26, 2023.

Meaddough EL, Olive DL, Gallup P, et al. Sexual activity, orgasm and tampon use are associated with a decreased risk for endometriosis. *Gynecol Obstet Invest* 2002; 53 (3): 163–69.

Skocaj M, Filipic M, Petkovic J, Novak S. Titanium dioxide in our everyday life; is it safe? *Radiol Oncol* 2011; 45 (4): 227–47.

U.S. Food and Drug Administration. CPG Sec. 345.300: Menstrual sponges. March 1995. https://www.fda.gov/regulatory-information/search-fda-guidance-documents /cpg-sec-345300-menstrual-sponges. Accessed April 10, 2023.

van Eijk AM, Zulaika G, Lenchner M, et al. Menstrual cup use, leakage, acceptability, safety, and availability: A systematic review and meta-analysis. *Lancet Public Health* 2019; 4 (8): e376–93.

Windler L, Lorenz C, von Goetz N, et al. Release of titanium dioxide from textiles during washing. *Environ Sci Technol* 2012; 46 (15): 8181–88.

Chapter 15: A Primer on Abnormal Bleeding

American College of Obstetricians and Gynecologists. The use of hysteroscopy for the diagnosis and treatment of intrauterine pathology: ACOG committee opinion, no. 800. *Obstet Gynecol* 2020; 135 (3): e138–48.

American College of Obstetricians and Gynecologists, Committee on Practice Bulletins—Gynecology. Practice bulletin no. 128: Diagnosis of abnormal uterine bleeding in reproductive-aged women. *Obstet Gynecol* 2012; 120 (1): 197–206.

Chapron C, Vannuccini S, Santulli P, et al. Diagnosing adenomyosis: An integrated clinical and imaging approach. *Hum Reprod Update* 2020; 26 (3): 392–411.

Chodankar R, Critchley HOD. Abnormal uterine bleeding (including PALM COEIN classification). *Obstet Gynaecol Reprod Med* 2019; 29 (4): 98–104.

De Silva NK. Abnormal uterine bleeding in adolescents: Evaluation and approach to diagnosis. UpToDate. https://www.uptodate.com/contents/abnormal-uterine -bleeding-in-adolescents-evaluation-and-approach-to-diagnosis. Accessed February 4, 2023.

Di Speizio Sardo A, Florio P, Sosa Fernandez LM, et al. The potential role of endome-trial nerve fibers in the pathogenesis of pain during endometrial biopsy at office hysteroscopy. *Reprod Sci* 2015; 22 (1): 124–31.

Magnay JL, O'Brien S, Gerlinger C, Seitz C. Pictorial methods to assess heavy menstrual bleeding in research and clinical practice: A systematic literature review. *BMC Women's Health* 2022; 20 (1): 24.

Marnach ML, Laughlin-Tommaso SK. Evaluation and management of abnormal uterine bleeding. *Mayo Clin Proc* 2019; 94 (2): 326–35.

Chapter 16: Heavy Periods

American College of Obstetricians and Gynecologists. ACOG committee opinion no. 557: Management of acute abnormal uterine bleeding in nonpregnant reproductive-aged women. *Obstet Gynecol* 2013: 121 (4): 891–96.

American College of Obstetricians and Gynecologists. Practice bulletin no. 136: Management of abnormal uterine bleeding associated with ovulatory dysfunction. *Obstet Gynecol* 2013; 122 (1): 176–85.

American College of Obstetricians and Gynecologists, Committee on Practice Bulletins—Gynecology. Management of symptomatic uterine leiomyomas: ACOG practice bulletin no. 228. *Obstet Gynecol* 2021; 137 (6): e100–115.

Beelen P, Reinders IMA, Scheepers WFW, et al. Prognostic factors for the failure of endometrial ablation: A systematic review and meta-analysis. *Obstet Gynecol* 2019; 134 (6): 1269–81.

Bulun SE. Uterine fibroids. *N Engl J Med* 2013; 369 (14): 1344–55.

Itriyeva K. The effects of obesity on the menstrual cycle. *Curr Probl Pediatr Adolesc Health Care* 2022; 52 (8): 101241.

Kaunitz AM. Abnormal uterine bleeding in nonpregnant reproductive-age patients: Terminology, evaluation and approach to diagnosis. UpToDate. https://www .uptodate.com/contents/abnormal-uterine-bleeding-in-nonpregnant -reproductive-age-patients-terminology-evaluation-and-approach-to-diagnosis. Accessed February 4, 2023.

Leminen H, Hurskainen R. Tranexamic acid for the treatment of heavy menstrual bleeding: Efficacy and safety. *Int J Women's Health* 2012; 4: 413–21.

Manyonda I, Belli A-M, Lumsden M-A, et al. Uterine-artery embolization or myomectomy for uterine fibroids. *N Engl J Med* 2020; 383 (5): 440–51.

Middleton LJ, Champaneria R, Daniels JP, et al. Hysterectomy, endometrial destruction, and levonorgestrel releasing intrauterine system (Mirena) for heavy menstrual bleeding: Systemic review and meta-analysis of data from individual patients. *BMJ* 2010; 341: c3929.

Schaff WD, Ackerman RT, Al-Hendry A, et al. Elagolix for heavy menstrual bleeding in women with uterine fibroids. *N Engl J Med* 2020; 382 (4): 328–40.

Upson K, Missmer SA. Epidemiology of adenomyosis. *Semin Reprod Med* 2020; 38 (2-03): 89–107.

Zhai J, Vannuccini S, Petraglia F, Giudice LC. Adenomyosis: Mechanisms and pathogenesis. *Semin Reprod Med* 2020; 38 (2-03): 129–43.

Chapter 17: Bleeding Bingo: When Periods Stop, When They Become Irregular, and Breakthrough Bleeding

Ackerman KE, Misra M. Functional hypothalamic amenorrhea: Evaluation and management. UpToDate. https://www.uptodate.com/contents/functional -hypothalamic-amenorrhea-evaluation-and-management. Accessed February 4, 2023.

American College of Obstetricians and Gynecologists. ACOG committee opinion no. 557: Management of acute abnormal uterine bleeding in nonpregnant reproductive-aged women. *Obstet Gynecol* 2013: 121 (4): 891–96.

American College of Obstetricians and Gynecologists. Committee opinion no. 702: Female athlete triad. *Obstet Gynecol* 2017; 129 (6): e160–67.

American College of Obstetricians and Gynecologists, Committee on Practice Bulletins—Gynecology. Practice bulletin no. 128: Diagnosis of abnormal uterine bleeding in reproductive-aged women. *Obstet Gynecol* 2012; 120 (1): 197–206.

Bij de Vaate AJM, Brölmann HAM, van der Voet LF, et al. Ultrasound evaluation of the cesarean scar: Relation between a niche and postmenstrual spotting. *Ultrasound Obstet Gynecol* 2011; 37 (1): 93–99.

De Souza MJ, Nattiv A, Joy E, et al. 2014 Female Athlete Triad Coalition consensus statement on treatment and return to play of the female athlete triad: 1st international conference held in San Francisco, California, May 2012 and 2nd international conference held in Indianapolis, Indiana, May 2013. *Br J Sports Med* 2014; 48 (4): 289.

Gibson MES, Fleming N, Zuijdwijk C, Dumont T. Where have the periods gone? The evaluation and management of functional hypothalamic amenorrhea. *J Clin Res Pediatr Endocrinol* 2020; 12 (Suppl 1): 18–27.

Huhmann K. Menses requires energy: A review of how disordered eating, excessive exercise, and high stress lead to menstrual irregularities. *Clin Ther* 2020; 42 (3): 401–7.

Karagiannis A, Harsoulis F. Gonadal dysfunction in systemic diseases. *Eur J Endocrinol* 2005; 152 (4): 501–13.

Kaunitz AM. Abnormal uterine bleeding in nonpregnant reproductive-age patients: Terminology, evaluation and approach to diagnosis. UpToDate. https://www .uptodate.com/contents/abnormal-uterine-bleeding-in-nonpregnant -reproductive-age-patients-terminology-evaluation-and-approach-to -diagnosis. Accessed February 4, 2023.

Makker V, MacKay H, Ray-Coquard I, et al. Endometrial cancer. *Nat Rev Dis Primers* 2021; 7 (1): 88.

Stuenkel CA, Gompel A. Primary ovarian insufficiency. *N Eng J Med* 2023; 388 (2): 154–63.

van der Voet LF, Bij de Vaate AM, Veersema S, et al. Long-term complications of caesarean section. The niche in the scar: A prospective cohort study on niche prevalence and its relation to abnormal uterine bleeding. *BJOG* 2014; 121 (2): 236–44.

Weiderpass E, Adami HO, Baron JA, et al. Risk of endometrial cancer following estrogen replacement with and without progestins. *J Natl Cancer Inst* 1999; 91 (13): 1131–37.

Chapter 18: Polycystic Ovarian Syndrome

American College of Obstetricians and Gynecologists. Screening and management of the hyperandrogenic adolescent: ACOG committee opinion, number 789. *Obstet Gynecol* 2019; 134 (4): e106–14.

American College of Obstetricians and Gynecologists, Committee on Practice Bulletins—Gynecology. ACOG practice bulletin no. 194: Polycystic ovary syndrome. *Obstet Gynecol* 2018; 131 (6): e157–71.

Azziz R. Polycystic ovary syndrome. *Obstet Gynecol* 2018; 132 (2): 321–36.

Azziz R, Carmina E, Dewailly D, et al. The Androgen Excess and PCOS Society criteria for the polycystic ovarian syndrome: The complete task force report. *Fertil Steril* 2009; 91 (2): 456–88.

Carmina E, Campagna AM, Lobo RA. A 20-year follow-up of young women with polycystic ovary syndrome. *Obstet Gynecol* 2012; 119 (2 Pt 1): 263–69.

Emanuel RHK, Roberts J, Docherty PD, et al. A review of the hormones involved in the endocrine dysfunctions of polycystic ovary syndrome and their interactions. *Front Endocrinol* (Lausanne) 2022; 13: 1017468.

Fessler DMT, Natterson-Horowitz B, Azziz R. Evolutionary determinants of polycystic ovary syndrome: Part 2. *Fertil Steril* 2016; 106 (1): 42–47.

Ismayilova M, Yaya S. "I felt like she didn't take me seriously": A multi-methods study examining patient satisfaction and experiences with polycystic ovary syndrome (PCOS) in Canada. *BMC Women's Health* 2022; 22 (1): 47.

Jayasena CN, Franks S. The management of patients with polycystic ovarian syndrome. *Nat Rev Endocrinol* 2014; 10 (10): 624–36.

Louwers YV, Stolk L, Uitterlinden AG, Laven JSE. Cross-ethnic meta-analysis of genetic variants for polycystic ovary syndrome. *J Clin Endocrinol Metab* 2013; 98 (12): E2006–12.

Teede HJ, Misso ML, Costello MF, et al. Recommendations from the international evidence-based guideline for the assessment and management of polycystic ovary syndrome. *Fertil Steril* 2018; 110 (3): 364–79.

Welt CK, Carmina E. Lifecycle of polycystic ovary syndrome (PCOS): From in utero to menopause. *J Clin Endocrinol Metab* 2013; 98 (12): 4629–38.

Chapter 19: Painful Periods

Altunyurt S, Göl M, Altunyurt S, et al. Primary dysmenorrhea and uterine blood flow: A color Doppler study. *J Reprod Med* 2005; 50 (4): 251–55.

American College of Obstetricians and Gynecologists. ACOG committee opinion no. 760: Dysmenorrhea and endometriosis in the adolescent. *Obstet Gynecol* 2018; 132 (6): e249–58.

Dawood MY. Primary dysmenorrhea. Advances in pathogenesis and management. *Obstet Gynecol* 2006; 108 (2): 428–41.

Elboim-Gabyzon M, Kalichman L. Transcutaneous electrical nerve stimulation (TENS) for primary dysmenorrhea: An overview. *Int J Women's Health* 2020; 12: 1–10.

Ferries-Rowe E, Corey E, Archer JS. Primary dysmenorrhea: Diagnosis and therapy. *Obstet Gynecol* 2020; 136 (5): 1047–58.

Kho KA, Shields JK. Diagnosis and management of primary dysmenorrhea. *JAMA* 2020; 323 (3): 268–69.

Lundström V, Gréen K. Endogenous levels of prostaglandins F2alpha and its main metabolites in plasma and endometrium of normal and dysmenorrheic women. *Am J Obstet Gynecol* 1978; 130 (6): 640–46.

Myers KM, Elad D. Biomechanics of the human uterus. *Wiley Interdiscip Rev Syst Biol Med* 2017; 9 (5).

Oladosu FA, Tu FT, Hellman KM. Nonsteroidal antiinflammatory drug resistance in dysmenorrhea: Epidemiology, causes, and treatment. *Am J Obstet Gynecol* 2018; 218 (4): 390–400.

Payne LA, Rapkin AJ, Saidman LC, et al. Experimental and procedural pain responses in primary dysmenorrhea: A systematic review. *J Pain Res* 2017; 10: 2233–46.

Proctor ML, Smith CA, Farquhar CM, Stones RW. Transcutaneous electrical nerve stimulation and acupuncture for primary dysmenorrhoea. *Cochrane Database Syst Rev* 2002; 2002 (1): CD002123.

Schoep ME, Adang EMM, Maas JWM, et al. Productivity loss due to menstruation-related symptoms: A nationwide cross-sectional survey among 32,748 women. *BMJ Open* 2019; 9 (6): e026186.

Tu C-H, Niddam DM, Yeh T-C, et al. Menstrual pain is associated with rapid structural alterations in the brain. *Pain* 2013; 154 (9): 1718–24.

Vincent K, Warnaby C, Stagg CJ, et al. Dysmenorrhoea is associated with central changes in otherwise healthy women. *Pain* 2011; 152 (9): 1966–75.

Wong CL, Farquhar C, Roberts H, Proctor M. Oral contraceptive pill as treatment for primary dysmenorrhoea. *Cochrane Database Syst Rev* 2009; (2): CD002120.

Chapter 20: Endometriosis

As-Sanie S, Harris RE, Harte SE, et al. Increased pressure pain sensitivity in women with chronic pelvic pain. *Obstet Gynecol* 2013; 122 (5): 1047–55.

Brawn J, Morotti M, Zondervan KT, et al. Central changes associated with chronic pelvic pain and endometriosis. *Hum Reprod Update* 2014; 20 (5): 737–47.

ESHRE Endometriosis Guideline Development Group. Endometriosis: Guideline of European Society of Human Reproduction and Embryology. February 2, 2022. https://www.eshre.eu/Guidelines-and-Legal/Guidelines/Endometriosis-guideline.

Giamberardino MA, Berkley KJ, Affaitati G, et al. Influence of endometriosis on pain behaviors and muscle hyperalgesia induced by a ureteral calculosis in female rats. *Pain* 2002; 95 (3): 247–57.

Grandi G, Barra F, Ferrero S. Hormonal contraception in women with endometriosis: A systematic review. *Eur J Contracept Reprod Health Care* 2019; 24 (1): 61–70.

Kalaitzopoulos DR, Samartzis N, Kolovos GN, et al. Treatment of endometriosis: A review with comparison of 8 guidelines. *BMC Women's Health* 2021; 21 (1): 397.

Mowers EL, Lim CS, Skinner B, et al. Prevalence of endometriosis during abdominal or laparoscopic hysterectomy for chronic pelvic pain. *Obstet Gynecol* 2016; 127 (6): 1045–53.

Orr NL, Huang AJ, Liu YD, et al. Association of central sensitization inventory scores with pain outcomes after endometriosis surgery. *JAMA Netw Open* 2023; 6 (2): e230780.

Shim JY, Laufer MR. Adolescent endometriosis: An update. *J Pediatr Adolesc Gynecol* 2020; 33 (2): 112–19.

Simko S, Wright KN. The future of diagnostic laparoscopy: Cons. *Reprod Fertil* 2022; 3 (2): R91–R95.

Zondervan KT, Becker CM, Koga K, et al. Endometriosis. *Nat Rev Dis Primers* 2018; 4 (1): 9.

Zondervan KT, Becker CM, Missmer SA. Endometriosis. *N Engl J Med* 2020; 382 (13): 1244–56.

Chapter 21: Alternative Therapies for Menstrual Pain

Baker M. Deceptive curcumin offers cautionary tale for chemists. *Nature* 2017; 541 (7636): 144–45.

Blumstein GW, Parsa A, Park AK, et al. Effect of Delta-9-tetrahydrocannabinol on mouse resistance to systemic *Candida albicans* infection. *PLoS ONE* 2014; 9 (7): e103288.

Brents LK. Marijuana, the endocannabinoid system and the female reproductive system. *Yale J Biol Med* 2016; 89 (2): 175–91.

Chavarro JE, Rich-Edwards JW, Gaskins AJ, et al. Contributions of the Nurses' Health Studies to reproductive health research. *Am J Public Health* 2016; 106 (9): 1669–76.

Ferries-Rowe E, Corey E, Archer JS. Primary dysmenorrhea: Diagnosis and therapy. *Obstet Gynecol* 2020; 136 (5): 1047–58.

Fonseca BM, Rebelo I. Cannabis and cannabinoids in reproduction and fertility: Where we stand. *Reprod Sci* 2022; 29 (9): 2429–39.

Huestis MA. Human cannabinoid pharmacokinetics. *Chem Biodivers* 2007; 4 (8): 1770–1804.

Khan KS, Champaneria R, Latthe PM. How effective are non-drug, non-surgical treatments for primary dysmenorrhoea? *BMJ* 2012; 344: e3011.

Liao S. Do seed oils make you sick? Consumer Reports, May 31, 2022. https://www .consumerreports.org/healthy-eating/do-seed-oils-make-you-sick-a1363483895 /. Accessed April 11, 2023.

National Academies of Sciences, Engineering, and Medicine. *The Health Effects of Cannabis and Cannabinoids: The Current State of Evidence and Recommendations for Research*. Washington, DC: National Academies Press; 2017.

Nodler JL, DiVasta AD, Vitonis AF, et al. Supplementation with vitamin D or ω-3 fatty acids in adolescent girls and young women with endometriosis (SAGE): A double-blind, randomized, placebo-controlled trial. *Am J Clin Nutr* 2020; 112 (1): 229–36.

Pattanittum P, Kunyanone N, Brown J, et al. Dietary supplements for dysmenorrhoea. *Cochrane Database Syst Rev* 2016; 3 (3): CD002124.

Sadeghi N, Paknezhad F, Rashidi Nooshabadi M, et al. Vitamin E and fish oil, separately or in combination, on treatment of primary dysmenorrhea: A double-blind, randomized clinical trial. *Gynecol Endocrinol* 2018; 34 (9): 804–8.

Sinclair J, Collett L, Abbott J, et al. Effects of cannabis ingestion on endometriosis-associated pelvic pain and related symptoms. *PLoS ONE* 2021; 16 (10): e0258940.

Smith CA, Armour M, Zhu X, et al. Acupuncture for dysmenorrhoea. *Cochrane Database Syst Rev* 2016, 4 (4): CD007854.

U.S. Food and Drug Administration. Scientific data and information about products containing cannabis or cannabis-derived compounds; public hearing. May 31, 2019. https://www.fda.gov/news-events/fda-meetings-conferences-and-workshops /scientific-data-and-information-about-products-containing-cannabis-or -cannabis-derived-compounds. Accessed June 28, 2023.

Chapter 22: The History of Hormonal Contraception

Bailey MJ, Hershbein B, Miller AR. The opt-in revolution? Contraception and the gender gap in wages. *Am Econ J Appl Econ* 2012; 4 (3): 225–54.

Centers for Disease Control and Prevention. Margaret Sanger. *MMWR Weekly* 1999; 48 (47): 1075. https://www.cdc.gov/mmwr/preview/mmwrhtml/mm4847bx.htm.

Dhont M. History of oral contraception. *Eur J Contracept Reprod Health Care* 2010: 15 Suppl 2: S12–18.

Eig J. *The Birth of the Pill: How Four Crusaders Reinvented Sex and Launched a Revolution*. New York: W.W. Norton; 2014.

Gregory Pincus and Enovid. Onview: Digital Collections and Exhibits. Center for the History of Medicine at Countway Library. https://collections.countway.harvard. edu/onview/exhibits/show/conceiving-the-pill/gregory-pincus-and-enovid. Accessed June 28, 2023.

Himes NE. Medical history of contraception. *N Eng J Med* 1934; 210: 576–81.

Katharine Dexter McCormick (1875–1967). *American Experience*, PBS. https://www
.pbs.org/wgbh/americanexperience/features/pill-katharine-dexter-mccormick
-1875-1967/. Accessed April 4, 2023.

Liu KE, Fisher WA. Canadian physicians' role in contraception from the 19th century
to now. *J Obstet Gynaecol Can* 2002; 24 (3): 239–44.

Malladi L. *United States v. One Package of Japanese Pessaries* (1936). *Embryo Project
Encyclopedia*, May 24, 2017. https://embryo.asu.edu/pages/united-states-v-one
-package-japanese-pessaries-1936.

McGill Johnson A. I'm the head of Planned Parenthood. We're done making excuses
for our founder. *New York Times*, April 17, 2021. https://www.nytimes.
com/2021/04/17/opinion/planned-parenthood-margaret-sanger.html. Accessed
March 26, 2023.

Milne J, Pincus G. An oral contraceptive. *Lancet* 1958; 271 (7032): 1230.

Pendergrass DC, Raji MY. The bitter pill: Harvard and the dark history of birth control.
Harvard Crimson, September 28, 2017. https://www.thecrimson.com/article/2017
/9/28/the-bitter-pill/. Accessed March 26, 2023.

Proceedings of a Symposium on 19-Nor Progestational Steroids. Chicago: Searle Research
Laboratories; 1957.

Roberts WC. "The pill" and its four major developers. *Proc (Bayl Univ Med Cent)* 2015;
28 (3): 421–32.

Seward S. The Comstock Law (1873). *Embryo Project Encyclopedia*, January 13, 2009.
ISSN: 1940-5030. http://embryo.asu.edu/handle/10776/1761.

Chapter 23: Estrogen-Containing Contraceptives: The Modern Pill,
Patch, and Ring

American College of Obstetricians and Gynecologists. Effectiveness of contraceptive
methods. https://www.acog.org/womens-health/infographics/effectiveness-of
-birth-control-methods. Accessed April 5, 2023.

Baker CC, Chen MJ. New contraception update—Annovera, Phexxi, Slynd, and Twirla.
Curr Obstet Gynecol Rep 2022; 11 (1): 21–27.

Centers for Disease Control and Prevention. US medical eligibility criteria for contraception use, 2015 (US MEC). https://www.cdc.gov/reproductivehealth/contraception
/mmwr/mec/summary.html. Accessed April 5, 2023.

Cwiak C, Edelman AB. Chapter 8: Combined oral contraceptives (COCs). In RA Hatcher,
AL Nelson, J Trussell, et al, eds. *Contraceptive Technology*, 21st ed. New York: Ayer;
2018: 263–316.

Dhont M. History of oral contraception. *Eur J Contracept Reprod Health Care* 2010:
15 Suppl 2: S12–18.

Estetrol/drospirenone (Nextstellis)—A new combination oral contraceptive. *Med Lett
Drugs Ther* 2021; 63 (1627): 101–2.

Gaspard UJ, Remus MA, Gillain D, et al. Plasma hormone levels in women receiving
new oral contraceptives containing ethinyl estradiol plus levonorgestrel or
desogestrel. *Contraception* 1983; 27 (6): 577–90.

Grandi G, Del Savio MC, Lopes da Silva-Filho A, Facchinetti F. Estetrol (E4): The new
estrogenic component of combined oral contraceptives. *Expert Rev Clin Pharmacol*
2020; 13 (4): 327–30.

London A, Jensen JT. Rationale for eliminating the hormone-free interval in modern oral contraceptives. *Intl J Gynaecol Obstet* 2016; 134 (1): 8–12.

Mishell Jr DR, Thorneycroft IH, Nakamura RM, et al. Serum estradiol in women ingesting combination oral contraceptive steroids. *Am J Obstet Gynecol* 1972; 114 (7): 923–28.

Morimont L, Haguet H, Dogné J-M, et al. Combined oral contraceptives and venous thromboembolism: Review and perspective to mitigate the risk. *Front Endocrinol* (Lausanne) 2021: 12: 769187.

Nanda K, Burke AE. Chapter 7: Contraceptive patch and vaginal contraceptive ring. In RA Hatcher, AL Nelson, J Trussell, et al, eds. *Contraceptive Technology*, 21st ed. New York: Ayer; 2018: 227–62.

Stanczyk FZ, Archer DF, Bhavani BR. Ethinyl estradiol and 17-estradiol in combination oral contraceptives: Pharmacokinetics, pharmacodynamics and risk assessment. *Contraception* 2013; 87 (6): 706–27.

Teal S, Edelman A. Contraception selection, effectiveness, and adverse effects: A review. *JAMA* 2021; 326 (24): 2507–18.

Twirla—A new contraceptive patch. *Med Lett Drugs Ther* 2021; 63 (1617): 17–18.

Chapter 24: Progestin-Only Methods

American College of Obstetricians and Gynecologists. ACOG practice bulletin no. 121: Long-acting reversible contraception: Implants and intrauterine devices. *Obstet Gynecol* 2011; 118 (1): 184–96.

American College of Obstetricians and Gynecologists. ACOG practice bulletin no. 206: Use of hormonal contraception in women with coexisting medical conditions. *Obstet Gynecol* 2019; 133 (2): e128–50.

American College of Obstetricians and Gynecologists. Effectiveness of contraceptive methods. https://www.acog.org/womens-health/infographics/effectiveness-of -birth-control-methods. Accessed April 5, 2023.

Baker CC, Chen MJ. New contraception update—Annovera, Phexxi, Slynd, and Twirla. *Curr Obstet Gynecol Rep* 2022; 11 (1): 21–27.

Bennink HJ. The pharmacokinetics and pharmacodynamics of Implanon, a single-rod etonogestrel contraceptive implant. *Eur J Contracept Reprod Health Care* 2000; 5 Suppl 2: 12–20.

Centers for Disease Control and Prevention. US medical eligibility criteria for contraception use, 2015 (US MEC). https://www.cdc.gov/reproductivehealth/contraception /mmwr/mec/summary.html. Accessed April 5, 2023.

Nelson AL, Crabtree Sokol D, Grentzer J. Chapter 4: Contraceptive implant. In RA Hatcher, AL Nelson, J Trussell, et al, eds. *Contraceptive Technology*, 21st ed. New York: Ayer; 2018: 129–56.

Polis CB, Hussain R, Berry A. There might be blood: A scoping review on women's responses to contraceptive-induced menstrual bleeding changes. *Reprod Health* 2018; 15 (1): 114.

Raymond EG, Grossman D. Chapter 9: Progestin-only pills. In RA Hatcher, AL Nelson, J Trussell, et al, eds. *Contraceptive Technology*, 21st ed. New York: Ayer; 2018: 317–28.

Teal S, Edelman A. Contraception selection, effectiveness, and adverse effects: A review. *JAMA* 2021; 326 (24): 2507–18.

Wu W-J, Bartz D. Chapter 6: Injectable contraceptives. In RA Hatcher, AL Nelson, J Trussell, et al, eds. *Contraceptive Technology*, 21st ed. New York: Ayer; 2018: 195–226.

Chapter 25: Emergency Contraception

Ella package insert. https://www.accessdata.fda.gov/drugsatfda_docs/label/2010/022474s000lbl.pdf. Accessed March 26, 2023.

Endler M, Li R, Gemzell Danielsson K. Effect of levonorgestrel contraception on implantation and fertility: A review. *Contraception* 2022; 109: 8–18.

Faculty of Sexual and Reproductive Healthcare. FSRH clinical guideline: Overweight, obesity and contraception (April 2019). https://www.fsrh.org/standards-and-guidance/documents/fsrh-clinical-guideline-overweight-obesity-and-contraception/. Accessed March 26, 2023.

Festin MPR, Peregoudov A, Seuc A, et al. Effect of BMI and body weight on pregnancy rates with LNG as emergency contraception: Analysis of four WHO HRP studies. *Contraception* 2017; 95 (1): 50–54.

Glasier A, Cameron ST, Blithe D, et al. Can we identify women at risk of pregnancy despite using emergency contraception? Data from randomized trials of ulipristal acetate and levonorgestrel. *Contraception* 2011; 84 (4): 363–67.

Glasier AF, Cameron ST, Fine PM, et al. Ulipristal acetate versus levonorgestrel for emergency contraception: A randomised non-inferiority trial and meta-analysis. *Lancet* 2010; 375 (9714): 555–62.

International Consortium for Emergency Contraception. *Emergency Contraceptive Pills: Medical and Service Delivery Guidance*, 4th ed. 2018. https://www.ec-ec.org/wp-content/uploads/2019/01/ICEC-guides_FINAL.pdf. Accessed March 26, 2023.

Trussel J, Cleland K, Schwarz EB. Chapter 10: Emergency contraception. In RA Hatcher, AL Nelson, J Trussell, et al, eds. *Contraceptive Technology*, 21st ed. New York: Ayer; 2018: 329–66.

Turok D. Emergency contraception. UpToDate. https://www.uptodate.com/contents/emergency-contraception. Accessed March 26, 2023.

World Health Organization. Emergency contraception. November 9, 2021. https://www.who.int/news-room/fact-sheets/detail/emergency-contraception. Accessed March 26, 2023.

Chapter 26: The History of the Intrauterine Device

Cates Jr W, Ory HW, Rochat RW, Tyler Jr CW. The intrauterine device and deaths from spontaneous abortion. *N Eng J Med* 1976; 295 (21): 1155–59.

Cox ML. The Dalkon Shield saga. *J Fam Plann Reprod Health Care* 2003; 29 (1): 8.

Hubacher D, Lara-Ricalde R, Taylor DJ, et al. Use of copper intrauterine devices and the risk of tubal infertility among nulligravid women. *N Engl J Med* 2001; 345 (8): 561–67.

Margulies L. History of intrauterine devices. *Bull NY Acad Med* 1975; 51 (5): 662–67.

McNicholas C, Madden T, Secura G, Peipert JF. The contraceptive CHOICE project round up: What we did and what we learned. *Clin Obstet Gynecol* 2014; 57 (4): 635–43.

Ortiz ME, Croxatto HB. Copper-T intrauterine device and levonorgestrel intrauterine system: Biological bases of their mechanism of action. *Contraception* 2007; 75 (6 Suppl): S16–30.

Segal SJ, Alvarez-Sanchez F, Adejuwon CA, et al. Absence of chorionic gonadotropin in sera of women who use intrauterine devices. *Fertil Steril* 1985; 44 (2): 214–18.

Sivin I. IUDs are contraceptives, not abortifacients: A comment on research and belief. *Stud Fam Plann* 1989; 20 (6 Pt 1): 355–59.

Sivin I, Batár I. State-of-the-art of non-hormonal methods of contraception: III. Intrauterine devices. *Eur J Contracept Reprod Health Care* 2010; 15 (2): 96–112.

Tatum HJ, Schmidt FH, Phillips D, et al. The Dalkon Shield controversy: Structural and bacteriological studies of IUD tails. *JAMA* 1975; 231 (7): 711–17.

U.S. Food and Drug Administration. History of the US Food and Drug Administration: Interview with Larry Pilot. December 21, 2004. http://www.fda.gov/media/81346/download. Accessed April 3, 2023.

Videla-Rivero L, Etchepareborda JJ, Kesseru E. Early chorionic activity in women bearing inert IUD, copper IUD and levonorgestrel-releasing IUD. *Contraception* 1987; 36 (2): 217–26.

Chapter 27: The Modern Intrauterine Device

American College of Obstetricians and Gynecologists. ACOG Practice Bulletin No. 121: Long-acting reversible contraception: Implants and intrauterine devices. *Obstet Gynecol* 2011; 118 (1): 184–96.

American College of Obstetricians and Gynecologists, Committee on Gynecologic Practice; Long-Acting Reversible Contraceptive Expert Work Group. Committee opinion no. 672: Clinical challenges of long-acting reversible contraceptive methods. *Obstet Gynecol* 2016; 128 (3): e69–77.

American College of Obstetricians and Gynecologists, Committee on Practice Bulletins—Gynecology, Long-Acting Reversible Contraception Work Group. Practice bulletin no. 186: Long-acting reversible contraception: Implants and intrauterine devices. *Obstet Gynecol* 2017; 130 (5): e251–69.

Dean G, Schwarz EB. Chapter 5: Intrauterine devices. In RA Hatcher, AL Nelson, J Trussell, et al, eds. *Contraceptive Technology*, 21st ed. New York: Ayer; 2018: 157–94.

Dina B, Peipert LJ, Zhao Q, Peipert JF. Anticipated pain as a predictor of discomfort with intrauterine device placement. *Am J Obstet Gynecol* 2018; 218 (2): 236.e1–9.

Foster DG, Grossman D, Turok DK, et al. Interest in and experience with IUD self-removal. *Contraception* 2014; 90 (1): 54–59.

Gemzell-Danielsson K, Jensen JT, Monteiro I, et al. Interventions for the prevention of pain associated with the placement of intrauterine contraceptives: An updated review. *Acta Obstet Gynecol Scand* 2019; 98 (12): 1500–513.

Lopez LM, Bernholc A, Zeng Y, et al. Interventions for pain with intrauterine device insertion. *Cochrane Database Syst Rev* 2015; 2015 (7): CD007373.

medSask. Comparison of copper intrauterine devices available in Canada. https://medsask.usask.ca/sites/medsask/files/2023-02/Comparison-Copper-IUD.pdf. Accessed March 4, 2023.

Nguyen L, Lamarche L, Lennox R, et al. Strategies to mitigate anxiety and pain in intrauterine device insertion: A systematic review. *J Obstet Gynaecol Can* 2020; 42 (9): 1138–46.e2.

Raifman S, Barar R, Foster D. Effect of knowledge of self-removability of intrauterine contraceptives on uptake, continuation, and satisfaction. *Women's Health Issues* 2018; 28 (1): 68–74.

Sivin I, Batár I. State-of-the-art of non-hormonal methods of contraception: III. Intrauterine devices. *Eur J Contracept Reprod Health Care* 2010; 15 (2): 96–112.

Teal S, Edelman A. Contraception selection, effectiveness, and adverse effects: A review. *JAMA* 2021; 326 (24): 2507–18.

Teal SB, Romer SE, Goldthwaite LM, et al. Insertion characteristics of intrauterine devices in adolescents and young women: Success, ancillary measures, and complications. *Am J Obstet Gynecol* 2015; 213 (4): 515.e1–5.

Chapter 28: Abortion

Abortion: Global perspectives and country experiences—Multiple choice answers vol. 62. *Best Pract Res Clin Obstet Gynaecol* 2020; 63: 120–26.

American College of Obstetricians and Gynecologists, Committee on Practice Bulletins—Gynecology, Society of Family Planning. ACOG Practice Bulletin No. 225: Medication abortion up to 70 days of gestation. *Obstet Gynecol* 2020; 136 (4): e31–47.

Bearak JM, Popinchalk A, Beavin C, et al. Country-specific estimates of unintended pregnancy and abortion incidence: A global comparative analysis of levels in 2015–2019. *BMJ Glob Health* 2022; 7 (3): e007151.

Benson J, Andersen K, Samandari G. Reductions in abortion-related mortality following policy reform: Evidence from Romania, South Africa and Bangladesh. *Reprod Health* 2011; 8: 39.

Cates Jr W, Grimes DA, Schulz KF. The public health impact of legal abortion: 30 years later. *Perspect Sex Reprod Health* 2003; 35 (1): 25–28.

Ciganda C, Laborde A. Herbal infusions used for induced abortions. *J Toxicol Clin Toxicol* 2003; 41 (3): 235–39.

Grossman D, Verma N. Self-managed abortion in the US. *JAMA* 2022; 328 (17): 1693–94.

Gunter J. Don't take advice from TikTok on herbal abortifacients. *The Vajenda*, June 29, 2022. https://vajenda.substack.com/p/dont-take-advice-from-tiktok-on-herbal.

Harris LH, Grossman D. Complications of unsafe and self-managed abortion. *N Engl J Med* 2020; 382 (11): 1029–40.

Hoyert DL. Maternal mortality rates in the United States, 2021. National Center for Health Statistics (U.S.), 2023. https://stacks.cdc.gov/view/cdc/124678.

Introduction to the Turnaway Study. ANSIRH. https://www.ansirh.org/sites/default/files/2022-12/turnawaystudyannotatedbibliography122122.pdf. Accessed March 28, 2023.

King H. Eve's herbs: A history of contraception and abortion in the West. *Med Hist* 1998; 42 (3): 412–14.

Shaw D, Norman WV. When there are no abortion laws: A case study of Canada. *Best Pract Res Clin Obstet Gynaecol* 2020; 62: 49–62.

Suran M. Treating cancer in pregnant patients after *Roe v Wade* overturned. *JAMA* 2022; 328 (17): 1674–76.

Trussell J, Aiken ARA, Micks E, Guthrie KA. Chapter 3: Efficacy, safety, and personal consideration: Combined oral contraceptives. In RA Hatcher, AL Nelson, J Trussell, et al, eds. *Contraceptive Technology*, 21st ed. New York: Ayer; 2018: 95–128.

World Health Organization. Self-management recommendation 50: Self-management of medical abortion in whole or in part at gestational ages < 12 weeks (3.6.2). Abortion Care Guideline. https://srhr.org/abortioncare/chapter-3/service-delivery-options-and-self-management-approaches-3-6/self-management-recommendation-50-self-management-of-medical-abortion-in-whole-or-in-part-at-gestational-ages-12-weeks-3-6-2/. Accessed March 26, 2023.

Chapter 29: Surgical Sterilization, Barrier Contraception, and Fertility Awareness Methods

Centers for Disease Control and Prevention. Classifications for fertility awareness–based methods. https://www.cdc.gov/reproductivehealth/contraception/mmwr/mec/appendixf.html. Accessed June 28, 2023.

Gunter J. Ricki Lake and the business of being wrong about birth control. *The Vajenda*, December 12, 2022. https://vajenda.substack.com/p/ricki-lake-and-the-business-of-being.

Hanley GE, Pearce CL, Talhouk A, et al. Outcomes from opportunistic salpingectomy for ovarian cancer prevention. *JAMA Netw Open* 2022; 5 (2): e2147343.

Hou MY, Roncari D. Chapter 16: Permanent contraception. In RA Hatcher, AL Nelson, J Trussell, et al, eds. *Contraceptive Technology*, 21st ed. New York: Ayer; 2018: 459–510.

Lindh I, Othman J, Hansson M, et al. New types of diaphragms and cervical caps versus older types of diaphragms and different gels for contraception: A systematic review. *BMJ Sex Reprod Health* 2020; 0: 1–8.

Park B. Phexxi, a vaginal pH regulator, approved for pregnancy prevention. MPR Medical Professionals' Reference, May 26, 2020. https://www.empr.com/home/news/phexxi-lactic-acid-citric-acid-potassium-bitartrate-vaginal-gel/. Accessed June 28, 2023.

Peragallo Urrutia R, Polis CB. Fertility awareness based methods for pregnancy prevention. *BMJ* 2019; 366: l4245.

Peragallo Urrutia R, Polis CB, Jensen ET, et al. Effectiveness of fertility awareness-based methods for pregnancy prevention: A systematic review. *Obstet Gynecol* 2018; 132 (3): 591–604.

Phexxi—A nonhormonal contraceptive gel. *Med Lett Drugs Ther* 2020; 62 (1605): 129–32.

Polis CB. How an unethical company (Daysy) responded to retraction of their study. Personal blog, June 9, 2019. http://chelseapolis.com/blog/how-an-unethical-company-daysy-responded-to-retraction-of-their-study. Accessed June 28, 2022.

Polis CB. Published analysis of contraceptive effectiveness of Daysy and DaysyView app is fatally flawed. *Reprod Health* 2018; 15 (1): 113.

Sheridan K, Ross C. In a defamation lawsuit, the hype around digital health clashes with scientific criticism. STAT, March 2, 2022. https://www.statnews.com/2022/03/02/health-fertility-thermometer-valley-polis/. Accessed December 12, 2022.

Teal S, Edelman A. Contraception selection, effectiveness, and adverse effects: A review. *JAMA* 2021; 326 (24): 2507–18.

USA Daysy. https://usa.daysy.me. Accessed Jun 28, 2023.

Warner L, Steiner MJ. Chapter 14: Male condoms. In RA Hatcher, AL Nelson, J Trussell, et al, eds. *Contraceptive Technology*, 21st ed. New York: Ayer; 2018: 431–50.

Wilson A, Ronnekleiv-Kelly SM, Pawlik TM. Regret in surgical decision making: A systematic review of patient and physician perspectives. *World J Surg* 2017; 41 (6): 1454–65.

Chapter 30: Contraception Potpourri

American College of Obstetricians and Gynecologists; Society for Maternal-Fetal Medicine. Obstetric care consensus no. 8: Interpregnancy care. *Obstet Gynecol* 2019; 133 (1): e51–72.

Anderl C, Li G, Chen FS. Oral contraceptive use in adolescence predicts lasting vulnerability to depression in adulthood. *J Child Psychol Psychiatry* 2020; 61 (2): 148–56.

Andersen JE. Nutrition and oral contraceptives. Fact sheet no. 9.323. Colorado State University Extension. https://extension.colostate.edu/docs/foodnut/09323.pdf.

Bailey MJ, Hershbein B, Miller AR. The opt-in revolution? Contraception and the gender gap in wages. *Am Econ J Appl Econ* 2012; 4 (3): 225–54.

Bernstein A, Jones KM. The economic effects of contraceptive access: A review of the evidence. Institute for Women's Policy Research, 2019. http://iwpr.org/wp-content/uploads/2020/07/B381_Contraception-Access_Final.pdf.

Business of Birth Control. BoGo Lifetime Membership Page. https://bizof.mykajabi.com/filmcircle. Accessed March 26, 2023.

Catlin R. The unknown designer of the first home pregnancy test is finally getting her due. *Smithsonian Magazine,* September 21, 2015. https://www.smithsonianmag.com/smithsonian-institution/unknown-designer-first-home-pregnancy-test-getting-her-due-180956684/.

Cwiak C, Edelman AB. Chapter 8: Combined oral contraceptives (COCs). In RA Hatcher, AL Nelson, J Trussell, et al, eds. *Contraceptive Technology*, 21st ed. New York: Ayer; 2018: 263–316.

Dr. Geogeanna Seegar Jones. Changing the Face of Medicine. Updated June 3, 2015. https://cfmedicine.nlm.nih.gov/physicians/biography_291.html. Accessed June 27 2023.

Fitzpatrick D, Pirie K, Reeves G, et al. Combined and progestagen-only hormonal contraceptives and breast cancer risk: A UK nested case–control study and meta-analysis. *PLoS ONE* 2023; 20 (3): e1004188.

Gallo MF, Lopez LM, Grimes DA, et al. Combination contraceptives: Effects on weight. *Cochrane Database Syst Rev* 2014; 1: CD003987.

Gilhar A, Etzioni A, Paus R. Alopecia areata. *N Engl J Med* 2012; 366 (16): 1515–25.

Gunter J. Ricki Lake and the business of being wrong about birth control. *The Vajenda,* December 12, 2022. https://vajenda.substack.com/p/ricki-lake-and-the-business-of-being.

Higgins JA, Kramer RD, Wright KQ, et al. Sexual functioning, satisfaction, and well-being among contraceptive users: A three-month assessment from the HER Salt Lake Contraceptive Initiative. *J Sex Res* 2022; 59 (4): 435–44.

Higgins JA, Sanders JN, Palta M, Turok DK. Women's sexual function, satisfaction, and perceptions after starting long-acting reversible contraceptives. *Obstet Gynecol* 2016; 128 (5): 1143–51.

Introduction to the Turnaway Study. ANSIRH. https://www.ansirh.org/sites/defaul/files/2022-12/turnawaystudyannotatedbibliography122122.pdf. Accessed March 28, 2023.

Iversen L, Sivasubramaniam S, Lee AJ, et al. Lifetime cancer risk and combined oral contraceptives: The Royal College of General Practitioners' Oral Contraception Study. *Am J Obstet Gynecol* 2017; 216 (6): 580.e1–e9.

Jones BC, Hahn AC, Fisher CI, et al. No compelling evidence that preferences for facial masculinity track changes in women's hormonal status. *Psychol Sci* 2018; 29 (6): 996–1005.

Kennedy P. Could women be trusted with their own pregnancy tests? *New York Times*, July 29, 2016. https://www.nytimes.com/2016/07/31/opinion/sunday/could -women-be-trusted-with-their-own-pregnancy-tests.html. Accessed June 27 2023.

Lopez LM, Grimes DA, Schulz KF. Steroidal contraceptives: Effect on carbohydrate metabolism in women without diabetes mellitus. *Cochrane Database Syst Rev* 2014; 4: CD006133.

Lundin C, Wikman A, Lampa E, et al. There is no association between combined oral hormonal contraceptives and depression: A Swedish register-based cohort study. *BJOG* 2022; 129 (6): 917–25.

Mørch LS, Skovlund CW, Hannaford PC, et al. Contemporary hormonal contraception and the risk of breast cancer. *N Engl J Med* 2017; 377 (23): 2228–39.

Morris MS, Picciano MF, Jacques PF, Selhub J. Plasma pyridoxal 5'-phosphate in the US population: The National Health and Nutrition Examination Survey, 2003–2004. *Am J Clin Nutr* 2008; 87 (5): 1446–54.

Nearly half of all pregnancies are unintended—a global crisis, says new UNFPA report. United Nations Population Fund press release, March 30, 2022. https://www.unfpa .org/press/nearly-half-all-pregnancies-are-unintended-global-crisis-says-new -unfpa-report#:~:text=Over%2060%20per%20cent%20of,reach%20the%20 Sustainable%20Development%20Goals.

Nichols HB, Schoemaker MJ, Cai J, et al. Breast cancer risk after recent childbirth: A pooled analysis of 15 prospective studies. *Ann Intern Med* 2019; 170 (1): 22–30.

Paterson H, Clifton J, Miller D, et al. Hair loss with use of the levonorgestrel intra-uterine device. *Contraception* 2007; 76 (4): 306–9.

Petersen N, Beltz AM, Casto KV, et al. Towards a more comprehensive neuroscience of hormonal contraceptives. *Nat Neurosci* 2023; 26 (4): 529–31.

Teal S, Edelman A. Contraception selection, effectiveness, and adverse effects: A review. *JAMA* 2021; 326 (24): 2507–18.

Williams NM, Randolph M, Rajabi-Estarabadi A, et al. Hormonal contraceptives and dermatology. *Am J Clin Dermatol* 2021; 22 (1): 69–80.

Final Thoughts

American Academy of Family Physicians. Education and training: Family physicians versus naturopaths. https://www.aafp.org/dam/AAFP/documents/advocacy /workforce/gme/ES-FPvsNaturopaths-110810.pdf. Accessed March 28, 2023.

American Academy of Family Physicians. Training requirements for family physicians. https://www.aafp.org/students-residents/medical-students/explore-career-in -family-medicine/training-requirements.html. Accessed March 28, 2023.

Bastyr University. Doctor of naturopathic medicine: Program overview. https://bastyr .edu/academics/naturopathic-medicine/doctoral/naturopathic-doctorate. Accessed March 28, 2023.

Crislip M. Naturopathic edumacation: A FAQ. Science-Based Medicine, May 12, 2017. https://sciencebasedmedicine.org/naturopathic-edumacation-a-faq/. Accessed March 28, 2023.

Ecker UKH, Lewandowsky S, Cook J, et al. The psychological drivers of misinformation belief and its resistance to correction. *Nat Rev Psychol* 2022; 1: 13–29.

Fazio LK, Brashier NM, Payne BK, Marsh EJ. Knowledge does not protect against illusory truth. *J Exp Psychol Gen* 2015; 144 (5): 993–1002.

Fazio LK, Rand DG, Pennycook G. Repetition increases perceived truth equally for plausible and implausible statements. *Psychon Bull Rev* 2019; 26 (5): 1705–10.

Fazio LK, Sherry CL. The effect of repetition on truth judgments across development. *Psychol Sci* 2020; 31 (9): 1150–60.

Gunter J. Response to Ricki Lake's claim about pheromones. https://www.tiktok.com /@drjengunter/video/7174870731568794922.

Henderson EL, Simons DJ, Barr DJ. The trajectory of truth: A longitudinal study of the illusory truth effect. *J Cogn* 2021; 4 (1): 29.

Hickey SE, Curry CJ, Toriello HV. ACMG practice guideline: Lack of evidence for MTHFR polymorphism testing. *Genet Med* 2013; 15 (2): 153–56.

Lacassagne D, Béna J, Corneille O. Is Earth a perfect square? Repetition increases the perceived truth of highly implausible statements. *Cognition* 2022; 223: 105052.

Navarro VJ, Khan I, Björnsson E, et al. Liver injury from herbal and dietary supplements. *Hepatology* 2017; 65 (1): 363–73.

U.S. Food and Drug Administration. FDA 101: Dietary supplements. https://www.fda .gov/consumers/consumer-updates/fda-101-dietary-supplements. Accessed March 28, 2023.

Index

functions, 59, 65
lack of, 236
and migraines, 132–33
misinformation about, 64–68, 251
during pregnancy, 76–77
progesterone and, 18, 45
removal from body, 66–67
and sexual identity, 55
testosterone and, 32
estrone (theelin), 58, 66, 85
estrus, 4, 7–8, 58–59
ethinyl estradiol, 312–13, 314, 340.
    See also estradiol
etonogestrel, 331
eugenics, 300
Evra, 321
exercise, 126–28, 226, 227–29, 246,
    287–88

fainting, 366
Fallopian tubes. *See* oviducts
Falloppio, Gabriele, 386
fatigue, 131, 274. *See also* anemia;
    endometriosis; PMS
FDA (US Food and Drug Administration)
    and contraceptives, 306, 334, 343,
        352–53
    and fertility tracking, 392
    and menstrual products, 153, 155–56,
        157, 168, 169
    and supplements, 420
FemCap, 388
fertility, 63–64, 242, 355. *See also*
    pregnancy
    awareness methods (FAMs), 389–93
    factors in, 90–91, 125
    tracking, 390–91
FHA (functional hypothalamic
    amenorrhea), 225–27
fiber (dietary), 66–68, 125
fibrinolysin, 45
fibroids, 195, 208–11, 220–21, 334, 363
fibromyalgia, 117, 258
fish oil, 288
Flex disc, 175–76
follicles, 17, 27, 30–31. *See also* ovaries;
    ovulation

antral, 16, 18
hormones and, 16, 32, 57, 63–64
menopause and, 83, 84–86
primordial, 15–16, 18, 73–74, 83,
    84–85
FSH (follicle-stimulating hormone), 16,
    29–30, 219–20, 238

gender, 55, 405–6. *See also* nonbinary
    people; trans people
gestodene, 314, 324
ginger, 288, 421
glyphosate (Roundup), 186
GnRH (gonadotropin-releasing hormone),
    28, 29–30, 31, 36, 135, 238
    for heavy bleeding, 219–20
    low levels of, 225, 227
    medications containing, 118–19, 278
    testosterone and, 31–32
gonad development, 73–74. *See also*
    HPG axis
gonadotropins, 28
gonorrhea, 200, 235, 355
grandmothers, 87, 88, 91
Greenspan, Louise, 78
gut microbiome, 66

Haas, Earle Cleveland, 151
Hadza people (Tanzania), 78, 148, 255
hair loss/excess, 409–10. *See also* PCOS
headaches, 132–33, 258
heart disease, 241, 317
hellebore, 381
herbal remedies, 378–82, 421
high blood pressure (hypertension), 241
Hippocrates' Women (King), 379
Hobby Lobby, 356
hormonal contraceptives, 24. *See also*
    ECCs; *specific hormones*
    for abnormal bleeding, 218–19, 235
    benefits, xiii, 307–8, 394
    and brain, 410–11
    and depression, 404–5
    discontinuing, 402, 407–8
    for endometriosis, 276–78
    history of, 299–309
    IUDs as, 249, 277, 354, 358–62